AF872714

"A stellar constellation of readers analyze two of Lacan's major seminars here, one on our relation to the object and the other on 'unconscious formations' like dreams, daydreams, and fantasies. Fascinating work will be found here on phobia, fetishism, and perversion more generally, as well as on witticisms, lack, metaphor, the phallus, castration, and clinical practice with children and adults."

Bruce Fink, Lacanian psychoanalyst, author of several books on Freud and Lacan, translator into English of Lacan's *Ecrits and Seminars VI: Desire and Its Interpretation, VIII: Transference, and XX: Encore*

"At last, a scholarly examination of Lacan's Seminars IV and V by practitioners who know how to read Lacan and show us the intimate link between conceptual developments and clinical work. This book couples two seminars, enabling us to trace the to and fro in Lacan's Seminar between subject and signifier, and here from lack to desire."

Ian Parker, Psychoanalyst, Secretary of Manchester Psychoanalytic Matrix.

"Studying Lacan's Seminars IV and V represents a fundamental breakthrough in the understanding of Jacques Lacan's thought. Through a series of fecund essays unpacking the intricacies of two of the more difficult early seminars, this volume sheds light on key problems like phobia, the phallus, and lack. Anyone who wants to know anything about the psychoanalytic project must view the collection that Carol Owens and Nadezhda Almquist have put together as utterly essential."

Professor Todd McGowan, University of Vermont

"As if live-streaming the seminars, this excellent collection highlights Lacan's contemporary relevance by putting it into action. Punctuated with clinical material, the book moves with ease between theory and practice, astutely deploying controversial psychoanalytic notions such as lack, desire, and the phallus. Drawing useful distinctions between phobias, fetishism, and perversion, the authors explain the clinical use of dreams and jokes. These forceful essays, all written with verve and clarity, set a model for the transmission of psychoanalysis while providing an indispensable companion to Lacan's seminars IV and V."

Patricia Gherovici, psychoanalyst and author, *Transgender Psychoanalysis: A Lacanian Perspective on Sexual Difference* (Routledge, 2017)

STUDYING LACAN'S SEMINARS IV AND V

This is the first collection of essays to offer a comprehensive analysis of, and reflection on, the major themes emergent in Jacques Lacan's seminars of 1955–56 and 1956–57: Seminar IV – the object relation, and Seminar V – formations of the unconscious.

Assessing the value of a clinical approach orientated around the question of the object lack in the contemporary clinic, the book comprises 16 chapters which follow the development of a range of concepts elaborated by Lacan in these seminars, including sustained engagement with his critique of object relations theory. It considers the effectiveness of these early ideas in clinical practice in relation to hysteria, phobia, fetishism, obsessional neurosis, and of the so-called "Borderline" case. Lacan's early concepts are also subjected to critique for engagement with Queer theory, and research on asexuality or the operation(s) of the signifier Phallus.

The chapters build to provide an invaluable resource to interpret and evaluate Lacan's early teaching, and to find in his early concepts a fresh utility and scope for both clinical work and psychoanalytic research and enquiry. The book will be of great interest to Lacanian scholars and students, as well as psychoanalytic therapists, and analysts interested in Lacan's early work.

Carol Owens and **Nadezhda Almqvist** are psychoanalytic practitioners in Dublin. They are the founders of the Dublin Lacan study group.

STUDYING LACAN'S SEMINARS IV AND V

From Lack to Desire

Edited by Carol Owens and Nadezhda Almqvist

Routledge
Taylor & Francis Group
LONDON AND NEW YORK

First published 2019
by Routledge
2 Park Square, Milton Park, Abingdon, Oxon OX14 4RN

and by Routledge
52 Vanderbilt Avenue, New York, NY 10017

Routledge is an imprint of the Taylor & Francis Group, an informa business

© 2019 selection and editorial matter, Carol Owens and Nadezhda Almqvist; individual chapters, the contributors.

The right of Carol Owens and Nadezhda Almqvist to be identified as the authors of the editorial material, and of the authors for their individual chapters, has been asserted in accordance with sections 77 and 78 of the Copyright, Designs and Patents Act 1988.

All rights reserved. No part of this book may be reprinted or reproduced or utilised in any form or by any electronic, mechanical, or other means, now known or hereafter invented, including photocopying and recording, or in any information storage or retrieval system, without permission in writing from the publishers.

Trademark notice: Product or corporate names may be trademarks or registered trademarks, and are used only for identification and explanation without intent to infringe.

British Library Cataloguing in Publication Data
A catalogue record for this book is available from the British Library

Library of Congress Cataloging-in-Publication Data
A catalog record has been requested for this book

ISBN: 978-0-367-02767-4 (hbk)
ISBN: 978-0-367-02768-1 (pbk)
ISBN: 978-0-429-39790-5 (ebk)

Typeset in Bembo
by Taylor & Francis Books

To my beautiful sister Noelle (Carol Owens)
На родителите ми (Nadezhda Almqvist)

CONTENTS

FIGURES

ACKNOWLEDGEMENTS

There is a story that we tell about the origins of the Dublin Lacan Study Group. In one version of this story, Carol responds to a desire of Nadezhda's to continue to read and study Lacan's works having recently completed a Masters degree in Psychoanalytic studies. In the other version, it is Nadezhda who supports the trajectory of Carol's desire to create a forum wherein the work of Lacan could be studied, interrogated, and critiqued, ideally from a trans-disciplinary perspective, and doubly ideally, without a master discourse. Both versions end in the same way: emerging out of our desire to continue to work and study Lacan together, a group of people began to meet on a regular basis, to read his work, in a non-doctrinaire, questioning, and lively (*aka* sometimes heatedly debated) manner. Beginning with *Seminar XVII, The other side of psychoanalysis* in order to tempt our Queer studies and philosophy friends, following up with *My Teaching* – the slender volume of essays from the late 60s published in English in 2008, we progressed onto *Seminar IX, Identification*; in those years following no particular trajectory other than the one reached by the consensus of the people meeting together during that particular year. Our work on *Identification* was interrupted by cancer; afflicting our dear colleague and friend Olga Cox Cameron who had consented to share with us her long-standing passion for that particular seminar in a short series of talks. We resumed the following year beginning with *Seminar I*, and have continued more or less chronologically since then, taking a seminar each year for our focus. Happily, Olga recovered completely from her illness and we want to acknowledge here our gratitude, and appreciation of her work with the group – especially over the past two years working on Seminars VI and VII – in the form of a set of wonderful talks on each seminar. Here, as everywhere else, Olga brings an exemplary scholarship to the work, noting the points and junctures in Lacan's teachings where theories are built, undermined, and rebuilt, as well as considering the effects of this kind of architecture and construction when taken as a whole. We are delighted to include in this collection Olga's piece on the phallus, long threatened, finally delivered!

Thanks to Colette Soler and colleagues at the Forums of the Lacanian field in Paris during the years of their English language seminars (2003–2010), we met and forged collegiate relationships and friendships with members of the APW (Affiliated Psychoanalytic Workgroups) including Bruce Fink, Patricia Gherovici, Manya Steinkoler, Rolf Flor, and Dan Collins, and other members of the Forums including Leonardo Rodríguez and Megan Williams, some of whom have essays in the present volume. Over the years the Dublin Lacan Study Group has worked in tandem with some of the APW study groups and this book emerges in part from their simultaneous study years of Seminars IV and V, and two conferences held in Dublin in 2014 and 2016 at which work on these seminars was presented. We therefore take this opportunity to thank all the colleagues who we met with and who spoke at each of these conferences and study days, and we especially acknowledge Dan Collins's part in mobilising and sustaining the study of Lacan across the US. Along the way, and because of these affiliations and new collegiate relationships, we met many others whose independent work was interesting and valuable to us and we are delighted to present some of that work here in this volume too.

This book thus represents a whole trajectory of desire and work embedded in a particular time in our history and relationships with numbers of colleagues; some psychoanalysts, some academics, some both, some neither. We gladly take this opportunity to thank all those who have participated in the work of the Dublin Lacan Study Group over the past eleven years. We thank Magda Kurzawska especially for her efforts in the running of the group's activities and study days. We thank Dr. Phil Hanlon and the DIT for giving us access to the beautiful Grangegorman venue for our meetings, and Dr. Gerry Moore and DCU for hosting our conferences and study days there. We also thank APPI for supporting the work of the study group by co-hosting many of our study days and conferences.

We wish to thank Rod Tweedy, our former editor at Karnac Books, for his warm receptiveness to the idea for this project, and are glad of this opportunity to wish him every success in his future endeavours. We fondly thank our new editors Charles Bath and Elliott Morsia at Routledge (Taylor & Francis Group) for their help and advice on a number of issues related to the preparation of this volume.

Over the course of the work of the group, Carol's children have grown up and are now college boys, and between the conception of this book and its delivery Nadezhda has had her first son. We acknowledge, with love and thanks, our husbands Carles and Olaf, and our beautiful loving sons, Tomàs, Oscar, and Nikolai.

Finally we gratefully acknowledge the permissions granted to include various elements in the book:

Chapter 1 "Drawing the urinary trait: Fantasy and analytic technique in Ruth Lebovici's treatment of a transitory perversion" by Dany Nobus was originally published as an article in the *Journal for Lacanian Studies,* Volume 2, Number 1 (published by Karnac Books in 2004) and is reprinted with kind permission of Karnac Books.

The article by Ruth Lebovici "Transitory sexual perversion in the course of a psychoanalytic treatment" appearing as Appendix to this volume, translated into English by Dany Nobus and with a new preface was also originally published as an article in the *Journal for Lacanian Studies* Volume 2, Number 1 (published by Karnac Books in 2004) and is reprinted with kind permission of Karnac Books.

The "Table of lack" adapted from the original appears as Figure 5.1 in chapter 5 with kind permission from Polity Books.

The lines from the Wallace Stevens poem in chapter 8 are quoted with the kind permission of Faber & Faber.

The "Graph" adapted from J. Lacan (2017) *Formations of the Unconscious: The Seminar of Jacques Lacan Book V*, appears as Figure 11.1 in chapter 11 with kind permission from Polity Books.

The "Schema of two waves" appears as Figure 13.1 in chapter 13 with kind permission from Colombia University Press.

The "First cell of the graph of desire" adapted from J. Lacan (2017) *Formations of the Unconscious The Seminar of Jacques Lacan Book V*, appears as Figure 13.3 in chapter 13 with kind permission from Polity Books.

The "First draft of the graph of desire" adapted from J. Lacan (2017) *Formations of the Unconscious The Seminar of Jacques Lacan Book V*, appears as Figure 13.4 in chapter 13 with kind permission from Polity Books.

The "Homology of the two triangles" adapted from J. Lacan (2017) *Formations of the Unconscious The Seminar of Jacques Lacan Book V*, appears as Figure 13.5 in chapter 13 with kind permission from Polity Books.

The cover image is courtesy of Dutch artist Anita Groener and is entitled "The Past is a Foreign Country" (2017, 28 x 28 cm, on polymer painted paper, copyright Anita Groener).

ABOUT THE EDITORS

Nadezhda Almqvist is a psychoanalyst in Dublin and member of the APPI (Association for Psychoanalysis and Psychotherapy in Ireland) and Асоциация Българско Психоаналитично Пространство (Bulgarian Psychoanalytic Association). Since its foundation in 2007, she has been a member of the Dublin Lacan Study Group and has presented papers on a number of occasions and subjects.

Carol Owens is a psychoanalyst and clinical supervisor in private practice in Dublin. She has lectured on psychoanalysis at Trinity College, Dublin City University, and Independent Colleges, Dublin. A registered practitioner member of the APPI and of the ICP (Irish Council for Psychotherapy), she is also a chartered member of the PSI (Psychological Society of Ireland). She is the founder and convenor of the Dublin Lacan Study Group. She edited *The Letter: Lacanian Perspectives on Psychoanalysis* from 2004–2006, and the *Annual Review of Critical Psychology* on Jacques Lacan in 2009. She has published articles and book chapters on the theory and practice of Lacanian Psychoanalysis and its various engagements with critical psychology, critical management theory, film studies, philosophy and Queer theory. She co-organises the annual Irish Psychoanalytic film festival. Her co-edited book with Stephanie Farrelly Quinn, *Lacanian Psychoanalysis with Babies, Children, and Adolescents Further Notes on the Child*, was published by Karnac Books in 2017.

NOTES ON CONTRIBUTORS

Lorenzo Chiesa is a philosopher who has published extensively on psychoanalysis. His works in this field include *Subjectivity and Otherness* (MIT Press, 2007); *Lacan and Philosophy* (Re.press, 2014); *The Not-Two* (MIT Press, 2016); and *The Virtual Point of Freedom* (Northwestern University Press, 2016). He serves as Director of the GSH – Genoa School of Humanities – and teaches at the Freud Museum, London. Previously, he was Professor of Modern European Thought at the University of Kent, where he founded and directed the Centre for Critical Thought.

Marcus Coelen is a psychoanalyst in private practice in New York and Berlin. He also teaches literature and literary theory, currently holding an appointment at the Psychoanalytic Studies Program at Columbia University. He has translated into German, and edited several volumes of texts, by the French novelist and theoretician Maurice Blanchot. Publications include: with Mark Hewson, *Georges Bataille – Key Concepts*, (Routledge, 2016), and with Jamieson Webster, *The Cambridge Introduction to Jacques Lacan* (forthcoming).

Dan Collins, PhD, MSW, of Buffalo, NY, is the founder of Affiliated Psychoanalytic Workgroups, a clinically oriented psychoanalytic organisation that puts on annual international conferences. Dan is a member of Lacan Toronto, where he gives seminars in their teaching program, and a guest member of the Toronto Psychoanalytic Society. He is also an associate member of the Association for Psychoanalysis and Psychotherapy in Ireland. Dan translates the works of Lacan, Miller, and other psychoanalysts, and he lectures widely on psychoanalytic topics.

Olga Cox Cameron has been a psychoanalyst in private practice in Dublin for the past thirty years. She lectured in Psychoanalytic Theory and also in Psychoanalysis and Literature at St. Vincent's University Hospital (UCD) and Trinity College Dublin from 1991 to 2013. She has published numerous articles on these topics in national and international journals. She is the founder of the annual Irish Psychoanalysis and Cinema Festival, now in its tenth year, held earlier this year at Dublin City University (DCU). The 2019 Festival will take place at DCU and will have for its theme: "Psychoanalysis on Celluloid; Same Time Next Week?"

Rolf Flor is a psychoanalytic practitioner in Massachusetts. He is the Clinical Director of the Eliot Center in Lynn and a founder and curator of the Boston Lacan Study Group. He has taught at Schiller International College, Heidelberg University, Mount Holyoke College, the University of Massachusetts at Amherst, Simmons University, and the Massachusetts Institute for Psychoanalysis.

Christine Gormley is a psychoanalyst practicing in Dublin. She is a member of APPI and ICP.

Ruth Lebovici (née Roos 1913–2003) was a French psychoanalyst. Coming from a Jewish family, she lived through the Nazi occupation of France where she lost many members of her family. After meeting her husband, Serge Lebovici, who was a psychiatrist, psychoanalyst, and at one time the president of the International Psychoanalytic Association, she changed her career from being a maths teacher and trained to become a psychoanalyst. She underwent analysis with Marc Schlumberger and was in supervision with Maurice Bouvet.

Sarah Meehan O'Callaghan is conducting PhD research with the School of Applied Languages and Intercultural studies at DCU. The research topic concerns an exploration of the body as a traumatic component of subjectivity from the perspective of Freudian/Lacanian theory and within a theatrical context. She is a member of the Dublin Lacan Study Group and has previously written on the body, sexuality, and the contemporary symptom.

Kevin Murphy is a psychoanalytic psychotherapist practicing in Dublin. His field is sexuality in both his private clinical practice and in his forensic work with sex offenders. He is currently a PhD candidate at Deakin University, Melbourne and his research topic is asexuality.

Dany Nobus is Professor of Psychoanalytic Psychology at Brunel University London and Chair of the Freud Museum, London. He is the author of numerous books and papers on the history, theory, and practice of psychoanalysis. His most recent book is *The Law of Desire: On Lacan's 'Kant with Sade'* (Palgrave, 2017).

Leonardo S. Rodríguez, PhD, is a psychoanalyst and founding member of the Australian Centre for Psychoanalysis and of the International School of Psychoanalysis of the Forums of the Lacanian Field, of which he is an Analyst Member. He is also in charge of the Master of Psychoanalysis program, Victoria University, and a former Senior Lecturer with the Department of Psychiatry, Monash University, Melbourne. He has published *Psychoanalysis with Children* (London and New York: Free Association Books, 1999) and numerous book chapters and articles on psychoanalytic theory and practice.

Manya Steinkoler, PhD, is a psychoanalyst in New York City and teaches English at Borough of Manhattan College, CUNY. She has co-authored, along with Patricia Gherovici, *Lacan, Psychoanalysis and Comedy* (Cambridge University Press, 2016), *Lacan on Madness: Madness Yes You Can't* (Routledge, 2014), *Psychoanalysis, Gender and Sexuality (*forthcoming Cambridge University Press, 2019) and *Angwash: Psychoanalysis and Violence* (forthcoming Routledge, 2019) with Vanessa Sinclair. She is an editor *of Division Review* (New York) and *La Clinique Lacanienne* (Paris). She has completed a manuscript, *The Uncoming Community: Trauma and the Cinema of War* with Prof. Jessica Datema and has authored many articles both in English and French. She is the co-organiser along with Dr. Michael Garfinkle of Psychoanalysis on Ice (Reykjavik 2015 and 2018). She is a competitive ballroom dancer and semi-professional opera singer.

Stephanie Swales is an Assistant Professor of Psychology at the University of Dallas and has a private psychoanalytic practice in Dallas, Texas. Her forthcoming book, co-authored with Dr. Carol Owens, on a Lacanian approach to ambivalence in the clinic and in contemporary times, will be published by Routledge in early 2019. She has also written the book *Perversion: A Lacanian Psychoanalytic Approach to the Subject* (Routledge, 2012) and numerous shorter works in the area of Lacanian psychoanalysis.

Peter Geoffrey Young is a faculty member and candidate psychoanalyst in the Lacanian School of Psychoanalysis (San Francisco, California), and a translator of Lacan's work into English. He is currently pursuing doctoral studies in clinical psychology in San Francisco and is in private practice in Berkeley. His translation of Pierre Legendre's *God in the Mirror* is scheduled for publication by Routledge in 2018.

Jamieson Webster is a psychoanalyst in New York. She has written for Artforum, Apology, Cabinet, The Guardian, Playboy, and The New York Times. She is the author of *The Life and Death of Psychoanalysis* (Karnac, 2011) and *Stay, Illusion!*, with Simon Critchley (Pantheon, 2013). She is currently working on *The Cambridge Introduction to Jacques Lacan*, with Marcus Coelen, and a new book, *Conversion Disorder* (Columbia, 2018).

Megan Williams is an analyst of many years' experience, practising in Melbourne. She is an Analyst of the School of the Freudian School of Melbourne, where she participates in the thinking of Lacanian psychoanalysis and the formation of analysts. She has presented her work internationally and published many articles on psychoanalysis in Australian and international journals and books. For several years she has conducted a seminar in Melbourne entitled "The Father in Psychoanalysis".

PREFACE

Essential to the formation of every Lacanian psychoanalyst has been the study of his early seminars: Seminar III, The Psychoses, in which the concept of foreclosure conclusively redraws the distinction between neurosis and psychosis; Seminar IV, Object Relations, with its analysis of phobia and perversion; and the monumental Seminar V, Formations of the Unconscious, which is necessary reading for understanding the Oedipus complex, the castration complex, the phallus as signifier and the Name-of-the-Father. *Seminar III* has been available in English since 1993, the English translation of *Seminar V* was published in 2017, and *Seminar IV* is currently available in a draft translation on the Internet.

In Seminar IV and Seminar V Lacan speaks with growing assurance and clarity on how to theorise a range of clinical and non-clinical issues. This collection of essays offers a comprehensive analysis of, and reflection on, the major themes of these two seminal works: phobia and fetishism; lack, the phallus and the Name-of-the-Father; neurosis, psychosis and perversion; obsessional neurosis and hysteria; and, last but not least, a fascinating return to wit and dreams as paradigmatic formations of the unconscious.

These seminars remain fundamental for clinicians and students of Lacan today, just as they have been for all analysts formed in the Lacanian orientation and who have learned to recognise in their practice the power of signifiers to resolve the imaginary basis that undergirds symptoms. In both seminars, Lacan demonstrates how a clinical approach which aims to restore missing significations in a clinical context is ultimately structured around the Name-of-the-Father as the founding signifier of the symbolic register. This approach, created by Lacan and inspired by the work of Claude Lévi-Strauss and Roman Jakobson, originally emerged with the Rome Report of 1953, was progressively refined over the course of these early seminars and reached its highest point in Seminar V. Indeed, we find in this latter seminar that many of the lessons draw on and illuminate several of the most important of Lacan's papers that were ultimately published in his *Écrits* in 1966.

The chapters in this excellent collection on Seminar IV and Seminar V thus mark a return to a crucial moment in Lacan's teaching, one in which he is already beginning to leave behind the systematic study of Freud and instead enter new territory in which he is in deep dialogue with post-Freudians, such as the British analysts Michael Balint and D. W. Winnicott, and the French-language analysts Ruth Lebovici and Maurice Bouvet.

This collection is a welcome companion to the at times breathtaking inventiveness and rigorous novelty of approach in these two very fertile seminars of a Lacan on the cusp of a more formal structuralism. Today we can appreciate the significance Lacan repeatedly attaches to the role of the image in the imaginary and, thereby, in the formation of the ego as narcissistic object, just as we can value the discussion of object choice – whether in little Hans or Gide or Leonardo da Vinci – for its relevance to today's clinical setting in which the discussion of object choice occurs in a less gendered environment than was the case at the time of these seminars. It is thus possible to follow the development of Lacan's teaching on the outcome of the Oedipus complex, with its discussion of the permutations of object choice, and assess the depth of its relevance to our contemporary clinical practice. Lacan also leads us through some very contemporary issues concerning the family and the child's place within it: the "unwanted" child and melancholia; the possibility of "devastation" (*ravages* in French) wrought on the child by the mother's desire; not to mention phobia, hysteria and obsessional neurosis.

Lacan's sustained critique of object relations and of the Kleinian approach, mounted here to devastating effect, is a convincing demonstration of the theoretical and clinical need to conceptualise that which, from the outset, lies "beyond" the mother-child relationship. No one who has made a serious study of these seminars will view the object-relations approach in quite the same light. Moreover, Lacan not only brilliantly chronicles contemporary family structures, but also anticipates the symbolic fragmentation and deconstruction of the concept of the family in our day.

The freshness and vivacity of these seminars strikes the reader from the first page and remains to the final word. What we find in both seminars, as the editor of these seminars, J.-A. Miller, has pointed out, is a clinical approach that is orientated by the question of object lack. This is a question that is not outdated by Lacan's later teaching, far from it. Even as we study and learn from the later seminars, a return to Seminar IV and Seminar V is no historical gesture but an opportunity to read Lacan's earlier work in the light of and, in some sense, against the later Lacan. These early seminars stand or fall in their own terms, of course; but just as when Lacan reads Freud, the initial revolutionary discovery of the unconscious is never lost, so Lacan's exploration of the discovery of the linguistic nature of the unconscious ramifies throughout his teaching unil the end. Moreover, these seminars treat concerns central to any and all clinical orientations: neurosis, psychosis and perversion; hysteria, phobia and obsessional neurosis.

The chapters in this collection by Lacanian scholars and analysts are to be read less as commentaries on these two seminars than as interpretations and evaluations of Lacan's contribution to the above topics in the context of his broader work. They form an excellent and comprehensive complement to these two great seminars.

Russell Grigg

INTRODUCTION

Carol Owens and Nadezhda Almqvist

Background to the volume

This volume of essays emerges from the work of the Dublin Lacan Study Group, its liaison with other study groups (most notably the Affiliated Psychoanalytic Workgroups in the US), and with independent psychoanalysts and academics actively studying the seminars of Jacques Lacan around the world. In 2014, some of these workgroups assembled in Dublin with the Dublin Lacan Study Group, having spent the previous year studying Lacan's 1956–57 seminar – *The Object Relation* – and presented papers engaging with, and critically examining, the seminar. Two years later, Lacan's 1957–58 seminar – *Formations of the Unconscious* – came under scrutiny in a similar way, again in Dublin. This volume presents a number of essays which were read for the first time at one or other of these meetings and which have been subsequently worked upon for this collection. Other essays were invited from colleagues who could not be at those meetings or who were independently working on these early seminars. At the time of these conferences we were working either from the French transcripts of the seminars or from various unofficial translations into English. As we finish work on this book, Russell Grigg's translation of *Seminar V* has already been published by Polity Press (2017) and Adrian Price's translation of *Seminar IV* (also Polity Press) is scheduled for publication during 2019.

For Lacanian scholars interested in Lacan's early work there has been very little dedicated study of these seminars from the mid-1950s. A couple of important works which are worth singling out are Bruce Fink's (2004) *Lacan to the Letter* in which his close reading of the *Écrits* comments most helpfully on the connections of parts of the *Écrits* with the seminars (especially IV and V), also Lorenzo Chiesa's erudite and scholarly cover of some of the material of these early seminars which takes place within the wider context of his analysis of the concept of subjectivity in Lacan's work (Chiesa, 2007). In a broader sense Roudinesco's (1999) comprehensive study of Lacan's life and times also proves useful in understanding the context of some of Lacan's arguments and discourse in some of the individual lessons of the seminars.

It is hoped therefore that this collection will provide Lacanian scholars and students, as well as psychoanalytic therapists, and analysts interested in Lacan's early work, a welcome opportunity to grasp and explore the key elements emergent in Lacan's work at this time in his teaching (1956–1958).

From lack to desire

The two seminars, IV and V – The Object Relation and Formations of the Unconscious, respectively – are regarded by Lacanians as "belonging together" in terms of the themes that emerge in the first and are elaborated upon in the second. It is for this reason that the subtitle "From Lack to Desire" will make sense to Lacanian readers whilst flagging an essential trajectory to those less familiar with his work. It is in Seminar IV that the paternal metaphor is introduced and in Seminar V that it is developed alongside the Oedipus complex. The "Table of lack" in IV, where Lacan articulates the distinctions between frustration, privation, and castration, and coordinates those with his registers of Imaginary, Symbolic, and Real, is elaborated in Seminar V in terms of his further development of the themes of desire and demand on the "graph of desire". His conceptualising of the phallus as signifier is consolidated in a certain way in IV and further worked through in V, and the structuring of the psyche by lack established in IV is illuminated in the clinical commentaries in IV on phobia and perversion, and in V on obsession and hysteria.

Rather than attempting to map a single essay onto a single session from either of the seminars, we believed that it would be interesting to frame the collection as a series of thematics emerging from the essays, in this way retroactively conferring salience upon the material. At the same time, we have tried to make sure that no obviously key element from either seminar has been omitted. The reader will also discover that certain motifs are underscored in essays for their overall importance in Lacan's theoretical and conceptual developments. Approaching the material in this way allows for readers to study a particular theme and follow it from its origin in Seminar IV through to its further elaboration in Seminar V, where applicable. In addition, some themes/motifs arise in Seminar IV and not in V, and vice versa, but a trajectory is immanent in the flow from IV to V nonetheless. For example, the section "Lack" is both logically and chronologically anterior to any considerations of the phallus.

Aside from providing what we very much hope will be a welcome supplement to commentaries on Lacan's teaching from the mid-1950s, the collection also aims to be radically contemporary with, for example, some focus on "Asexuality" (Chapter 7), and Queer Theory (Chapter 10). It aims to be clinically astute with considerations of the utility of early Lacan for working with the so-called "borderline" case (Chapter 8), obsessional neurosis (Chapters 16 and 17), phobia (Chapters 4 and 5), and children (Chapter 3). Each essay takes its starting point in one or other of the seminars and engages with the theoretical and conceptual claims advanced there by Lacan, providing a thoroughgoing exegesis of a theme (e.g., Cox Cameron on the archaeology of the phallus in Lacan's early work and consequences for his later teachings, Young on *Witz* in Freud and Lacan), while at the same time indicating the particularity of the individual scholar's desire and research (e.g., Collins on the graph of desire, Coelen and Webster on meaning and metaphor, Murphy on the a/sexual).

We are delighted to be able to include in this collection Dany Nobus's English translation of the Ruth Lebovici case[1]. Nobus's commentary on the Lebovici case also appears here highlighting some of the nuances Lacan brought out in relation to this case and his formulation of the distinction between the phobic and fetish objects on the one hand, and his hard critique of French object-relations theories and practice on the other.

The frame

The collection comprises 16 essays which we have arranged in seven sections and an appendix.

The first section "Phobia/Fetish" has four essays.

The first of these, Chapter 1, is Dany Nobus's commentary on Ruth Lebovici's case of a "transitory sexual perversion", which Lacan remarks upon both in Seminar IV and in his presentation at the 1958 Royaumont conference (later appearing in his *Écrits* as "The Direction of the Treatment and the Principles of its Power"). Nobus points out that when commenting on the case, Lacan expressed his appreciation for Lebovici's clinical honesty, and also showed how her continuous self-critical reflection upon the validity of her interpretations had testified to her cautious application of object-relations theory. However, Nobus argues, whilst agreeing with Lebovici's diagnosis of Yves's condition as a phobia, Lacan also re-interpreted her patient's "transitory sexual perversion", which revolves around the desire to observe women urinating, as the outcome of a series of technical *faux-pas*. Nobus reconstructs Lacan's argument with particular emphasis on his proposition that the analyst's interpretation of the transference triggers the acting out of the patient's fantasy. The chapter thus functions as an introduction to the Lebovici case (which appears – translated by Nobus – as an appendix to this volume), and provides a guide for re-reading it through the lens of Lacan's critique of psychoanalytic practice during the 1950s.

In Chapter 2 Leonardo Rodríguez highlights the importance given by Lacan to Freud's "little Hans" case enabling him to find in Hans an essential reference point for his theses on the object relation and the birth of desire in Seminar IV. Rodríguez argues that Lacan's examination of little Hans introduced a new perspective in psychoanalysis on the aetiology of phobias, as well as a conceptual framework to identify the family's historical constellations that determine particular neurotic formations. Rodríguez explains how in Seminar IV, Lacan was interested in identifying the function that the phobia has for the subject, and why and how it serves as an organising principle, a kind of compass that "tells" the subject the paths to follow and those to avoid. As such, as Rodríguez makes clear, phobia reveals an order that resembles the symbolic order of a myth; a neurotic order that attempts to restore or create a compensation for the failure in the installation of the paternal metaphor, the result of which entails the human law of castration being improperly introduced.

Chapters 3 and 4 both follow Lacan's considerations of phobia and fetish in the early sessions of Seminar IV in order to tease out the distinctions, conjunctions, and disjunctions between the two types of "objects". Carol Owens examines the "principles" Lacan establishes in Seminar IV to distinguish the phobic object as "an all-purpose signifier to make up for the Other's lack [from] the fundamental fetish in every perversion as an object perceived in the signifier's cut" (cf. Lacan, 1958, p. 510). In Chapter 3 she traces the pathway in Seminar IV along which Lacan lays down these guiding principles, in order to consider their utility for analysts and how they may benefit in their clinical work from the distinction he is making between phobia and fetishism. Staying very close to the steps Lacan takes in the seminar, and in order to illustrate moments in the development of his ideas, Owens makes use of material from the *cases* of three little boys plagued by phobia, and in some way tormented by fetishism: Freud's little Hans case especially as this is the pivotal case Lacan takes for examination in this respect in the seminar; the character Jack from the novel Room by Irish/Canadian novelist Emma Donoghue; and the exemplary case of Jean by René Tostain.

In Chapter 4 Stephanie Swales points out that phenomenologically speaking, the two objects – phobia and fetish – seem quite different at first. After all, she remarks, the phobia elicits intense fear and is avoided by the subject, whereas the fetish elicits sexual jouissance and is actively sought out. What could the two objects have in common? Lacan makes the case that both the fetish and the phobic object function to protect the subject from castration anxiety and they are linked by virtue of their relationship to the father, the Other's desire, and the law. Swales comments on this connection as well as their differences.

The second section of the book "Lack" has three essays.

Chapters 5, 6, and 7 are each engaged with considerations of "lack", the exemplary concept at the very core of Lacan's formulation of human subjectivity developed rigorously in his Seminar IV, and its continuing effectiveness in the "Lacanian" psychoanalytic clinic. In Chapter 5 Rolf Flor situates his examination of lack referring to Lacan's critique of post-Freudian takes on castration and frustration and his introduction of a distinct type of lack, which he calls "privation". Demonstrating Lacan's nuancing of the three kinds of lack as contextualised within the three registers of experience (Imaginary, Symbolic, Real), Flor explains Lacan's essential underscoring of the function of symbolic castration which, in turn, conditions the pivotal notion of demand in Lacan's metapsychology of need, demand and desire which he establishes in Seminar V.

In Chapter 6, Kevin Murphy uses the concept of lack as theorised by Lacan in Seminar IV to approach the theorisation of asexuality. Lacan's critique of post-Freudian object relations theories of the 1950s and attendant emphases upon the notion of a harmonious relationship of subject, object, and Other allowed Lacan to introduce the concept of lack as a rectification of, and return to, Freud's formulation of an essential gap at the core of human sexual desire. In Freudian terms, as a result of this gap, the sexually desiring subject is driven to re-find the object. In asexuality, however, Murphy remarks, it appears that the object as "nothing" is that which is sought. Murphy goes on to explore asexuality in terms of this relation to an object – that can sustain the subject – as absence.

In Chapter 7 Steinkoler argues that Lacan's theorisation of lack as phallic may allow us to theorise cases (such as the so-called "borderline") – characterised by acting out, mad jouissance, nonsensical claims, uncanny repetition, and seemingly incessant demand – thanks to the conceptual advances he makes in Seminar IV with regard to the mother, the phallus, and the elaboration of modalities of lack. She points out that, in this seminar, arguing counter to what was more and more popular at the time, Lacan specifically emphasised that analytic technique was not about "frustrating the patient". In Lacan's critical formulation, a challenge to object relations theory, an object is an object insofar as it lacks, not insofar as it "satisfies", or answers, a demand. By linking early theorisations from Seminar IV with later elaborations in Lacan's work, and with reference to a clinical case, Steinkoler shows how these early concepts actually develop and become more nuanced, allowing us to work more efficiently with what are often the clinical impasses of such difficult cases.

The third section of the book "Phallus" also has three essays. The function and importance of the concept phallus in Lacan's work cannot be overstated. Here in this volume the three essays that focus specifically on the phallus each attest in their own way to the challenges for Lacanian scholars and practitioners faced with the phallus in its myriad shape and form in Lacan's teachings, especially as he appears to contradict himself at times in his early seminars even as he insists on its precise signification.

In Chapter 8 Olga Cox Cameron takes on the challenge of examining the successive moves by which Lacan, over the course of Seminars IV *and* V, establishes the phallus as "the single signifier upholding the whole world of meaning". In terms of Lacanian scholarship, Cox Cameron insists that it is always worth asking; how does Lacan build a given theory, and having built it when and how does he begin to undermine the edifice he has created? In these terms, Cox Cameron reflects upon how the mesh of the symbolic order, the world of pact and law held together by the play of signifiers, as developed by Lacan in his first three seminars, is gradually compressed into what she calls a "totalitarian structure" maintained in existence by a single signifier, the Name-of-the-Father. Cox Cameron goes on to argue that Seminars IV and V represent the apogee of masculinism in Lacanian theory and despite notable revisions regarding this bias she claims that he never quite succeeded in flying the nets of masculinist fantasy. However, she points out, as the world we live in is still imbued with masculinism, and that for many heterosexual men the trajectory sketched out by Lacan rings absolutely true, Seminars IV and V remain important and relevant.

In Chapter 9 Sarah Meehan O'Callaghan explores the concept of the phallus and its relation to considerations of unconscious desire and sexual identity categories, within the context of Lacan's Seminar V. Meehan O'Callaghan emphasises that the phallus is a concept within Lacan's theoretical framework open to interpretation, rather than a signifier with static signification. Whilst acknowledging that critiques of the phallus as "signifier of desire" foreground its patriarchal overtones, in her chapter she argues that the phallus, though targeted as an agent of the binary conception of male-female relations, is actually a signifier which leads to the undoing of this binary. This exploration of the crossroads of the phallus opens out a pathway for Meehan O'Callaghan to consider unconscious desire as something not reducible to sexuality and ultimately beyond any categorisation of identity.

In Chapter 10 Christine Gormley critically examines Lacan's reading of Jean Genet's comedy *Le Balcon*, which he remarked upon at length in Seminar V during his discussion of Joan Riviere's *Womanliness as Masquerade,* and Jean Delay's *The Youth of André Gide*; the latter two texts offering him particular opportunities to refine his conceptualisation of the phallus (specifically on "having it") and its function as semblance (as mobilising of phallic jouissance). Gormley's chapter scrutinises, and critiques, the coincidence of these texts in Lacan's thought coordinated by him with comedy. By way of offering a reading of Oscar Wilde's *The Importance of Being Earnest*, Gormley discusses Alenka Zupančič's theory of comedy and finds there the possibility to consider how the phallus may be "demystified" via comedy, and the very contingency of the subject's identification brought to light.

The next section "*Witz*" has two chapters. The first of these, Chapter 11, by P. G. Young, offers an introductory examination of how, over the course of Seminar V, Lacan's reference to Freud's analysis of jokes supports reformulation of the phallus as signifier. As such, the chapter proposes a reading of Freud's text which renews emphasis upon his articulation of three distinct yet linked dimensions – the joke, humour, and the comic – as fundamental registers of the clinical encounter. In this close reading of Lacan's own reading of Freud's book on jokes, Young comments upon the punctuating cuts and scansions of analytic discourse that induce momentary transformation of the economy of jouissance at stake in the treatment. When analytic discourse cracks the joke of interpretation, the phallus is functioning as the signifier of a lack. In such moments, Young claims, analyst and analysand are experiencing phallic jouissance.

In Chapter 12, Webster and Coelen also reflect on Lacan's reading of Freud's book on jokes, especially on the joke that Lacan spends a good deal of time on in the early part of Seminar V, namely, Heinrich Heine's joke about the *famillionaire.* This paradigmatic *Witz* for Freud in Lacan's hands is examined not only for how the *Witz* condenses and economises language in uncanny, upsetting ways, but also for how it may reveal the object as diverse and arbitrary, and potentially dissolvable in language. Investigating the mechanisms of metaphor and metonymy in relation to the *Witz* lead Webster and Coelen in two directions: towards a discussion of the concept of transmission in psychoanalysis and towards an examination of the concept of cure.

The next two sections have one essay each. The first is "Graph of desire" and the second is "Paternal metaphor". The essays in each section are, in their own right, fully exegetic of each concept. In Chapter 13 Dan Collins traces the early stages of the development of Lacan's graph of desire in Seminar V. He explains that the definitive and canonical version of the graph of desire appearing in Lacan's "Subversion of the Subject" – a talk given in 1960 but revised for the *Écrits* (1966) – differs in many ways from the versions of the graph that were incremental steps in its development. The early versions of the graph – and Lacan's commentary on them – featured many elements that were dropped or obscured in the final version. Most notably, Collins claims, Lacan's emphasis on the connection between the metonymic object and the place of the code in the developmental versions of the graph are crucial for understanding what he has to say about formations of the unconscious, even though this connection doesn't appear in the final version of the diagram. This connection prevents the graph from being merely a linguistic model of communication. In fact, Collins argues, this link between the metonymic object and the code goes a long way towards explaining how language *means*.

The Oedipus complex as defined by Freud involved the prohibition of unconscious, incestuous desire. In Chapter 14 Megan Williams elaborates the structural analysis which Lacan made of this in his Seminar V, framed by the recurring theme of father-love in Freud and Lacan. What had been thought of as a privation of the child is analysed by Lacan as a detachment of the child from his or her subjection to the desire of and for the mother. The child who had been helplessly captivated by trying to be the phallus for the mother is freed to take up a masculine or feminine relation of having or desiring the phallus. Prohibited from being an object *a* of the mother and from finding its own object *a* in the mother, the child becomes subject of a desire caused by the loss of the object. It moves from an imaginary to a symbolic position, in which the real of sexual jouissance, as prohibited, becomes that which the phallus signifies. This occurs via a linguistic operation called by Lacan the "Paternal Metaphor", in which the signifier Name-of-the-Father metaphorically substitutes for what represents to the child the desire of the mother, resulting in the new signification of the phallus. Williams then goes on to sketch an outline of the changes in this theory in Lacan's later work.

The final section of the book is given over to an examination of the "Obsessional". The first of the two essays which comprise this section is by Nadezhda Almqvist. In Chapter 15, Almqvist takes the example of Bernard Shaw's fictional Professor Higgins as an illustration of someone who inhabits the obsessional mode of existence. The chapter explores Lacan's thought on the obsessional's relation to the signifier according to his teachings in Seminar V and explores a number of related questions. How does an obsessional man love and desire and what are the effects of castration on his love life? How can a highly civilised man obsessed with proper speech fall in love with an uneducated flower girl who has an accent that is painful to his ears? How can women become so problematic and make many such men discontented and what are the conditions revealed behind this situation?

In Chapter 16, the concluding essay in this collection, Lorenzo Chiesa provides an in-depth reading of obsessional desire as treated by Lacan in Seminar V. There Lacan defines obsessional desire as marked by a profound contradiction and as eventually an impasse. On the one hand, the obsessional looks for his desire in a "beyond" that corresponds with "desire as such" (Lacan, 1957–1958, p. 393, p. 400). On the other hand, this very movement is inextricable from an attempted "destruction of the Other" (ibid., pp. 401–403, p. 468, p. 472, p. 484), and, more specifically, of his desire. Chiesa remarks that as such, the obsessional can thus only subjectivise himself as "a Tantalus" (ibid., p. 412), condemned to eternal non-satisfaction all the more satisfaction appears to be within his grasp. Chiesa goes on to show how, for Lacan, the analyst should always bear in mind this general contradiction when, in directing the cure, he observes the phenomenology of obsessional desire and its revolving around a set of recurrent destructive behaviours

The collection concludes with an Appendix in which the reader can enjoy the Ruth Lebovici case translated into English by Dany Nobus. Ruth Lebovici's case study "Transitory Sexual Perversion in the Case of a Psychoanalytic Treatment" was first published in *Bulletin d'activités de l'Association des Psychanalystes de Belgique* in 1956. In this paper she discussed what she regarded as a treatment of neurosis with phobic elements in a young man, Yves, which continued for about five years with sessions three times weekly for most of the time. Yves suffered from anxieties such as thinking that he was too tall and that people would laugh at him. Yves's fear prevented him from pursuing his career. He came from a family where his mother was the dominant figure and this, among other things, led Lebovici to conceptualise Yves's mother as phallic. In the treatment Lebovici interpreted Yves's fear of a man in armour and linked it with his fear of the phallic mother. The way Lebovici dealt with the transference and her interpretation led to two critical discussions by Lacan between 1956 and 1958. While Lebovici believed that the treatment was dominated mostly by pre-genital relations, Lacan disagreed and criticised the direction which this treatment had taken.

We hope the reader will appreciate the individual chapters and experience the collection as indicating the value of Lacan's early work for contemporary psychoanalytic practice and research.

Note

1 The case and commentary first appeared in the Journal for Lacanian Studies (Vol. 2(1), 2004) and are reprinted here with a new introduction by Nobus to his commentary.

References

Chiesa, L. (2007). *Subjectivity and Otherness: A Philosophical Reading of Lacan*. Cambridge, Massachussetts: MIT Press.

Fink, B. (2004). *Lacan to the Letter: Reading Écrits Closely*. Minneapolis & London: University of Minnesota Press.

Lacan, J. (1958). The Direction of the Treatment and the Principles of its Power. In: *Écrits: The First Complete Edition in English* (pp. 489–542). B. Fink (Trans.). London & New York: W.W. Norton & Company, 2006.

Lacan, J. (1957–1958). *Le séminaire. Livre V. Les formations de l'inconscient*. Paris: Seuil, 1998.

Roudinesco, E. (1999). *Jacques Lacan: An Outline of a Life and a History of a System of Thought*. Cambridge: Polity Press.

PART 1

Phobia/Fetish

1

DRAWING THE URINARY TRAIT

Fantasy and analytic technique in Ruth Lebovici's treatment of a transitory perversion

Dany Nobus

Lacan discussed Ruth Lebovici's case-study of Yves in his 1956-1957 seminar on object-relations (Lacan, 1956–1957), and again in one of two presentations at the Royaumont conference of July 1958, which would subsequently be published as "The Direction of the Treatment and the Principles of Its Power" (Lacan, 1961). On both occasions, he expressed his appreciation for Lebovici's clinical honesty, and showed how her continuous self-critical reflection upon the validity of her interpretations had testified to her rather cautious application of object-relations theory. However, whilst agreeing with her diagnosis of Yves' condition as a phobia, Lacan also re-interpreted her patient's "transitory sexual perversion", which revolved around the desire to observe women urinating, as the outcome of a series of technical faux-pas. In this chapter, I shall reconstruct Lacan's argument, with particular emphasis on his proposition that the analyst's interpretation of the transference triggers the acting out of the patient's fantasy. The chapter may serve as a critical introduction to Lebovici's case, and as a guide for re-reading it through the lens of Lacan's own conception of psychoanalytic practice during the late 1950s, yet the reader will undoubtedly also benefit from comparing and contrasting my own commentary to other discussions of the case (Berenguer, 2015; Bonnet, 2008, pp. 52–62; Bruno, 2003, pp. 50–53; Grose, 2017, pp. 13–15; Krajzman, 1986; McAleese, 2015).

On the twelfth of December 1956, during the fourth session of his seminar on object-relations, Lacan mentioned to his audience that a copy of the *Bulletin d'activités de l'Association des Psychanalystes de Belgique* had fallen into his hands, containing several papers by representatives of the French object-relations movement in psychoanalysis (Lacan, 1956–1957, p. 64). At that time, French object-relations theorists found their main source of inspiration in the works of Maurice Bouvet (1967, 1968), and they attempted to formulate, much like Lacan himself, a solid alternative to the reigning doctrine of ego-psychology. Aversive to Anna Freud's pedagogical outlook on psychoanalysis, yet equally critical of Melanie Klein's "preformationist" conception of the drives and the Oedipus complex, the French object-relations group endeavoured to circumvent the controversy that had torn apart the British psychoanalytic community, by endorsing a nativist point of view without losing track of the possibilities for growth and development. Lacan hated it. He hated it so much that he devoted the first months of his 1956-1957 seminar entirely to an exposition of the fallacies, inconsistencies and stupidities pervading the movement's key texts, such as the collectively edited volumes *La psychanalyse d'aujourd'hui* (Nacht, 1956). Lacan's dismissal of French object-relations subsequently dominated a lengthy intervention on the direction of the psychoanalytic treatment at the Royaumont conference of July 1958. Here, his ruthless attack on the movement's proposed programme of emotional re-education and genitalisation made his former critique of ego-psychology seem rather gentle and kind (Lacan, 1961).

When presenting the contents of the *Bulletin d'activités de l'Association des Psychanalystes de Belgique*, Lacan commended the fact that its contributors, although permeated by object-relations principles, had been more nuanced in their assumptions and less arrogantly self-confident about the value of their interpretations. This tentative and self-critical stance he especially highlighted in the case-study of a perversion emerging during the psychoanalytic treatment of a phobic patient by Ruth Lebovici (1956), which Lacan singled out both during his seminar and at the Royaumont conference as a worthy object of clinical investigation. As if trying to show that this paper deserved more attention than any of the chapters included in *La psychanalyse d'aujourd'hui*, whose authors he refused to mention by name because he believed that they had not actually made any significant, "properly scientific" contribution to psychoanalysis (Lacan, 1961, p. 537), Lacan included its author in the bibliography of his Royaumont presentation as "R.L." (ibid., p. 540).

In this chapter, I wish to reconstruct the backbone of Lacan's comments on Lebovici's case-study as they appear in Seminar IV and, more succinctly, in the Royaumont text. Although the reader does not need to endorse Lacan's remarks in order to make sense of Lebovici's account, my chapter may nonetheless draw attention to some particularly thorny issues in Yves' analysis, and it will hopefully also demonstrate how Lacan's conception of psychoanalytic practice during the early 1950s differed from other approaches.

The first thing to note is that Lacan fully agreed with Lebovici's diagnosis of Yves as a phobic patient, even though his "fear of being too tall" did not seem to revolve around an external object (Lacan, 1956–1957, p. 88; Lacan, 1961, p. 510). Lebovici herself had realised this complication when, in bringing her case-study to a close, she reflected upon the clinical-diagnostic aspects of her patient's condition:

> The obsessive worry for which Yves had consulted [the fear of being too tall and therefore laughable] seems indeed to enter the framework of the phobias, in particular because all anxiety is displaced onto the idea of height and because it is not annulled by a series of obsessional mechanisms. Nonetheless,

> in mainstream phobias, the anxiety is displaced onto an external phobogenic object.
>
> *(Lebovici, 1956, pp. 216–217)*

Yet whereas Lebovici simply registered (and accepted) the absence of the external object, Lacan pointed out that, although this object may not have been "exterior" in the traditional sense, it had been conspicuously present in a repetitive dream which Yves reported during the first year of his analysis (Lacan, 1956–1957, pp. 88–89). In Lebovici's case-study, this dream is presented as follows: "[A] man in armour attacks him [Yves] from behind with a kind of gasmask, which brings to mind a fly-tox spray and which would suffocate him" (Lebovici, 1956, p. 205). For Lacan, the man in armour "is a perfectly recognizable phobic object, a splendidly illustrated substitute for a paternal image that is altogether lacking" (Lacan, 1956–1957, p. 89).

Lacan's interpretation of Yves' dream, here, does not only reflect his profound scepticism towards psychoanalytic frameworks in which exteriority is conflated with the outside world—it is not because the object appears in a dream that it is therefore less exterior—but also his budding theory on the nature and function of a phobia, which would come to full fruition during the Spring of 1957, in a sustained commentary of Freud's case-study of little Hans (Lacan, 1956–1957, pp. 199–435; Freud, 1909b). Lacan theorised the phobic object (or the phobic signifier, as he later designated it) as a symptomatic compensation for the failing Name-of-the-Father, which thus averts the overwhelming anxiety of the unmediated maternal presence. The development of the phobia paradoxically allows the subject to live a relatively anxiety-free life, because the anxiety resulting from the anticipated confrontation with the mother's desire is bound to an object-signifier which can be identified and avoided (Lacan, 1960–1961, p. 259).

From Lebovici's perspective, the "man in armour" did not feature as a phobic object nor, for that matter, as a substitute for the paternal image. Instead she interpreted "him" as an avatar of the phallic mother whom she believed to preside over the life of her patient. And indeed, Yves' mother seemed to have exercised control over most of her son's activities, even providing him with a mistress with a view to relieving his fear of being too tall. Yet Lebovici's interpretation did not stop there, for she also used it as a template for gauging the position that she herself was being accorded within the transference: man in armour = phallic mother = analyst. Witness the following passage from Lebovici's comments on the transference:

> [H]e talked about his fear of being mugged in the dark: the treatment gave him the impression that he was left in the dark and his associations prompted him to make explicit his fear of being attacked in the darkness from behind. We were able to remark that it was us that was precisely behind him. A couple of sessions later, he explained that he had the impression of suffocating during the session and he returned to his dream in which he had been sprinkled by the fly-tox spray of the man in armour. He actually associated it

> with the sensations of suffocation he would have experienced when he came down with faux croup around the age of six. Our second intervention was situated there, according to which his fear of us reminded him of his fear of the man in armour.
>
> *(Lebovici, 1956, p. 211)*

This is probably the most explicit instance of the analyst forging a link between her patient's dreams, the dominant image of the phallic mother, and her own position in the transference, yet it is by no means the only point at which Lebovici actively manoeuvred herself into a phallic position. At crucial moments, she tried to convince Yves that she was even more untouchable, more unshakeable, more phallic than his mother. For example, when, during the third year of his analysis, Yves asked his analyst to cancel a session, the analyst decided to interpret his passivity by telling him "that he would not obtain any satisfaction from us and that he would in this way be forced to come to the session as before" (Lebovici, 1956, p. 207). The effect seems to have been that Yves started thinking that his analysis would only be over when he had finally succeeded in having sex with his analyst, to which the latter replied "that he was playing a game of making himself afraid of an event which he knew would never happen" (ibid., p. 207). During the fourth year of Yves' analysis, Lebovici told her patient "that he feels the analyst to be more authoritarian than his mother, because the latter supported his regressive activities: jokes concerning anality, encouragement to go hunting" (ibid., p. 208). Lebovici was very much aware of how she was intermittently frustrating her patient (ibid., p. 209), and of how he experienced his mother as "infinitely more tolerant" than herself (ibid., p. 216), yet she pursued her strategy of transference handling with utter conviction, although she was not entirely sure of the validity of her own interpretations. Lacan (1956–1957, p. 89; 1961, p. 510) drew attention to how Lebovici expressed an element of doubt after having interpreted the "man in armour" as the oneiric representation of the analyst/phallic mother: "The question arises whether this interpretation was appropriate" (Lebovici, 1956, p. 211).

Lebovici's justification for her own doubt is quite remarkable here:

> [W]e had indeed explained to him some time before that he would have preferred being treated by our husband and one could suppose that he was encouraged to defend himself against the fear of a positive maternal transference by the outcome of material indicating a passive homosexual fear transferred onto our husband.
>
> *(Ibid., p. 211)*

This comment only makes sense in light of the way in which Yves came to be Ruth Lebovici's patient, and of how her husband's clinical reputation cast a shadow over the analytic treatment. When, in the opening sentences of the paper, it is stated that "The twenty-three-year-old patient … was referred to Dr Lebovici by Dr Mignot" (ibid., p. 201), "Dr Lebovici" should not be understood here as a self-referential term in the third person, but as a reference to Ruth Lebovici's husband, Serge Lebovici, a renowned psychiatrist-psychoanalyst, personal adversary of Lacan, and the initiator of child psychiatry in France, who would become the first French president of the International Psychoanalytic Association, from 1973 to 1977 (Coblence, 1996; Saladin & Casanova, 2003). Hence, for reasons impossible to determine, Ruth Lebovici accepted Yves as a patient after he had been referred by her husband. Whether the young man was aware of the fact that his analyst's husband, his "original" psychoanalyst, enjoyed a reputation far exceeding that of his analyst is not clear from the case-study, yet the analyst herself sporadically reminded her patient within the transference of her husband's significance. When Yves reported a dream in which he was not taking the train to Paris, where the consultations were taking place, but was going to Caen instead, where a good friend of his resided, the analyst told him that "seeing our husband would have been more pleasant and less dangerous" (Lebovici, 1956, p. 210). Subsequently, she persisted in pointing out to Yves how he harboured a passive homosexual transference towards her husband, which would explain why he wanted to defend himself against a positive transference towards herself, i.e., why he wanted to sustain a negative transference relationship with his analyst.

In his Royaumont paper Lacan suggested that in continuously referring to her husband, Lebovici inadvertently stitched the Oedipal situation back into the fabric of the analytic sessions, thus compensating for the patient's "faltering Oedipus complex" with an "entirely forced" analytic Oedipality (Lacan, 1961, p. 510). And it is indeed extraordinary how, after Lebovici's interpretation of his presumed defence against the positive transference, Yves started to integrate the image of her husband into his psychic landscape. During the fourth year of his analysis he imagined that Serge Lebovici had died (Lebovici, 1956, p. 208). Around the same time, he revealed to his analyst that he was afraid of being caught in the act by her husband during one of the analytic sessions. The more he expressed his desire to sleep with his analyst, the more he became afraid of her spouse. He told his analyst that the only reason why her husband chose to see female patients was to cheat on her (ibid., p. 212).

If Lebovici doubted the value of her interpretation of the "man in armour" as an image of the phallic mother, this doubt would thus have been instilled by her intimation that the appearance of the armed figure may also have been triggered by the patient's repressed homosexual transference towards her husband. The interpretive doubt does not conceal an insecurity as to the clinical value of interpreting the transference, but rather reflects a profound ambivalence as to the relative importance of the analyst and the analyst's husband within the transference. The following passage bears witness to this ambivalence:

> Since he tried to perceive us as severe, demanding and prohibitive, we suggested to him—concerning the fear of a man who might strangle him in the dark, and the repeated evocation of the man in armour associated with a feeling of being suffocated during the sessions—that he was scared of us just as he had been scared of the man in armour. This interpretation of the transference-situation merits discussion: we can indeed ask ourselves whether the material that alluded to a fear of being attacked by a man could be translated as a transference of the paternal type, as the flight into homosexuality mentioned above seemed to

> suggest, or rather concerned a maternal transference in which the fear of a phallic mother was relived.
>
> *(Ibid., pp. 210–211)*

It bears repeating here that up until then the patient had not mentioned the analyst's husband in any of his associations; it is the analyst who introduces him into the sessions, after which the patient accords him the place of a rival in his thought processes.

Despite her doubt, Lebovici decided to pursue the "phallic mother" approach, a technical decision which, according to Lacan, leads to the crystallisation and acting out of Yves' "perverse fantasy" (Lacan, 1956–1957, pp. 89–90). Again, Lebovici herself is vaguely aware of her own contribution to the emergence of Yves' transitory perversion. Charting Yves' sexual history, she concedes:

> During adulthood, his sexual life was definitely not satisfying. Nonetheless, we can indeed say that before the psychoanalytic treatment there was no such thing as a distinct perversion. Yves' sexual life, as we were able to reconstruct it before the treatment, was much more that of a neurotic than that of a pervert … In our opinion, the voyeuristic perversion thus appeared during the course of the treatment itself, and it has developed within the framework of the transference neurosis. It is remarkable that this transference neurosis was essentially structured around the displacement of the maternal imago onto the analyst, yet it appears clearly enough that the patient did not talk about his perverse fantasies until his transference onto the analyst had been interpreted to him in terms of the displacement of the phallic mother onto her (as an identification of the man in armour with the phallic woman analyst).
>
> *(Lebovici, 1956, p. 215).*

Although Lebovici offered all the elements here that could possibly lead her to consider her own implication in the patient's perversion, she did not as such take responsibility for its emergence. Would it have been as remarkable for the patient's transference neurosis to revolve around the analyst's identification with the (phallic) maternal image, had Lebovici acknowledged that she herself suggested this link? Whilst she admitted that the interpretation of the patient's transference seems to have elicited his perverse fantasies, she simultaneously failed to ascertain that her interpretation reveals less about the patient's transference than about her own counter-transference.

The merit of Lacan's commentary on Lebovici's case-study lies in his meticulous reconstruction of the relationship between the analyst's technical faux-pas—her interpretation of the transference as a blueprint of the patient's position vis-à-vis the phallic mother, implying a reduction of his symbolico-imaginary sphere to the real of the analytic situation—and the analysand's manifestation of an increasingly dramatic perverse fantasy, of seeing women urinating. The crystallisation and acting out of this fantasy follows a three-tiered process, whereby each of the transitions from one level to the next hinges around a specific analytic intervention (Lacan, 1956–1957, pp. 89–92).

As Lebovici herself underscored, Yves did not start to recount dreams and fantasies involving urine until the second year of the treatment, after she had interpreted his dream of the "man in armour" as a representation of his fear towards the phallic mother. The first time Yves talked about his urethral eroticism he told his analyst how urinating women occupied his dreams, how his masturbatory fantasies were often supported by drawings of women who are urinating, and how he imagined being watched by a woman whilst masturbating in a urinal. Lebovici added that at the same time he also started to express a compulsion to urinate on the couch, and fantasised about urinating on the analyst's faeces. In these fragments, we can observe a mixture of passive (being watched) and active positions (watching), yet for Lacan it was beyond doubt that the patient's original fantasmatic scenario had placed the subject in a passive role, and that the actual transition from passive to active had already been triggered by the analyst's interpretations.

The first stage of the fantasy would thus entail the subject imagining being watched by a woman whilst he is urinating. This original passivity could also be justified on the basis of one of Yves' childhood memories, in which he was being reprimanded by his mother for urinating on the floor (Lebovici, 1956, p. 203). Likewise, the two dreams Yves brings to the sessions during the first year (of the man in armour, and of him lying naked on the floor under a blanket whilst Yves Montand is standing naked in front of his mother), could be regarded as formations of the unconscious in which he is passive—being attacked from behind, being reduced to an object on the floor. For Lacan, the transformation of these scenarios to circumstances in which the subject plays an active part did not follow a natural, intrinsic course of development but constituted a reaction to the analyst's interventions. In other words, if Yves reported dreams and fantasies in which he was actively observing women who are urinating, or in which he was urinating on the analyst's couch, this would have been an outcome for which no one but the analyst herself had been responsible.

Through her interpretations, the analyst had inadvertently controlled, and thereby annihilated, her patient's desire, just like his mother had always done, and this analytic strategy had been fortified by her explicit wish to relate her patient's materials back to the transference relationship, in which she had tried to convince him that he was perceiving her as a super-phallic mother. Confronted with his analyst's attempt at neutralising his desire, Yves reacted with a more vehement, active expression of his fantasy. This is exemplified by a dream he reported at the end of his second year of analysis:

> [D]ream: he wants to ask the fishmonger, who is a family friend, to have sex with him, but he is stopped by the sight of her maid. In the course of his associations he will tell us that he had seen the fishmonger urinating … He tells us that he was in love with the maid in the dream, but that he was afraid

> of her husband. We were thus able to give him the following interpretation: it was less dangerous for him to watch, as he had done, this woman urinate than to desire having sexual intercourse with a woman whose husband scared him.
> *(Ibid., p. 206)*

In the dream, Yves appeared in a much more active position (he wanted to ask a woman to have sex with him), yet he was stopped in his activity by the intervention of a third party (the maid). His love for this third party had in itself been thwarted owing to the presence of a "second" third party (notably, the husband). In her interpretation, Lebovici endeavoured to "Oedipalise" and "re-genitalise" Yves' sexual interest. In doing so, however, she was less concerned with producing an interpretation of it, than with articulating a rationale for its preferable replacement with a more mature attitude. What Lebovici called an interpretation of Yves' desire for passivity effectively comes down to its rejection as a *non sequitur.*

Consequently, and for Lacan, this was the third stage in the crystallisation of the fantasy; Yves started to act out his "perversion" both within and outside the treatment. When, during the third year, Lebovici "interpreted" Yves' first request to cancel a session as a futile desire for passivity, since "he knew very well that he would not obtain any satisfaction from us and that he would in this way be forced to come to the session as before" (ibid., p. 207), he eventually decided to tell his analyst that he would only be able to finish his analysis the day he had had sex with her. To which Lebovici responded categorically with a variation on what she had told him before: "[H]e was playing a game of making himself afraid of an event which he knew would never happen" (ibid., p. 207). At this point, the analyst again asked herself whether her intervention was justified, yet again this did not stop her from pursuing her path and confirming herself in her phallic position. And the more she allowed Yves' fantasies to enter the transference, the more he reacted to it by substantiating their value. During the fourth year, he expressed a desire to drink the analyst's urine, he told her that he could smell her urine in the consultation room, he enjoyed spying on her legs, etc. Interestingly, Lebovici "interpreted" these occurrences as signs that the analysis was moving in the right direction. Although she discerned her own implication into their emergence, she did not regard them as indications of clinical failure, but as clear indices of therapeutic progress. Lacan was prepared to excuse Lebovici for entertaining this belief, which he attributed to her being misguided by the supervision she had received (from Maurice Bouvet): "[T]his analysis was, in supervision, given a direction that inclined her to constantly harass the patient to bring him back to the real situation" (Lacan, 1961, p. 510). Lacan accused Bouvet of orienting his supervisee towards the worst the object-relations movement had to offer (a reduction of the distance between the analyst and the analysand; genitalisation etc.), yet he at once applauded Lebovici's recurrent self-reflexivity as an indication of her clinical insight. Her acumen would have prevented her from letting the analysis go astray, had she not been taught to recognise the analysand's "sniffing" of the analyst as a firm sign of analytic progress.

Outside the treatment, Yves responded to his analyst's interventions with the acting out of voyeuristic fantasies. Judging by Lebovici's account, the acting out itself started off in a passive way and gradually incorporated more active elements. Initially, Yves masturbated in a cinema toilet, fantasising about how he was observing women who are urinating. After a while he discovered a cinema on the Champs-Elysées whose women's toilets had a cubicle with a hole in the wall, so that he could really observe the woman on the other side urinating. When he told his analyst about his new hobby, she reacted with a statement whose analytic truth remains totally inconsequential: "[W]e pointed out to him that he found a compensation there for the frustrations we imposed upon him" (Lebovici, 1956, p. 209). Again, these developments do not bother Lebovici. On the contrary, she treated them as analytically productive phenomena. For her, Yves was actively reliving his pre-genital drives inside and outside the transference, in direct contact with the analyst, which would be a prerequisite for their subsequent genitalisation. In accordance with Bouvet's conception of the end of analysis—the realisation of a dual, genital object relationship through the fantasy of the incorporation of the phallus—Lebovici even welcomed Yves' desire to drink her urine, which for her symbolised the benign return of the extra-transferential acting out towards the transference relationship, and the start of a genitalised exchange of objects.

Of course, in Lacan's reading of this case, matters are completely different. Rather than seeing the crystallisation of Yves' fantasy as an analytically productive development, he conceptualised it as a progressively worsening acting out, elicited and aggravated by the analyst's "constantly intervening in a castrating manner" (Lacan, 1961, p. 510). It should be noted, here, that Lacan did not so much criticise Lebovici for preferring the phallic mother over the weak (invalidated) father. Rather, he criticised her for interpreting the transference as such, and thereby "killing" her patient's desire, to which the latter could only react by showing it more forcefully. Through her interpretive actions Lebovici literally drew the urinary trait in and from her patient's fantasy.

The reader who studies Lebovici's case and Lacan's critique of it will quickly discover that his comments do not exhaust the richness of the paper. Lacan highlighted certain aspects to the detriment of others and his entire reading was conditioned by his own attempt at formulating a set of principles that could help the analyst direct the treatment. Here and there Lacan also remained very allusive, so that it is difficult to measure the precise significance of his remarks. This is especially true for his notes on the way in which Yves' treatment ended. Lebovici reported the events as follows:

> After the summer holidays, he insisted on his desire to end the treatment. He said that he had nothing to learn about himself anymore. We stopped at a mutually agreed date: about six weeks from then. He had been treated for varicose veins and he did not pay for the last session—with the money he went to see a prostitute. The treatment ended then.
>
> *(Lebovici, 1956, p. 210)*

This account is quite mysterious in its own right. How did Lebovici know that he used the money to see a prostitute? Did the patient tell her during the last session that he would be unable to pay her, because he had already spent his money somewhere else? Why didn't she elaborate on this extraordinary decision? However, Lacan's comments make things even more intriguing. In his Royaumont paper he posited that "the patient's joke—probably not devoid of malice—about the fee for the last session being misappropriated to pay for debauchery is not a bad omen for the future" (Lacan, 1961, p. 511). I have pondered the meaning of this phrase numerous times over, yet I must admit that I am still not entirely sure how to situate it.

In any case, Lebovici's paper has much more to offer than what Lacan extracts from it. Theoretically, it can stimulate further reflection on the relationship between phobia and fetishism. After all, we could be justified in the belief that Yves' original phobia disappeared into the background as the analysis gets underway, and is being replaced, whether or not artificially, with a urine-fetish. In this context, Lebovici's paper deserves to be compared with other cases addressing the relationship between phobia and fetishism, such as that by Tostain (1980). Clinically, it can reopen interesting questions on the incidence and vicissitudes of urethral eroticism, a vastly under-theorised realm in the field of psychoanalysis, despite imaginative contributions by Sadger (1910) and Freud (1932a) himself. Given Lacan's emphasis on Yves' acting out of the fantasy as a response to the analyst's interpretations, Lebovici's paper may also be studied in conjunction with Ernst Kris's famous case of the "man with the fresh brains" (Kris, 1951), to which Lacan regularly returned as a paradigmatic text on the vicissitudes of an analytically induced acting out.

Finally, I should mention that this case-study appears to be the only clinical publication by Ruth Lebovici. In 1958, she published a small piece on the role of the psychotherapist in a child welfare organisation in a professional journal (Lebovici, 1958), and much later she co-authored with her husband some remarks on the status of reality in psychoanalysis, as part of a conference discussion (Lebovici & Lebovici, 1971), yet these are the only other contributions by her that are in the public domain. The *Bulletin* in which her case-study was published stopped appearing in 1959, when Fernand Lechat, one of its founding editors, passed away (Haber, 1992; Nobus & Libbrecht, 1997), yet after her 1956 paper Lebovici did not contribute anything else to the journal. Some additional biographical details on the person Lacan called "R.L." may nonetheless be of interest to the readers, if only because they may assist them when it comes to situating Lacan's interest in the case within a broader historical perspective. Ruth Lebovici (*née* Roos) (1913–2003) originally trained as a maths teacher, but after her marriage to Serge Lebovici (1915–2000) in 1942 she decided to train as a psychoanalyst (Missonnier, 2003). Lebovici did her training analysis with Marc Schlumberger (1900–1977) (Roudinesco, 1986, p. 206), a respected member of the *Société Psychanalytique de Paris* (SPP), which was the only psychoanalytic organisation in France at the time. During the first years of her clinical practice, she was supervised by Lacan (Miller, 2013), which may explain why her case-study attracted his attention when he came across it. However, by the time the case-study was published, an acrimonious split had occurred within the French psychoanalytic movement, which had turned old allies into new enemies, and which had resulted in Lebovici choosing the side of her husband (Missonnier, 2003), against the newly formed *Société française de Psychanalyse*, where Lacan had rapidly established himself as the intellectual figurehead. As Lebovici indicated at the very beginning of her paper, the case of Yves had been supervised by Maurice Bouvet (1911–1960), one of Lacan's adversaries in the SPP. As such, one could also read Lacan's commentary on the case as a supra- or *ex post facto* supervision, with which Lacan intended to show how the treatment had been steered in the wrong direction by his opponent, and how some of its unexpected twists and turns could have been prevented had he himself still been in a position to supervise it.

References

Berenguer, M. (2015). Una Crítica Clínica, Epistémica y Política. *Nodus*, 45, 60–64.

Bonnet, G. (2008). *La Perversion: Se venger pour survivre*. Paris: Presses Universitaires de France.

Bouvet, M. (1967). *Œuvres Psychanalytiques – Tôme 1: La Relation d'objet, Névrose obsessionnelle, Dépersonnalisation*. Paris: Payot.

Bouvet, M. (1968). *Œuvres Psychanalytiques – Tôme 2: Résistances, Transfert, Écrits didactiques*. Paris: Payot.

Bruno, P. (2003). *La passe*. Toulouse: Presses Universitaires du Mirail.

Coblence, F. (1996). *Serge Lebovici*. Paris: Presses Universitaires de France.

Freud, S. (1909b). Analysis of a Phobia in a Five-Year-Old Boy. *S.E.*, 10: 3–149. London: Hogarth Press.

Freud, S. (1932a). The Acquisition and Control of Fire. *S.E.*, 22: 183–193. London: Hogarth Press.

Grose, A. (2017). *From Anxiety to Zoolander: Notes on Psychoanalysis*. London & New York: Karnac.

Haber, M. (1992). Belgium. In P. Kutter (Ed.), *Psychoanalysis International: A Guide to Psychoanalysis Throughout the World. Vol. 1: Europe* (pp. 25–33). Stuttgart: Frommann-Holzboog.

Krajzman, M. M. (1986). À propos d'un cas dit de perversion transitoire. *Quarto*, 24: 16–19.

Kris, E. (1951). Ego Psychology and Interpretation in Psychoanalytic Therapy. *The Psychoanalytic Quarterly*, 20(1): 15–30.

Lacan, J. (1956–1957). *Le Séminaire. Livre IV: La relation d'objet*. (J.-A. Miller, Ed.). Paris: Le Seuil, 1994.

Lacan, J. (1960–1961). *The Seminar of Jacques Lacan. Book VIII. Transference*. (J.-A. Miller Ed.) & B. Fink (Trans.). Cambridge UK & Malden MA: Polity Press, 2015.

Lacan, J. (1961). The Direction of the Treatment and the Principles of its Power. In: *Écrits: The first complete edition in English* (pp. 489–542). B. Fink (Trans.). London & New York: Norton & Co., 2006.

Lebovici, R. (1956). Transitory Sexual Perversion in the Course of a Psychoanalytic Treatment. D. Nobus (Trans.). In C. Owens, & N. Almqvist (Eds.), *Studying Lacan's Seminars IV and V: From Lack to Desire* (pp. 201–220). London & New York: Routledge, 2018.

Lebovici, R. (1958). Le personnel des organismes de Sauvegarde de l'Enfance – l'Assistant de Psychothérapie. *Sauvegarde de l'enfance*, 1/2/3: 136–139.

Lebovici, R., & Lebovici, S. (1971). À propos de la névrose actuelle: Contribution à la discussion sur la réalité en psychanalyse. *Revue française de psychanalyse*, 35(5–6): 983–992.

McAleese, A. (2015). An Incorrect Interpretation. *The Letter: Irish Journal for Lacanian Psychoanalysis*, 59/60: 63–68.

Miller, J.-A. (2013, March 19). Les pères ont mangé des raisins verts, et les dents des enfants en ont été agacées. *La règle du jeu*. Retrieved from: https://laregledujeu.org/2013/03/19/12799/«-les-peres-ont-mange-des-raisins-verts-et-les-dents-des-enfants-en-ont-ete-agacees-»/.

Missonnier, M. (2003). Hommage à notre amie Ruth Lebovici. *Le Carnet Psy*, 7(84): 27.

Nacht, S. (Ed.) (1956). *La psychanalyse d'aujourd'hui, 2 vols*. Paris: Presses Universitaires de France.

Nobus, D., & Libbrecht, K. (1997). De Franse connectie: Een geschiedenis van de psychoanalyse in België. *Tijdschrift voor Psychoanalyse*, 3(3): 132–149.

Roudinesco, É. (1986). *Jacques Lacan & Co.: A History of Psychoanalysis in France, 1925–1985*. J. Mehlman (Trans.). London: Free Association Books, 1990.

Sadger, I. (1910). Über Urethralerotik. *Jahrbuch für Psychoanalytische und Psychopathologische Forschungen*, 2: 409–450.

Saladin, M., & Casanova, A. (Eds.). (2003). *Serge Lebovici par lui-même et ceux qui l'ont connu*. Paris: Bayard.

Tostain, R. (1980). Fetishisation of a Phobic Object. In S. Schneiderman (Ed.), *Returning to Freud: Clinical Psychoanalysis in the School of Lacan* (pp. 247–260). New Haven CT & London: Yale University Press.

2

THE LESSONS OF LITTLE HANS

Leonardo S. Rodríguez

> Well done, little Hans! I could wish for no better understanding of psycho-analysis from any grown up.
>
> *Sigmund Freud (1909b, p. 72, fn.2)*

Preamble: The youngest pioneer

Freud was grateful to "his" hysterics for having contributed so much, through their body and soul, to the invention of psychoanalysis. His recognition of the young Herbert Graf's contribution to the establishment of a new modality of practice of psychoanalysis – psychoanalysis with children – is a testimony of the trust he had in his analysands and in the formations of the unconscious. However, he had reservations as to what could be analysed with a child, or how "far" the analysis could go in the treatment of very young patients (Freud, 1909b, p. 5; 1918b, pp. 8–9; Jones, 1953–1957, vol. 2, p. 292; Nunberg & Federn, 1967; Rodríguez, 1999, pp. 11–14). But he also respected the validity and authenticity of the evidence provided by the inaugural case of Hans, and then the work of the pioneers in the analysis of children: Hermine Hug-Hellmuth, Melanie Klein and Anna Freud (Freud, 1925d, p. 70 and p. 70 fn.1).

Lacan had his own reservations – not about the practice of psychoanalysis with children in general, which he always supported, but rather as to whether the analysis of little Hans was really an analysis, a "proper" analysis. In the twelve sessions of his seminar on the object relation devoted to the case, he referred to it as the "observation" of Hans's phobia, rather than to its "analysis" (Lacan, 1956–1957, pp. 197–435). Perhaps this was because in this case *princeps* it is easier to tell who the analysand was than who the analyst was. But then, who could tell in 1908 what the "proper" analysis of a child would be like, namely, an analysis conducted by an analyst who assumes the ethical and technical responsibility for the treatment, propelled by what Lacan called the analyst's desire? Freud refers to Hans's father as the analyst, but Hans himself regarded the Professor as the object of his transferences, as *the subject supposed to know*. Hans perceived his father as one who did not know how to analyse properly (although he could consult with the Professor, he suggested; then his father would know how to proceed; Freud 1909b, p. 72). Beyond all assumptions and expectations, Hans worked as a proper analysand, and appeared to be more confident in what he was doing than his father, and even than Freud – Freud, who was still trying to find his way not just in the treatment of a child but also in all other cases, in the new clinical praxis he had created only a few years earlier. The case study of Hans preceded by a few years the collection of essays gathered in the *Standard Edition* under the title of "Papers on Technique".

Despite his reservations, the case history of little Hans shows Freud at his best as a researcher and a builder of knowledge. The concept of the castration complex, the nosological category of anxiety hysteria and an aetiological theory of phobias appear for the first time in the "Analysis of a Phobia". The text is also a testimony of Freud's extraordinary capacity to learn: this time from listening to a child with the psychoanalytic ear and from reading the father's reports with the psychoanalytic eye (Freud 1909b, p. 8; pp. 114–141; Rodríguez 2016, pp. 11–13). Freud also intervened in Hans's life in a decisive way when he advised Max Graf, the young patient's father, against having the boy converted to Catholicism – which would have constituted a *real* castration for him, a horrendous price to pay for the sake of a supposed elevation of his social standing (Graf, 1942).

It is in direct relation to Freud's conceptual developments as presented in the case history of Hans, that Jacques Lacan introduced in his seminar of 1956–1957 a few original and fundamental theses, on which he continued to work over the years, concerning the function of castration and the structuring power of lack among humans; the paternal metaphor; the mother's desire and her jouissance, and the psychoanalytic conception of the object. Faithful to the writings and the praxis that Freud conceived, Lacan questioned nevertheless fundamental aspects of Freud's interpretation of the clinical data, selected by Freud himself from the reports of Hans's father. For Lacan's re-interpretation of the case relied entirely on Freud's written case history. His return to Freud through a careful, critical reading of Freud's texts is not just an homage to Freud's works but, more importantly, a creative, dialectical opposition to the texts of the creator of psychoanalysis, a case of "Freud against Freud" (*sit venia verbo*). In his essay on the experience with Hans, Freud's theoretical deductions contradict his clinical findings at some crucial points, with conceptual implications that go beyond the case. Since the moment of inception of psychoanalysis, its creator, guided by an incorruptible intellectual honesty, did not hesitate to recognise inconsistencies in his most fundamental formulations and to remain faithful to the persuasive power of the experience that he created.

Lacan's questioning of Freud addresses the core of what makes the case of Hans foundational for psychoanalysis as a clinical practice and as a theory: the concepts of the castration complex and of the Oedipus complex, and of their formative effects for the human subject. The logical consequences of Lacan's critical revision of Freud in Seminar IV practically affect all the theoretical constructions in psychoanalysis after 1956. More specifically, Lacan's examination of Freud's conclusions introduces a new perspective on the aetiology of phobias, as well as a conceptual framework to identify the family's historical constellations that determine these neurotic formations. Lacan's original approach to the study of family constellations within the frame of the psychoanalytic discourse leads him to recognise structural conditions and effects of the human family that are beyond the scope of Lévi-Strauss's studies – studies which are certainly an inspirational source for his critique of Freud's perspective on the origins of the prohibition of incest and its subjective impact, the Oedipus complex (Lévi-Strauss, 1969; Rodríguez, 1996b; 2016).

Freud returned several times to the case of Hans. Of particular interest is his review of the case in "Inhibitions, Symptoms and Anxiety" (Freud, 1926d). Freud's re-formulation of the aetiological link between anxiety and symptoms had consequences for his interpretation of the genesis of phobias. From a notion of anxiety as the symptomatic manifestation of unsatisfied libido, Freud moved to a concept of anxiety according to which anxiety operates as a signal that sets in motion defensive operations and the constitution of symptoms. Lacan's revision of the case of Hans in *Seminar IV* on the object relation (Lacan, 1956–1957), prepared him (among other elaborations) for his theses on anxiety six years later, in *Seminar X* (Lacan, 1962–1963).

These are only a few abbreviated acknowledgements of the lessons taught by the case history of little Hans, the first child analysand – lessons that those indefatigable scholars, Freud and Lacan, learned and re-worked creatively, posing new questions that still inspire our own research, more than a hundred years later.

A paradigmatic case

The case of little Hans is paradigmatic in more than one sense. The search for an explanation for that enigmatic, uncanny symptom, the phobia, took Freud to a detailed historical reconstruction of Hans's life circumstances and family relations. He could identify the fundamental temporal milestones of the case within the frame of the life of the child's family and the changing subjective position of the young patient in response to critical events in his existence. Those events affected him uniquely, singularly, and they all concerned the familial Other as incarnated by his significant others: in particular, the discovery of the phallic value of his sexual organ – a value that is "transindividual", as Lacan said, of the unconscious itself (Lacan 1953, p. 214); but also the pregnancy of his mother and subsequent birth of his sister, and the unhappy relation between his parents.

His loving parents did not, or could not, do much to assist Hans in his assimilation of the law of castration. As Lacan (1957) put it in "The Instance of the Letter in the Unconscious" (published at the time of *Seminar IV*), the boy was "left in the lurch at the age of five by the failings of his symbolic entourage", and had to face "the suddenly actualized enigma to him of his sex and his existence" (Lacan,

1957, p. 432). As any other human being at that crucial point during the process of humanisation, he had to face that enigma all by himself. Now, parents are normally expected to support the child in his solitude when confronted with the puzzling questions posed by sex and existence. That parents tend to "normally" fail in their task at those decisive and historically constitutive moments that Freud identified as the onset and the decline of the Oedipus complex, is an almost universal finding in the clinical history of neurotic children who have been through the psychoanalytic experience.

The best response that Hans found for those vital enigmas was the use of "all the possible permutations of a limited number of signifiers in the form of a myth, around the signifying crystal of his phobia" (Lacan, 1957, p. 432). That is Lacan's thesis: the phobia is a response, not a mere "disorder" or pathological effect; not an "irrational" fear; and as a human response, it is supported by a symbolic structure moulded upon the form of a myth. The symbolic structure in question is that of a "limited number of signifiers" arranged according to "all the possible permutations" (ibid.).

In phobias, as in the other neurotic symptoms, there is a convergence of the symbolic and the real orders of the subject's experience. The imaginary order participates of the construction, and not only as a series of effects of the entanglements and collisions between the symbolic and the real: the phobic experience is an experience *of* and *in* the body; it *impresses* the senses; it affects the integrity of the body *qua* imaginary scenario of the subjective drama, and its characteristic affective component – *Angst*, anguish, anxiety, fear – invades and shakes the bodily ego.

Lacan's definition of the phobic object as an "all-purpose signifier" that makes up for the Other's lack (Lacan, 1958a, p. 510) implies the inscription of the signifier in *both* the symbolic and the real registers of the subject's experience. In the symbolic: because, as a signifier, it must operate within the structural constraints, or rules, that ordain this order. In the real: because its operation depends on what Lacan called its *motérialisme* ("materialism"), a neologism that condenses *mot* ("word") and *materialité* ("materiality") (Lacan, 1975, p. 14), i.e., the materiality of the signifier as such. In what constitutes a historical milestone of modern linguistics, Ferdinand de Saussure underlined the significance of the materiality of the signifier (de Saussure, 1916). This materiality of the signifier is also the basis for its capacity to become frozen in actual situations of discourse (and not only in the psychoses), when its dialectic versatility becomes suspended, with the concomitant affective turmoil that culminates in the phobic fear. There is an intimate link between the materiality of language, the Lacanian concept of *lalangue* and the genesis of discourse (Rodríguez, 2013).

Freud discovered in the analysis of Hans's case a nosological paradigm:

> Anxiety-hysterias are the most common of all psycho-neurotic disorders. But, above all, they are those which make their appearance earliest in life; they are *par excellence* the neuroses of childhood.... It seems to me that of all neurotic disorders it is the least dependent upon a special constitutional predisposition and that it is consequently the most easily acquired at any time of life.... An

> anxiety-hysteria tends to develop more and more into a 'phobia'. In the end the patient may have got rid of all his anxiety, but only at the price of subjecting himself to all kinds of inhibitions and restrictions.
>
> *(Freud, 1909b, pp. 116–117)*

In clinical psychoanalysis it is difficult to deduce formulations of general validity on the basis of one's clinical experience alone. On the other hand, we must regard our psychoanalytic clinical experience, if properly directed, as epistemologically sound and fertile, as there are human realities which are only accessible within the frame of the social bond that Lacan called the psychoanalytic discourse (Lacan, 1969–1970). As an ethical condition for our epistemological developments, we must retain a critical perspective on our conceptual tools and productions. On the basis of my own practice, the supervision of many cases and the clinical presentations of colleagues, I believe that Freud's assertion about anxiety hysteria as being the most common form of neurosis and the neurosis of childhood *par excellence* continues to be valid (Rodríguez, 2015a, pp. 11–15). I have referred elsewhere to the frequent demands for analysis by children of about the same age as little Hans (Rodríguez, 2017, p. 65).

In their article on anxiety hysteria, after tracing the history of the expression in Freud's work, J. Laplanche and J.-B. Pontalis emphasise the distinction between anxiety hysteria and phobia:

> '[A]nxiety hysteria' and 'phobic neurosis' cannot, strictly speaking, be treated as completely synonymous terms. 'Anxiety hysteria' is used less descriptively, concentrates attention on the constitutive mechanism of the neurosis in question and stresses the fact that displacement onto a phobic object is secondary to the emergence of a liberated anxiety which is not bound to an object.
>
> *(Laplanche & Pontalis, 1980, p. 38)*

These authors argue, however, that phobia is a central symptom in this form of neurosis, which Freud called "hysteria" because of its structural affinity with conversion hysteria. They also say that the terminological innovation introduced by Freud is justified because although there is structural common ground between anxiety hysteria and conversion hysteria the effects of the mechanism of repression, common to both forms of neurosis, is different in each one. They follow Freud in his first theory of anxiety, and quote Freud's statement that "the libido which has been liberated from the pathogenic material by repression is not *converted* … but is set free in the shape of *anxiety*" (Freud, 1909b, p. 115).

Laplanche and Pontalis (1980) also point out that phobic symptoms can be found in other neurotic and psychotic clinical structures, but it is in anxiety hysteria that phobia becomes the principal symptom.

Lacan was interested in identifying the function that the phobia has for the subject, and why and how it serves as an organising principle, a kind of compass that "tells" the subject the paths to follow and those to avoid. The dangers that the paths to avoid present to the subject appear to be the product of an irrational perception. Yet the work of analysis, as the analysis of Hans shows, reveals an order that resembles the symbolic order of a myth; a neurotic order that attempts to restore or create a compensation for the failure in the installation of the paternal metaphor. As a result of this failure, the human law of castration is improperly introduced, to the point of not being recognised as a law: its effects are perceived by the subject as being arbitrary, as affecting him or her unjustly, depriving him or her of a jouissance to which he or she appeared to have an unrestricted right. The typical neurotic feeling of "having been hard done by" is the direct affective expression of this misrecognition of castration. The universal law of castration is then reduced to being a particular and arbitrary rule, imposed by parents (and occasionally by others) who leave the subject "in the lurch" (to use Lacan's expression), as they fail to transmit to the child the rationale of the law and its benefits – as the law of castration not only deprives, but also establishes the right to jouissance within the parameters imposed by the cultural order (Lacan, 1957, p. 432).

In *Seminar IV*, Lacan also discusses the case of Sandy, reported by Anneliese Schnurmann, in which the child's phobia was resolved by the introduction of the girl to the law of castration and the realisation that the absence of the penis on her body is a condition present in all girls and women, not just an unfortunate accident in her life (Lacan, 1956–1957, pp. 71–75; Schnurmann, 1949).

The cultural imposition of the law of castration via the agency of the parents always induces an adverse affective reaction on the part of the subject, as it entails the renunciation of a jouissance that was at the subject's disposal from birth. It splits the subject: it demands that the subject opposes and suppresses his/her jouissance, thus becoming alien in relation to him/herself. But if the law of castration – castration as a human law – is adopted by the subject as his own law, it is because it imposes not only prohibitions and privations, but also the promise of a portion of jouissance that is compatible with human life.

Little Hans had a hard time in accommodating himself to the law. His parents did not neglect him; they loved him and cared for him. But if Lacan says that they left Hans in the lurch, it is because they themselves had a problematic relation with the law and a very problematic relation with each other. Lacan speaks of Hans's mother as an "unsatisfied" mother (Lacan, 1956–1957, p. 179), and his father appears in the case history as an impotent father: impotent as regards his wife and powerless *qua* father. In fact, the impotence of Hans's father makes him also unsatisfied, although his lack of satisfaction is not the same as his wife's.

In Seminar IV, Lacan presented a first perspective on his original concept of the "paternal metaphor" (Lacan, 1956–1957, pp. 389–408). He developed this concept in greater detail during the following year of seminars (*Seminar V*, on the formations of the unconscious; Lacan, 1957–1958). This was another chapter of his return to Freud, this time to critically revise and expand on the thesis that Freud had regarded as the *shibboleth* of psychoanalysis: the Oedipus complex (Freud, 1905d, p. 226, fn 1; Rodríguez, 2016).

Family constellations and the aetiology of phobias

Thirteen years after his seminar on the object relation, Lacan addressed a brief note to Jenny Aubry that in a very succinct form contains a few fundamental aetiological theses that link specific clinical structures and the subjectivity of child and parents. This seminal text can be regarded as a post-script to Lacan's study of the case of little Hans in Seminar IV. In particular, it touches on the question of the function that the child's symptom has as a response to the malaise of the parental relations: it is "in a position of answering to what is symptomatic in the family structure" and represents the truth of the family couple (Lacan, 1969, p. 7).

This familial constellation fits in with Lévi-Strauss's notion that for any society families are both its condition and its negation (Lévi-Strauss, 1985, 62). It is the tension between those two poles, between the Biblical mandate of leaving one's father and one's mother, and the incestuous attraction towards them and from them, that makes the human species so prone to neurosis. This tension begins at an early age, when the *infans* is introduced into the dialectic of the phallic order: to be or not to be the phallus; to have or not to have the phallus. It was left to Lacan to make explicit, and clearly so, the "signification of the phallus" in the process of human sexuation, a concept whose foundations Freud had established (Lacan, 1958b). Years later, Lacan added his theses on sexuation to his theory of the phallic order, thus de-completing the signification of the phallus and postulating the incompleteness of human sexuality, whether this is considered from the point of view of the individual subject or from the perspective of a couple of individuals, or more than a couple (Lacan, 1971–1972; 2011).

In his seminar on the object relation, Lacan prepared the ground for his ulterior contributions to the understanding of human sexuality. The emphasis of the last few years on the conceptual innovations that Lacan introduced during the last period of his life (the so-called "later" Lacan), necessary as it may be, should not obscure the fact that the theoretical and clinical body of knowledge that he built until the early 1970s are not only a prerequisite for his later developments: for a good number of problems are already present in his earlier writings and seminars in relation to the fundamental concepts of psychoanalysis. Lacan revised, modified and expanded his works prior to the 1970s, but those works cannot be considered as superseded.

The concept of the paternal metaphor introduced in Seminar IV condenses major and original conceptual contributions: the functions of the father at the three levels of subjective inscription (Symbolic, Imaginary and Real) and the signifier of the Name-of-the-Father; the structural link between human desire and the law; the desire for and of the mother, and the mother's position in the Symbolic, Imaginary and Real registers; the effects of the *unsatisfied* mother; the paternal superego and the archaic maternal superego; and the structural connections between phobias and perversions – in this respect following the contributions of Hanns Sachs and Helene Deutsch (Deutsch, 1965; Sachs, 1986; Rodríguez, 1996a, 2015b).

Inspired by the fine clinical studies of Helene Deutsch (Deutsch, 1965), in Seminar XVI Lacan proposed a succinct yet significant contribution to the elucidation of phobias. In this seminar he argues that the phobia is not a clinical entity in its own right, but a *turning plate*: it commonly turns towards the two principal neuroses, hysteria and obsessional neurosis, but it may also establish a junction with the structure of perversion, and appear in "infinitely diverse" clinical contexts (Lacan, 1968–1969, pp. 305–307; Rodríguez, 2015b). This can be understood, in my view, as an extension of the notion that the phobia is constituted by an "all-purpose" signifier: dialectically mobile and polysemic in its function.

It was at the time of Seminar XVI that Lacan wrote his "Note" to Jenny Aubry, in which he also made pertinent clinical remarks on a set of aetiological determinants other than the constitution of a symptom by the child as a response to what does not work in the family couple. This occurs when the child *realises* (i.e., incarnates in the real) the object *a* in the mother's fantasy. Depending on the mother's subjective position and her dominant clinical structure, the child may come to incarnate a different object: testimony of guilt, fetish or primordial refusal (Lacan, 1968–1969, p. 7). Re-reading Lacan's discussion of the case of Hans in *Seminar IV*, and applying the insights of the note to Jenny Aubry retrospectively, one can argue that little Hans was open to the two modes of psychopathological induction described in the later text. Being "left in the lurch" by his symbolic entourage, little Hans was at a loss as to *his phallic value as object*. He came to realise his mother's object cause of desire through his very existence. Removed from the phallic position he occupied for his mother, he was concomitantly dispossessed of the phallic value of his sexual organ, and perplexed as to the jouissance that this organ could provide. Anxiety was the corresponding affective response:

> The anxiety is correlative of the time in which the subject is suspended between a moment when the subject no longer knows where he is and a moment when he is going to be something where he is never going to be able to find himself again.
>
> *(Lacan, 1956–1957, p. 226)*

Hans's very good father fails to present himself as a real father in charge of enforcing the law of castration. This failure leaves Hans in the lurch:

> For little Hans it is a question of finding a suppletion as a compensation for this father that obstinately insists in not wanting to castrate him. This is the key of the observation. It is a question of knowing how little Hans is going to be capable of supporting his real penis, precisely in so far as his penis is not under any threat. This is the basis of the anxiety. What is intolerable in Hans's situation is this lack on the side of the castrator.
>
> *(Lacan, 1956–1957, p. 365)*

His phobia was an attempt, however insufficient, to establish an order that resembled the normative order of the law of castration. For the phobia establishes an *order* in the subject's life; it is not merely a *disorder*, as contemporary nosological classifications would have it (e.g., "Diagnostic and Statistical Manual of Mental *Disorders*"). Since its inception, psychoanalysis has regarded symptoms and psychopathological formations as following, and imposing, an order: they are *productions*, rather than *deficits*. When little Hans calls his phobia "a nonsense" (Freud, 1909b, p. 28), he is right, as it defies conventional sense. But Freud demonstrated that there is sense in nonsense when the unconscious is at work – in the formations of the unconscious and in the products of our clinical instrument, the rule of free association.

The object relation and the birth of desire

In his seminar on the object relation, Lacan elaborates on a concept that was already present in his writings since the 1930s (Lacan, 1938), namely, the *structuring* function of *lack* in the genesis of human desire. Both terms in the seminar's title are problematic in Lacan's usage: questions, or fields of enquiry, rather than descriptive words. Since Freud, the *object*, the human object, is approached outside the parameters that epistemological, philosophical and psychological critique had imposed for its apprehension. Lacan identifies the specificity of the human object – be it object of desire, object of love or object of the drive or of jouissance in general – as being supported by a lack. In Seminar IV – which precedes his later development of the concept of the object *a*, for which it is a principal antecedent – the lack assumes three modalities: *castration, frustration* and *privation*, depending on whether the object appears in the register of the Imaginary, the Real or the Symbolic.

The study of the object in phobias and of the fetish as an object, "bizarre" as these objects are, offers a privileged opportunity for research into not only the structure and phenomenology of human desire, but also of its genesis in the subject's history. A human subject is first and foremost a *desiring* subject. It is precisely the failure in the constitution of the subject as desiring that the psychoanalytic clinic found in the most serious forms of psychopathology: the psychoses and autism. What Freud identified in the treatment of neurotics can also be regarded as pathologies of desire: hysterical desire and obsessional desire. Even when it is "normal", desire unsettles the subject by splitting him/her: a human subject is someone who does not want what he desires (Lacan, 1960).

Where there is a fear, there is a wish, says Freud (Freud, 1909d, pp. 179–180). For Lacan, the case of Hans illustrates clearly his assertion that desire is the other side of the law. Hans is literally *dis*oriented in relation to both, as a result of clear guidance by those in charge of guiding him. He had to find a solution, an orientation, all by himself, which he did. It is fortunate that he came across Freud, who could help him to make sense of his nonsense, raising the child's phobia to the dignity of a human production from which a lesson can be learnt.

As for the term *relation*, Lacan examined the clinical facts (in Seminar IV and on numerous occasions later) in the light of what human relations reveal when considered in the context of the *discourses* in which they emerge and which they sustain. In the Lacanian conception, a discourse is a social bond inscribed in language and specified by a set of primordial statements (Lacan, 1969–1970, pp. 11–24). So, without ignoring the significance of biological and psychological attachments, Lacan highlighted that the relations into which the human subject is born belong in the order of culture and the field of language, through the function of speech to which that subject is exposed even before he/she becomes an *infans*.

Psychoanalysis *with* children

From the point of view of a clinical practice that intends to serve the community at large, and not only a few patients, the most important lesson that little Hans has taught us concerns the position and subjectivity of children in our culture. Hans demonstrated that a child can become, if he/she so wishes, an analysand in his/her own right and in the full sense of the term (my loose translation of the felicitous expression of Rosine and Robert Lefort: *l'enfant: un analysant à part entière*; Lefort & Lefort, 1984). The practice that Hans, his devoted father and Sigmund Freud inaugurated is not only an extension of psychoanalytic praxis. More importantly, it is a major contribution to our culture, to our conceptions of what a child is, to our acknowledgement that a child is a human subject and has to be respected as such. The implications of this acknowledgement have not only affected the field of education: it is a contribution to human ethics, that field of reflection on human affairs at whose centre is desire itself and the human law that supports it.

The lessons of little Hans behove us to regard psychoanalysis *with* children as an integral part of psychoanalysis; to address the child, not as a child, but as a subject and an analysand *à part entière*; and to treat his/her parents also as subjects – which is how they present to us when they come for our assistance. Despite his reservations, Freud was able to verify that a child is capable of conducting an analysis as an analysand independently and without the need of any pedagogical influence. Melanie Klein pursued this clinical and ethical orientation, and then Jacques Lacan demonstrated why psychoanalysis with a child is not only possible, but also necessary, if analysand and analyst agree to work together.

References

de Saussure, F. (1916). *Course in General Linguistics*. C. Bally and A. Sechehaye (Eds.). New York: MacGraw-Hill. 1966

Deutsch, H. (1965). *Neuroses and Character Types: Clinical Psychoanalytic Studies*. New York: International Universities Press.

Freud, S. (1905d). Three Essays on the Theory of Sexuality. *SE.*, 7: 125–245. London: Hogarth.

Freud, S. (1909b). Analysis of a Phobia in a Five-Year-Old Boy. *SE.*, 10: 3–149. London: Hogarth.
Freud, S. (1909d). Notes Upon a Case of Obsessional Neurosis. *SE.*, 10: 153–318. London: Hogarth.
Freud, S. (1918b). From the History of an Infantile Neurosis. *SE.*, 17: 3–122. London: Hogarth.
Freud, S. (1925d). An Autobiographical Study. *SE.*, 20: 1–74. London: Hogarth.
Freud, S. (1926d). Inhibitions, Symptoms and Anxiety. *SE.*, 20: 77–175. London: Hogarth.
Graf, M. (1942). Reminiscences of Professor Sigmund Freud. *Psychoanalytic Quarterly*, 11: 465–476.
Jones, E. (1953–1957). *Sigmund Freud, Life and Works.* (Three volumes). London: Hogarth.
Lacan, J. (1938). Les Complexes familiaux dans la formation de l'individu. In *Autres écrits.* Paris: Seuil, 2001.
Lacan, J. (1953). The Function and Field of Speech and Language in Psychoanalysis. In: *Écrits* (pp. 197–268). B. Fink (Trans.). New York and London: W. W. Norton & Company, 2006.
Lacan, J. (1956–1957). *Le Séminaire. Livre IV: La relation d'objet.* Paris: Le Seuil, 1994
Lacan, J. (1957). The Instance of the Letter in the Unconscious, or Reason Since Freud. In: *Écrits* (pp. 412–444). B. Fink (Trans.).New York and London: W. W. Norton & Company, 2006.
Lacan, J. (1957–1958). *The Seminar of Jacques Lacan: Book V, Formations of the Unconscious.* J.-A. Miller (Ed.) & R. Grigg (Trans.). Cambridge, UK and Malden, MA: Polity Press, 2017.
Lacan, J. (1958a). The Direction of the Treatment and the Principles of its Power. In: *Écrits: The First Complete Edition in English* (pp. 489–542). B. Fink (Trans.). New York and London: W. W. Norton & Company, 2006.
Lacan, J. (1958b). The Signification of the Phallus. In:*Écrits: The First Complete Edition in English* (pp. 575–584). B. Fink (Trans.). New York and London: W. W. Norton & Company, 2006.
Lacan, J. (1960). The Subversion of the Subject and the Dialectic of Desire in the Freudian Unconscious. In: *Écrits: The First Complete Edition in English* (pp. 671–702). B. Fink (Trans.). New York and London: W. W. Norton & Company, 2006.
Lacan, J. (1962–1963). *The Seminar, Book X, Anxiety.* J.-A. Miller (Ed.) and A.R. Price (Trans.). Cambridge, UK and Malden, MA: Polity Press, 2014.
Lacan, J. (1968–1969). *Le Séminaire, Livre XVI, D'un Autre à l'autre, 1968–1969.* Paris: Seuil, 2006.
Lacan, J. (1969). Note on the Child. R. Grigg (Trans.). *Analysis*, 1990, 2: 7–8.
Lacan, J. (1969–1970). *The Other Side of Psychoanalysis: The Seminar of Jacques Lacan: Book XVII.* J.-A. Miller (Ed.) & R. Grigg (Trans.). New York & London: W. W. Norton & Company, 2007.
Lacan, J. (1971–1972). *The Seminar, Book XIX, …or Worse.* Cambridge, UK & Medford, MA, USA: Polity Press, 2018.
Lacan, J. (1975). Geneva Lecture on the Symptom. *Analysis, 1*: 13.
Lacan, J. (2011). *Je parle aux murs: Entretiens de la chapelle de Sante-Anne.* Paris: Seuil.
Laplanche, J. & Pontalis, J.-B. (1980). *The Language of Psycho-Analysis.* London: Karnac.
Lefort, R. & Lefort, R. (1984). L'enfant: un Analysant à Part Entière. *L'Ane*, 16: 3.
Lévi-Strauss, C. (1969). *The Elementary Structures of Kinship.* Boston: Beacon Press.
Lévi-Strauss, C. (1985). *The View from Afar.* New York: Basic Books; London: Blackwell.
Nunberg, H. & Federn, E. (Eds.). (1967). *Minutes of the Vienna Psychoanalytic Society. Volume II: 1908–1910.* New York: International Universities Press.

Rodríguez, L. (1996a). The Archaic Maternal Superego. *Journal of the Centre for Freudian Analysis and Research*, 7: 25–43.
Rodríguez, L. (1996b). The Family and the Subject: a Lacanian Perspective. *Analysis*, 7: 21–33.
Rodríguez, L. (1999). *Psychoanalysis with Children*. London and New York: Free Association Books.
Rodríguez, L. (2013). Discourse and lalangue. *Analysis*, 18: 151–166.
Rodríguez, L. (2015a). Hysterics today. In A. Grosse (Ed.), *Hysteria Today* (pp. 1–25). London: Karnac and CFAR Library.
Rodríguez, L. (2015b). Notes on the Analysis of Perversions. *Analysis*, 20: 101–110.
Rodríguez, L. (2016). The Oedipus Complex from Freud to Lacan. *Australasian Journal of Psychotherapy*, 34(2), 7–30.
Rodríguez, L. (2017). Psychoanalysis with Children, the Work with Parents and the Clinical Structures. In C. Owens and S. Farrelly Quinn (Eds.), *Lacanian Psychoanalysis with Babies, Children, and Adolescents: Further Notes on the Child* (pp. 65–80). London: Karnac.
Sachs, H. (1986). On the genesis of perversions. *Psychoanalytic Quarterly*, 55: 477–488.
Schnurmann, A. (1949). Observation of a Phobia. *Psychoanalytic Study of the Child*, 3/4: 253–270.

3

"ONCE BITTEN, FOREVER SMITTEN"

Phobias, fetishes, and small boys

Carol Owens

Phobia and/or fetish

In his commentary on transference in his 1958 "Direction of the Treatment paper" Lacan invites his students to find it deplorable that in her treatment of a case of transitory perversion Ruth Lebovici didn't have the chance to benefit from his establishment of the principles that distinguish the phobic object from the fetish. These were the "*principles*" (Lacan, 1958a, p. 510) he claimed he had laid down in Seminar IV, just a year before, to distinguish the phobic object as "an all-purpose signifier to make up for the Other's lack [from] the fundamental fetish in every perversion as an object perceived in the signifier's cut" (ibid.). That he never conceptualises this distinction in these precise terms in Seminar IV is already of interest, but what is also remarkable is how the two objects come into focus as constituted at certain moments which are contingent, structured, and structuring. Indeed, in "The Signification of the Phallus" – the paper being the unchanged text of a talk given a couple of months earlier in May 1958 – he claims that while interesting transmutations of the phobic object into the fetish object occur, what makes such transmutations interesting is the place each object occupies in the structure (Lacan, 1958b, p. 577). In this essay I want to trace the pathway in Seminar IV along which Lacan lays down these guiding principles, and from which we can, as analysts, benefit from the distinction he is making between phobia and fetishism. I will stay very close to the steps he takes and, in order to illustrate moments in the development of his ideas, I will make use of material from the *cases* of three little boys plagued by phobia, and in some way tormented by fetishism: Freud's little Hans case especially as this is the pivotal case Lacan takes for examination in this respect in the seminar; the character Jack from the novel *Room* by the Irish novelist Emma Donoghue; and the exemplary case of John (Jean) by René Tostain.

Here then is Lacan's first consideration from *Seminar IV*:

> The question is to know whether there is something in common between the phobic object and the fetish.
>
> *(Lacan, 1956–1957, lesson of 21 November 1956, p. 16)*

Lacan very quickly advances that the common ground between the two is functional since, as he puts it: "one and the other are centred upon the same ground of a fundamental anxiety, against which one and the other may be invoked as a measure of protection or as a guarantee for the subject" (ibid., pp. 16–17). This statement simply recasts Freud's late remarks on the splitting of the subject from 1938:

> [T]here is a conflict between the demand by the instinct and the prohibition by reality. But in fact the child takes neither course, or rather he takes both simultaneously, which comes to the same thing. He replies to the conflict with two contrary reactions, both of which are valid and effective. On the one hand, with the help of certain mechanisms he rejects reality and refuses to accept any prohibition; on the other hand, in the same breath he recognises the danger of reality, takes over the fear of that danger as a pathological symptom and tries subsequently to divest himself of that fear.
>
> *(Freud, 1938, p. 275)*

From his article "Science and Truth" of 1965 – (actually) the typescript of the opening lecture from his thirteenth seminar, The Object of Psychoanalysis – Lacan claims that the division of the subject is at the same time a knot. He remarks that Freud unties this knot in his discussion from 1938 of the lack of the mother's penis, where the nature of the phallus is revealed. What the phallus reveals is the site of lack it indicates in the subject. Here the subject divides: faced with this privation in the real, he protects himself with a phobia and at the same time covers over this real with a surface upon which he erects a fetish (Lacan, 1965, pp. 744–745).

As it is sketched here by both Freud and Lacan there is an essential doubling: either there is the constitution and coming into being of the object/signifier functioning as phobia, then there is the constitution and coming into being of the object/signifier functioning as fetish, *or*, they happen "in the same breath" for Freud (ibid.), and in Lacan's interpretation of this Freudian moment, they happen "at the same time" (Lacan, 1965, p. 745). However, Freud's famous footnote to the little Hans case would appear to inscribe the place of the phobia second, with the precondition for the existence of the fetish first: "what is today the object of phobia was in the past the object of a sharp pleasure" (Freud, 1909b, p. 59). In Seminar IV, although it is the fetish object which structurally appears in first place, Lacan's comments regarding the possible transmutation of the phobic object into the fetish logically implies the emergence of the phobic object first. In terms of his introduction to the two types of objects qua signifiers, he alternates in his discussion of the two in quite an ambiguous way during the first few months of the seminar. There are many levels on which he wants to work and many new and rich concepts which he wants to formulate: the phobia and the fetish come to serve as exemplary objects of his critique of object relations on the one hand, but on the other hand, at times, it can be difficult to piece together the precise moments of constitution of each and indeed their relation to each other, especially, as he and Freud testify, they can appear in the same breath, and/or, one can transmute into the other.

Dialectic of frustration

I am going to attempt a simplification of the moments of the trajectory of the subject towards the Oedipus complex as Lacan handles it in the seminar in order to arrive at bearings on how and when the fetish appears and how and when the phobia appears.

In the beginning there is a child and another subject, one who is already installed in the symbolic order. We call her the mother and she is a being who is divided. She is marked with a double lack: symbolic and imaginary. Because she is a woman she is deprived of the symbolic phallus. That is to say, the real absence of a penis is symbolically registered in her. Her minus of phallus is at the same time an inscription in the symbolic order as presence. (She partakes of the symbolic, phallicised order with her lack, which – among other things – make her beloved for what she does not have). Because she is a castrated subject, she desires the phallus that she is missing, to use Lacan's term, the imaginary phallus. This is not a desire that can be sated as it is metonymic. But she may well have a go at doing that with her child.

That is the mother.

Now, the child.

In the beginning there is need and there is a real object, for example there is hunger and thirst, and there is the breast, nipple (or bottle). Attached to that object there is the mother who is referred to in this moment by Lacan as symbolic for the child. Why symbolic? Because she comes and goes, she is "on" and "off", there and gone. In the novel *Room* by Emma Donoghue, the little protagonist Jack is the son of "Ma" and "Old Nick". Old Nick is the man who captured and raped Ma and kept her and then her baby – the result of the rape – imprisoned in his garden shed. The entire novel is told in Jack's voice. He is five years old when we first hear it. He sleeps in a wardrobe and when Old Nick comes to *visit*, from behind the wardrobe door, he is only able to hear and count the creaks of the bed, until there is quiet. When Old Nick has left and Ma is asleep, Jack sometimes finds himself still "on" – switched on – while Ma is "off" (i.e., asleep, or not available to him). The moments of anguish are accentuated when Ma and Jack are alone and she is sometimes "off" or "gone". Her inexplicable absence even while she is there, only feet away from him, is sketched in this extract:

> Today is one of the days when Ma is Gone. She won't wake up properly. She's here but not really. She stays in Bed with the pillows on her head.... I wonder did Old Nick come in the night. Maybe Ma's not just Gone. Maybe he squished her neck even harder and now she's – I go up really close and listen till I hear breath. I'm just one inch away, my hair touches Ma's nose and she puts her hand up over her face so I step back. There's hours and hours, hundreds of them. Ma gets up to pee but no talking, with her face all blank.... Ma's never Gone more than one day. I don't know what I do if I wake up tomorrow and she's still Gone. Then I'm hungry, I have a banana even though it's a bit green.
>
> *(Donoghue, 2010, pp. 62–63)*

In a simplified take on this encounter, the symbolic mother is ideally there when the child is hungry and gone when he isn't. However it doesn't always happen this way. She doesn't always come when he cries (indeed she doesn't always go away when he is full up). This not coming when he demands brings about a transformation, a switching of the characteristic of object and the agency of the mother. The object now becomes symbolic, a sign of something that can be given and taken away, actually her love. And she as agent becomes real, omnipotent, power (Lacan 1956–1957, lesson of 12 December 1956, p. 70). This moment marks the experience of primordial frustration for the child and inaugurates the dialectic of frustration. The child experiences the imaginary and fundamentally narcissistic injury of having had something robbed from him. Therefore he demands. This is the domain of the claim: I want it! I want it back! In addition, his frustration encounters only the blank face of the mother's absence or rather the deaf ear. This is why the analyst doesn't respond to the demand, frustrating the subject so that the archaic signifiers of demand emerge. In her omnipotence, she does not lack, neither does she desire. She simply isn't there when he wants. And she doesn't always give what he needs. Like the Calvinist the child has to believe himself to be loved for what he receives. However, the dialectic of frustration is asymmetrical, for the mother is divided. As such, her own search for the phallus is calmed somewhat through the child, while at the same time the child cannot entirely match up to the missing phallus, which remains irreducible in the mother.

Emerging from the experience of the frustrated demand for love, the child regresses to a degraded satisfaction – taking the opportunity to grasp, swallow, and devour the object of need as a compensation for the frustrations in love. "I eat when I've had a bad day" we hear in the clinic. And the whole "Because you're worth it" campaign targets the frustrated demand for love, compensating the subject with an array of other little items which can be elevated to items of need/satisfactions. Of note here is the constitution of the symbolising of the real object after frustration since it compensates for the structural lack which accompanies the symbolic object as an insufficient sign of love. Here's Lacan:

> The term regression is applicable to what happens when the real object and at the same time the activity which is designed for attaining it, come to be substituted for the symbolic demand. The fact that the child crushes his disappointment in his saturation and satiation in contact with the breast or any object at all is what will permit him to enter into the necessity of the mechanism, which has it that a symbolic frustration can always be followed by a regression.
>
> *(Lacan 1956–1957, lesson of 27 February 1957, p. 217)*

And indeed this is well observed in the novel *Room* where Jack reaches for the Banana when Ma is *Gone,* but also for her breast (especially the left one which has become his favourite).

Now we will take the "jump" (ibid., p. 218) that Lacan himself describes in the seminar and consider with him how the phallus is introduced into the dialectic of frustration.

Phallus, mother, child, privation

A multitude of questions accompany the jump from the dialectic of frustration to the cut of privation. Why does the child more or less occupy the place of the mother with regard to the phallus? Or sometimes the position of the phallus with respect to the mother? Why is he led there? To what extent does he put something of himself there?

And again, is the relation mother-phallus given to the child in a way that is spontaneous and direct? Does everything happen simply because he looks at his mother and perceives that it is a phallus that she desires? What happens to the extent that the image of the phallus is not completely absorbed for the mother by the image of the child?

Lacan says here then that the question is to know at what moment, and how, the child can be introduced directly into the structure of Symbolic-Imaginary-Real, as it is produced for the mother. At what moment can the child feel himself dispossessed of something that he demands from the mother, in perceiving that it is not he who is loved, but a certain image?

Privation is the operation by which the imaginary father – a function rather than a real person - interrupts the dialectic of frustration with some intervention that emphasises a new piece of knowledge. Mothers, sisters, daughters don't have penises, never did, never will. And the penis they don't have won't get bigger, ever. As such, not only do they not have a penis, they do not nor ever will have a phallus. But how is this missing – minus – object to be comprehended as a symbolic object? Only by establishing by law or some other agreed upon code can we say that something should be in a certain place and therefore can be missing from that place. I will attempt a simplification of this operation by saying that just as the real object of need becomes a symbolic object or gift from the real mother due to the vagaries of her being, the real penis becomes a symbolic phallus due to the intervention of a function which unequivocally states that a vagary of human existence means that men have penises and women don't and that's just how it is.

Now, finally, the jump! At the precise moment when the subject discovers that this imaginary phallus is lacking to the mother, he can find himself engaged in coming to be a substitute for it. In other words, the moment of understanding isn't necessarily commensurate with the explanation. In still other words, if the mother is omnipotent it can be a real pain in the ass and you may never know where you stand with her, but if after all that she turns out to be impotent, lacking, decaying, sick, degraded, or just plain different, what will it take to ever know if you are on solid ground again. So you try out a couple of other options first. This is how Lacan proceeds from symbolic phallus to imaginary phallus in the blink of an eye. That's how little moment is involved in privation all going well. Then there's this very stretched out moment involved in privation not going well, and all the incidents and accidents in the whole mother, child, and phallus affair, which send little boys (and girls) looking for a phobia or a fetish.

Back in *Room*, little Jack's penis stands to attention every morning. He keeps putting his finger in his mouth, and Ma keeps telling him not to. He has kept Ma's rotten tooth that fell out and sleeps with it at night and wears it in his sock during the day. He thinks his nose will grow bigger when he grows up or maybe it will fall off and an adult one will grow in its place.

On the other side of the world, a little boy called John lives with his mother and his father. His mother heats him up like a massive dildo (Tostain, 1980, pp. 251–252). She calls his real little penis "*ton bout*", her own sexual organ is called a *bouton* by John's father. John feels something in his own penis when he has to fasten *les boutons* on her dress but is nauseated and upset when faced with a single one (ibid., pp. 248–250).

Little Hans is disgusted by his mother's black culottes when they are off her body and not disgusted when they are on her body. He sees her widdler when she is all nude in her chemise. He would like for her to share in the fun of touching his widdler. But, because he's afraid, *because of the horse*, he has already found a substitute for castration, which will suffice until the "real thing" comes along (Lacan 1956–1957, lesson of 13 March 1957, p. 263).

In the same lesson Lacan makes the statement that will allow us to understand how and when what begins with a game ends in anxiety:

> The child presents himself to the mother by offering her the phallus in itself, to different degrees and in different positions. He can identify with the mother, identify with the phallus, identify with the mother as bearer as the phallus, or present himself as bearer of the phallus.
>
> *(Ibid., p. 258)*

Let us take these four identifications and suggest that while the former two belong to the fetishist, the latter two belong to the phobic.

Privation –> phobia

When precisely does this business of playing the game with the mother of "where's the phallus?" become problematic? Well, Lacan says, just before Oedipus, between the primary relation of primitive frustration and the Oedipus complex (Lacan 1956–1957, lesson of 27 February 1957, p. 223), at the end of the pre-Oedipal period and the border of the Oedipus (ibid., lesson of 6 March 1957, p. 228). In other words, it occurs during, in, or around, privation. And it must occur during the phallic phase – i.e., when the real little penis is a major player in the game, and at a time when questioning that lack is itself contingent upon the child's specular identification with the image of his own body, providing a matrix by which he can realise what is lacking in the mother. Hans in this way considers that his mother must have a widdler as big as a horse because she herself is so big. At this point, where the real penis is experienced as inadequate, and as such of potential disappointment to the real mother, and in so far as the child is engaged with this, bringing in himself and his own lack to fulfil this specific lack in the mother, the game may fall apart. It turns out that no satisfaction by any real object can match the mother's lack. So the inevitable experience of inadequacy, impotence, and anxiety that will accompany his not measuring up to the task with his real little penis engages him in a game of lure/deception and trickery with the mother, with all of the anxiety that will eventually entail. Ultimately he can be led to the shattering conclusion that it isn't his penis she is after but his entire being. And if the real object, *child as real*, isn't enough for the mother – it never is – will she feed on him, bite him, devour him, just the way he attempts to on, and of, her, when his demand is frustrated?

Like all unsatiated beings, she is seeking whom she may devour; Lacan quotes the Latin "*Querens, quem devoret*" from the First Epistle of Peter (Lacan 1956–1957, lesson of 27 February 1957, p. 224). Maternal castration, Lacan says, implies for the child the possibility of being devoured by the mother's "bite" (ibid., lesson of 5 June, 1957, p. 433); being bitten by the insatiable, menacing mother due to her own privation (ibid., lesson of 15 May 1957, p. 386). Paternal castration is to be thought of as not merely a substitute, but *the* substitute for maternal castration. No less terrible, but whereas with the "father" a dialectic is possible – some kind of rivalry, murderous fantasies and so on – it is on the other hand impossible to castrate the mother because she has nothing that one could castrate (ibid., lesson of 5 June 1957, p. 434).

As such, it is an accident of development or an historic incident that damages the links of the mother child relation with regard to the phallus which is what the woman lacks and the child discovers as lacking in the mother. When the harnessing of these three objects is broken there is more than one solution possible. One of these possible outcomes is that the father intervenes as a fourth term and paves the way towards Oedipus via his menace of castration and second privation of the mother, a symbolic operation that allows the child to renounce being the imaginary phallus for the mother. When this path is not available, as in the case of little

Hans whose *Vatti* is too kind to be sufficiently menacing, when as Lacan says later in the seminar - there is no exit from the game of the lure, the game of big Giraffe/little Giraffe - a phobia constitutes a call to rescue. This is why Lacan formulates the phobia as the signifier in the place of the missing father (ibid., lesson of 13 March, 1957, p. 263). The horse that bites, like the biting dog in the nightmare of the little girl Lacan mentions early on in the seminar, is – because of regression on the oral-sadistic plane – the real mother biting and devouring. As Lacan puts it:

> the horse bites ... that is to say ... since I can no longer satisfy my mother in anything, she will satisfy herself on me the way I satisfy myself on her when she does not satisfy me at all, that is, she will bite me the way I bite her, since it's my last recourse when I am not sure of her love.
>
> *(Ibid., lesson of 5 June 1957, p. 423)*

The bite is on the one hand linked to the surging of something that happens each time the mother's love is lacking (ibid., lesson of 22 May 1957, p. 408) but also linked to the excitement Hans experiences in his own penis, *it bites him*. The phobia displaces anxiety from the biting mother (and perhaps indeed away from the biting penis) onto the biting horse. This ultimately, I believe, is what Lacan is getting at when he says that the only real relation with the mother is the relation of devoration (ibid., lesson of 19 June 1957, p. 449).

Because of his reasoning thus far in the seminar, Lacan says that all phobic objects in childhood are signifiers belonging to the same genre: lions, tigers, and bears, etc. But ... some phobic objects from childhood transmute into fetish objects, having had their origin in a childhood pleasure/jouissance. Indeed, it is even thinkable that behind the phobia of the biting horse there is the original phobic object as displaced, that is to say the biting penis, the widdler, the thing that gives pleasure but becomes a source of anxiety. The very thing that can be seen and not seen when mum is all nude in her chemise, veiled by the fringe of the chemise, characteristic of the fetishist's apprehension.

Privation-> fetish

Nothing of the phenomenology of the perversions is conceivable in a direct way, Lacan argues, unless we start with the idea that the phallus is implicated:

> This is an idea that is much simpler than what you are usually given, an obscurity of identifications, of re-identifications, of projections, a knit of every stitch which produces a labyrinth in which one is lost. It is a matter of the phallus and of knowing how the child more or less consciously realises that his omnipotent mother fundamentally lacks something, and it is always a question of knowing how he will give her this object which she lacks, and which he still lacks himself.
>
> *(Lacan 1956–1957, lesson of 27 February 1957, p. 222)*

As such:

> [T]here is here a high degree not of abstraction, but of generalization of the imaginary relation which I call one of lure, through which the child attests to the mother that he can fulfil her, not only as child, but also in her desire ... *in what she is lacking*. This situation is certainly structuring, since it is uniquely around it that the relation of the fetishist to his object is articulated.
>
> *(Ibid., lesson of 13 March 1957, p. 258)*

This latter identification for Lacan is the exemplary situation structuring of fetishism which is well illustrated in the case of little six year old John as reported by his analyst René Tostain (1980, pp. 247–260). John recalls having to do up his mother's *boutons* (buttons) as a child and feeling an intense excitement in his penis at the same time. Tostain remarks that as a child John was frequently ill and became the object of an "attentive maternal care" and reports that the insertion of the rectal thermometer held inside by the mother's fingers caused erections and arousal for young John (ibid., p. 251). As an adult John reflects that he took some pleasure in this, but there was also, finally, the anxiety correlated with what Tostain describes as John's part in his mother's game of lure and seduction, involving her treatment of his entire body as a living dildo: a position in which he served as imaginary phallus for his mother "her lack, a toy to inflate" (ibid., p. 252). John's response was to become sick again, this time with an acute appendicitis. This is a moment of privation in which he ends up in hospital to have his appendix removed: what is taken is a little inessential bit of him (*un petit bout*). He wakes to find his father, previously absent in his life, jiggling his appendix in a jar. According to Tostain's analysis of the case (*après-coup*, so to speak), it is at this point that the father fulfils a certain essential function, registering for John his support of his imaginary dis-identification with being the phallus for his mother. John at this moment, separated from his little appendix, takes the opportunity to identify with it, and he passes from the "no-one wins game" of lure with his mother to a new period in which he no longer fastens (or indeed we could say, presses) his mother's buttons. But now, John forges a phobia, since as he no longer is the phallus for the mother, neither can he be the bearer of the phallus for her. Underscoring this deficiency, his mother referred to his own little penis as "*ton bout*" or "*ton petit bout*" emphasising its inadequacy (and indeed perhaps its inessential aspect to her). How then, Tostain asks, did the button pass from a horrifying singularity to an erotic plurality (ibid., p. 258)?

In his discussions in *Seminar IV* Lacan says he will avoid the "forest" of the analytic literature on fetishism (not wishing to beat around the bush no doubt) (Lacan, 1956-1957, lesson of 30 January 1957, p. 170). What does he claim then? The child identifies with the mother; via an imaginary displacement he makes a phallic choice in her place and realises for her the assumption of her longing towards the phallic object, and/or, he identifies with the object and via a regression on the oral-sadistic plane considers himself to be a destructive, devouring object (ibid., lesson of 19 June 1957, p. 449). This latter position we saw in little Hans' preoccupation, and identification, with the horse that bites. In the former position the child finds an inanimate object deprived of subjective, inter-subjective, trans-subjective properties. In fetishism, the signifier *as a fetish object* is in the place of the mother's imaginary phallus. And here we arrive at what John tried to put together from the "bits" and "pieces" of his childhood jouissance and anxiety. In John's case, the *bouton* is the name given to his mother's sexual "bit" (her imaginary phallus) by John's father, but it is a horrific name for it reverses *ton bout* in an unbearable way for this boy. After all, what kind of wrong can there be in having your bits and your mum's bits reversed? If the *boutons*, the many buttons – plural – together make up the fetish object we may well wonder what of the mother's imaginary phallus is present in this? We may well, along with Tostain, be amazed that:

> the object of horror and fright, the object of repulsion and of insurmountable disgust, an object bringing evil and an object of death ... will also be a love object, irresistibly attractive, the object of all seeking, the apparently elected object of desire.
>
> *(Tostain, 1980., p. 249)*

It is only if we make the error of descending to the place of the signified, i.e., these countable little objects, that we miss something crucial in this case (and perhaps in others). What, in fact Tostain, despite his erudite and interesting analysis of his case, also misses entirely; caught up as he was with the idea that the object "button" when singular was the object of phobic anxiety, and when multiplied, put into the plural, became a fetish (ibid., p. 250). For, it is not so simple as one button = phobia, many buttons = fetish. What does Lacan give us to work with? In fetishism the signifier as a fetish object is in the place of the mother's imaginary phallus, and the fetish object is loved for what it lacks. We will find everything we need at the level of the signifier, not at the place of the signified. *Bouton, boutons.* They sound exactly the same in French, only John knows when it is *bouton*, or when it is *boutons*. It is in this way that *boutons*, in the plural, as fetish object qua signifier, symbolises the imaginary phallus of the mother by including what she lacks: the little appendix, the "s" which pluralises the single *bouton*. In his excellent commentary on the case Bruce Fink has argued that pluralising the single *bouton* supplements the symbolic action by John's father (cf. Fink, 1999, p. 183), but the point I am trying to establish is different. Furthermore, what is brought into excellently sharp focus is Lacan's 1958 statement about the fetish as the "object perceived in the signifier's cut" (Lacan, 1958a, p. 510). Applied to the signifier *ton bout*, we can see that in between the successive iterations of *ton* and *bout*, there is the phobic object – *bouton* – but, in the cut of the signifier, multiplied, over and over, there is the fetish object – all the *boutons* – as many as it takes.

Ton ... bout... ton ... bout ... ton... bout ... ton... bout... ton ... bout ... ton... bout ... ton ... bout ... ton ... bout ... ton ... bout ... ton ... bout ... ton ... bout ... ton ... bout ... ton ... bout ... ton ... bout ...

References

Donoghue, E. (2010). *Room*. London: Picador.

Fink, B. (1999). *A Clinical Introduction to Lacanian Psychoanalysis Theory and Technique*. Harvard: First Harvard University Press.

Freud, S. (1909b). Analysis of a Phobia in a Five-Year-Old-Boy. *S.E.*, 10: 3–149. London: Hogarth Press.

Freud, S. (1938). Splitting of the Ego in the Process of Defence. *S.E.*, 23: 273–278. London: Hogarth Press, 1940e.

Lacan, J. (1956–1957). *The Seminar of Jacques Lacan Book IV; The Object Relation, 1956–1957*. L.V.A. Roche (Trans.). Unpublished.

Lacan, J. (1958a). The Direction of the Treatment and the Principles of its Power. In: *Écrits: The First Complete Edition in English* (pp. 489–542). B. Fink (Trans.). London & New York: W.W. Norton & Company, 2006.

Lacan, J. (1958b). The Signification of the Phallus. In: *Écrits: The First Complete Edition in English* (pp. 575–585). B. Fink (Trans.). London & New York: W.W. Norton & Company, 2006.

Lacan, J. (1965). Science and Truth. In: *Écrits: The First Complete Edition in English* (pp. 726–745). B. Fink (Trans.). London & New York: W.W. Norton & Company, 2006.

Tostain, R. (1980). Fetishization of a Phobic Object. In S. Schneiderman (Ed. & Trans.), *Returning to Freud: Clinical Psychoanalysis in the School of Lacan* (pp. 247–260). New York: Yale University Press.

4

THE PHOBIC AND FETISH OBJECTS

Stephanie Swales

At the end of the very first session of Seminar IV Lacan poses the question of whether or not there is a relation between the phobic and the fetish object. Phenomenologically speaking, the two seem quite different at first. After all, the phobia elicits intense fear and is avoided by the subject, whereas the fetish elicits sexual jouissance and is actively sought out. What could the two objects have in common? In Seminar IV, Lacan makes the case that both the fetish and the phobic object function to protect the subject from castration anxiety. What is more, Lacan links the two objects by virtue of their relationship to the father, the Other's desire, and the law. It is this connection, as well as their differences, that I will elucidate in this chapter, following what Lacan says about it in Seminar IV.

In the first session of Seminar IV, Lacan (1956–1957) says that the "object's role is to push anxiety into the background" (p. 11) and that it is fundamental to the "different stages of the development of the subject" (ibid., p. 11). What is this object? At this stage in Lacan's work, Lacan is referring not to the object *petit a*, which he did not begin to develop until his sixth seminar, but instead to a kind of hybrid between Freud's lost object (ibid., p. 4) and the imaginary phallus (ibid., p. 17). Lacan uses these concepts to substantially reinterpret Freud's Oedipus complex. As such, both the phobic and the fetish objects become ways to deal with the Other's desire and attain subjectivity. Instead of the lynchpin of castration anxiety and penis envy having to do with the actual penis, as it does in Freud's work, Lacan here warns us not to "confuse phallus and penis … [and] to distinguish the penis as a real organ with functions that we could describe through certain real coordinates, and the phallus within its imaginary function" (ibid., p. 19). Rather, what is crucial in the re-envisioned Oedipus complex is that the imaginary phallus is the object of the mother's desire. Castration relates to an imaginary object (ibid., p. 25), to the loss of the imaginary phallus (which means giving up an identification with the imaginary phallus).

The central tasks of the Oedipus complex thus understood involve coming to grips with the trauma of the discovery of sexual difference and of the Other's desire. The child in this process realises that the mOther is lacking and wonders if she or he can be the imaginary phallus or if the mOther's desire extends irremediably beyond the child. In Lacan's formulations of the graph of desire in Seminar V and in "The Subversion of the Subject and the Dialectic of Desire in the Freudian Unconscious" (Lacan, 1960), he said that the child poses a related question: "*Chè vuoi*?" (ibid., p. 690) or "What does the Other desire?" This is the question that Lacan said in psychoanalysis "best leads the subject to the path of his own desire" (ibid., p. 690) insofar as the subject models her or his desire in the fashion of the interpretation of the Other's desire. Initially, however, how the child answers this question can have structural consequences in terms of whether she becomes perverse or neurotic. This can be understood alongside Lacan's (1962–1963) final treatment of the question "*Chè vuoi*?" in Seminar X, when he spoke to "the essential relationship concerning anxiety and the desire of the Other" (p. 5). The child who believes that he is what the Other wants, that he is equated with the imaginary phallus, is subjected to substantial anxiety. In contrast, the child who passes through the Oedipus complex, separating from the mOther and believing that the Other desires the symbolic phallus, has less anxiety and more subjective space for himself.

Little Hans and the paternal metaphor

In Seminar IV Lacan said, "A mother always requires her child to have (or be) the phallus, which the child symbolizes or realizes more or less" (Lacan, 1956–1957, p. 56). The young child, for example little Hans—whose case Lacan discussed at great length in this seminar—who experiences himself to be identified with the imaginary phallus, is someone who is subjected to great anxiety. We might say in our day and age that Hans had a mother who was lacking in good "boundaries" with her son. On this account, Freud observed that as a four-year-old, Hans's mother gave him a daily bath and then dried and powdered him (Freud, 1909b, p. 19); she often took him into the bathroom with her (ibid., p.57); and she let him get into bed to "coax" (his word for "cuddle") with her despite protests from her husband (ibid., p. 39). She also gave Hans a guilt trip when he expressed a desire to separate from her and sleep at night with the neighbour's fourteen-year-old daughter, Mariedl:

HANS: "Oh, then I'll just go downstairs and sleep with Mariedl."
MOTHER: "You really want to go away from Mummy and sleep downstairs?"
HANS: "Oh, I'll come up again in the morning to have breakfast and do number one."
MOTHER: "Well, if you really want to go away from Daddy and Mummy, then take your coat and knickers and— good-bye!"

> Hans did in fact take his clothes and go towards the staircase, to go and sleep with Mariedl, but, it need hardly be said, he was fetched back.
>
> *(Ibid., p. 17)*

Hans made fruitless attempt after fruitless attempt to separate from his mother, and so his anxiety persisted. Freud, in his intervention, mistakenly tried to convince Hans that his father was not angry with him for being in love with his mother. Freud's intervention was based on the assumption that Hans's anxiety was rooted in a fear of castration rather than a wish for it.

Optimally, Hans's father would have intervened, separating the child from his mother by being convincingly angry, jealous, or authoritative in his prohibition of the mother-child over-proximity. It is in making just that point that Lacan (1956–1957), in his fourth seminar, first coins the term "paternal metaphor" (p. 379). The paternal metaphor is what enables the child to separate from the mother's desire and successfully pass through the Oedipus complex. The metaphor's structure is that the Name-of-the-Father stands in for the mother's desire, represented by the "*Chè vuoi?*", what does the mOther want from me? At this point in Lacan's work, the metaphor is the structure of the symptom, in which one signifier stands in for another which is repressed. Similarly, with the installation of the paternal metaphor, the signifier which is repressed or under the bar has to do with the mother's insatiable desire for the child, whereas the signifier above the bar is the paternal "No!", or prohibition. And, as Lacan pointed out in Seminar III (1981) and in "On a Question Prior to Any Possible Treatment of Psychosis" (Lacan, 1959), the paternal function can be carried out by someone other than a father. Nevertheless, Lacan used the term "paternal" to indicate that in his day and age it was most commonly the father who took on this function. Further, the father does not have to be especially fearsome in order to help his child undergo Oedipalisation. His role as an authoritative voice that can at least sometimes change the mother's mind is what counts. The mother herself also has authority and can have the phallus (Lacan, 1956–1957, p. 191). If the mother, in her discourse about the father to the child, respects his point of view, then whatever prohibition the father may make—even very politely—should have a sufficient effect on the child.

In the case of little Hans, Lacan commented that Hans reached an impasse in trying to separate from his mother. "He cannot get out [of the grip of his mother] because there is no father, there is nothing to metaphorize his relations with his mother" (ibid., pp. 379–380). For example, Mrs. Graf rendered Mr. Graf's protests weak and unsuccessful that Hans not share the bed with Mrs. Graf. Mr. Graf was anxious to be loved and not feared by Hans—so much so that he said he never hit or scolded Hans. It was on this account that Mr. Graf even interrupted Freud's speech to Hans:

> 'But why do you think I'm angry with you?' his father interrupted me at this point; 'have I ever scolded you or hit you?' Hans corrected him: 'Oh yes! You have hit me.' 'That's not true. When was it, anyhow?' 'This morning,'

> answered the little boy; and his father recollected that Hans had quite unexpectedly butted his head into his stomach, so that he had given him as it were a reflex blow with his hand.
>
> *(Freud, 1909b, p. 42)*

In this scene, Hans is actually eager to believe his father was angry with him. It may have been that Hans used the unconscious mechanism of disavowal, which might be formulated as follows: "I know very well that my father was not angry (or was not angry enough) but nevertheless I prefer to believe that my father was angry and hit me so that I would not continue to be so close with my mother."

Following Freud's own recommendation to interpret an expressed fear as a wish, we can re-interpret the following exchange: "Hans (aged four and three-quarters) woke up one morning in tears. Asked why he was crying, he said to his mother: 'When I was asleep I thought you were gone and I had no Mummy to coax [his expression for "to caress"] with'" (Freud, 1909b, p. 23). It was the mother's lack of lack, or rather her seeming fixation on Hans to exclusion of other desires, that was so terrifying for Hans. Anxiety appears when there seems to be no possibility of separation.

The phobic object

Lacan (1956–1957) referenced an "insatiable, unsatisfied mother" (p. 195) that the child encounters in the "crucial" pre-Oedipal stage (ibid., p. 194) and in relation to whom he becomes a split subject and constructs a stable ego.

> This insatiable, unsatisfied mother ... she is there, and like all unsatiated beings, she is seeking what she can devour, *querens quem devoret* ... That is the great danger his fantasies reveal, being devoured. We find it at the origin, and we find it again at this detour, where it gives us the essential form in which phobia is presented.
>
> *(Ibid., p. 195)*

The child's anxiety is the signal of a dangerous situation, one in which the mother's enigmatic desire has to do with his very being, and as such, a being that could be devoured. It is no wonder, then, that some children develop phobias of crocodiles, sharks, zombies, or witches who eat children in a stew. The invention of the phobia is at root a protection for the child. *The phobia makes up for a deficiency in the paternal metaphor.* "The establishment of the phobia is thus written with the same formula" (ibid., p. 380) that Lacan gave for the paternal metaphor except with "that element of metaphoric mediation which is for Hans the horse" (ibid., p. 380). The child can feel safe when a nightlight is turned on to show that there is no witch hiding in the corner of the room. The phobic object functions to crystallise the child's generalised anxiety (related to being identified with the imaginary phallus) into a feared object. For Hans, he transformed his fear of being devoured by his mother into a fear of being bitten by a horse. This construction, or "myth," as Lacan called it (ibid., p. 343), allowed Hans to feel safe as long as there were no horses present—even when he was in the company of his mother. The mother's dangerous insatiability was thereby cancelled out.

Lacan pointed out that "horse" did not become a sufficient signifier to play the role of a temporary paternal function until it became associated with two crucial elements: the bite and the fall. With the former, Hans had masturbated at night since he was three, and had ignored his mother's castration threats, admitting to her that despite her warnings he had put his hand to his "widdler" all the same (Freud, 1909b, pp. 7–8; p. 23). Hans traced the origin of his well-named "nonsense" (ibid., p. 30)—as Lacan emphasised the non-meaning in the kernel of the symptom—or horse phobia to March 1st, when he noticed "at the head of the luggage cart that is to take little Lizzie's luggage, the horse can turn around and bite" (Lacan, 1956–1957, p. 380). Lacan pointed out that the horse's linkage with its bite threatens Hans's masturbation much more effectively than his mother. What is more, the bite of the horse connected the horse to the "possible bite of the mother" (ibid., p. 380), to her "devoration" (ibid., p. 380), so that from then on the mother's bite or insatiability for Hans was transferred to the horse. The other crucial piece of the ability of the horse to function as a phobia, or as a temporary paternal metaphor, began on April 5th when Hans, while out with his mother, saw an omnibus horse fall.

> *From now on, all horses will always fall.* Now, the function of the fall is precisely the term common to all of what figures in the lower part of the equation [of the Oedipal complex facilitated by the paternal metaphor]. M—we have underlined the element fall-of-the-mother. φ—the mother's phallus, which is what is no longer tenable, is no longer in the game.
>
> *(Ibid., p. 381)*

Finally, Freud's intervention was also crucial in allowing the horse phobia to crystallise because Freud made the connection between Mr. Graf and the kind of horse that scared Hans. The horse that fell seemed convincingly angry—the way Hans wanted to see his father angry with him—on account of making "*a row with its feet*" (Freud, 1909b, p. 50; italics in original). The horse in that way gained an important connection to the paternal function. The horse phobia, then, is made possible through the horse's anger, its bite, and its ability to fall. As such, it does the work of signification central to a substitute for the paternal metaphor.

The phobic object is a signifier; indeed, as Lacan said in Seminar VI and in "The Direction of the Treatment", it can play the role of "an all-purpose signifier" (Lacan, 1958–1959, June 10, 1959, Session XXIV) "to make up for [*suppléer*] the Other's lack" (Lacan, 1957, p. 610). In Seminar IV, Lacan (1956–1957) noted that the phobic object, the horse in Hans's case, is "a phallus that takes on the value of all signifiers, that of the father if need be" (p. 425). It is worth pointing out that in Seminar IV Lacan's conceptualisations of the imaginary phallus are paired with statements that the phallus is a signifier (ibid., p. 191) and a symbolic object (ibid.,

p. 152). In Seminar V, Lacan went on to develop what became the standard notion of the symbolic phallus in "The Signification of the Phallus" (Lacan, 1958) and thereafter the symbolic phallus is a signifier of the Other's desire or of the Other's jouissance. The phobic object is best understood to be the symbolic phallus, as that which names the Other's desire. As Lacan (1966) emphasised, "the letter kills" the real (p. 719). In other words, by putting the mOther's enigmatic desire into words (and naming it as desire instead of it remaining a demand fixated on the child), the child can breathe more easily. The horse for little Hans does the work of signification, of plugging up the anxiety-provoking lack in the Other, allowing the subject "to protect himself against the emergence of an anxiety that is far more dreadful than the fear that is localized by the phobia" (Lacan, 1958–1959, p. 503).

In the last session of Seminar IV, Lacan suggested that the phobic solution is but a temporary one rather than a firmly established paternal metaphor. Instead, "the whole situation is resolved for him by an identification with the maternal desire" (Lacan. 1956–1957, p. 414) or the "maternal phallus" (ibid., p. 415). Instead of losing his status as imaginary phallus and becoming the symbolic phallus, there "is no phase of symbolization" (ibid., p. 415). Lacan commented that Hans "will have no father" (ibid., p. 416). Lacan continued, saying that he did "not believe that anything new in the experience of [Hans's] existence will ever give him one" (ibid., p. 416). In the absence of a firmly instantiated Name-of-the-Father, Lacan concluded that little Hans will become "something like a fetish object" (ibid., p. 414). Little Hans, he said, "has not passed by the castration complex, but by another route" (ibid., p. 408). The horse "phobia gradually vanish[ed], which made the signifier of the horse superfluous" (ibid., p. 408), the paternal metaphor only having been propped up as long as the horse phobia remained. Instead, little Hans will become perversely structured.

What, then, is the status of the phobia in terms of a structural position? In Seminar VI, Lacan (1958–1959) referred to the phobia both as "the fertile moment of neurosis" and as "the simplest form of neurosis" (p. 503). The latter gestures toward phobia being its own substructure of neurosis alongside hysteria and obsessional neurosis. The former, however, indicates that a phobia may have a developmental role in helping children become neurotic. Along those lines, Catherine Vanier has argued that the development of phobias in early childhood is extremely common and provides a pathway to separation and working through the encounter with sexual difference.

> During the infantile neurosis, fears and phobias normally accompany the castration complex. When all goes well, they are left behind at the end of the Oedipal period. This moment, when the child finds himself confronted with his lack, is the logical time for the constitution of his desire. Seized with panic if nothing comes to reassure him at that moment, the child institutes repression and phobia appears. If the parents are too nice, they may be transformed into terrifying monsters playing the part of agents of castration, like the wolf.
>
> *(Mathelin-Vanier, 2008, p. 181)*

From this perspective, a phobia is a symptom—like any other, perhaps—but one that is specifically constructed to deal with the problems of the castration complex. As such, if the phobia "works" it allows the child to become a neurotic subject. If it fails the child could become perversely or psychotically structured.

Bruce Fink asserts that phobia is "not so much 'in between' hysteria and obsession or a third independent structure, as in some sense prior to the other neuroses" (Fink, 1997, p. 163). Fink points out that phobia, unlike hysteria and obsession, has to prop up the Name-of-the-Father, which has a "precarious status" (ibid., p. 163), by negating the mother's desire with something other than the father's prohibition or name. Nevertheless, Fink maintains that phobia successfully installs the paternal metaphor, such that phobics might subsequently attain an obsessional or hysteric structure. On the other hand, Fink comments that little Hans, who initially had a phobic symptom, did not succeed in becoming phobic or neurotic because his phobic symptom did not manage to successfully instate the paternal metaphor. Some phobias, then, are sufficient in strength to permanently shore up the Name-of-the-Father while others are not. Of further interest is Fink's comment that phobia does not "have a full set of defining characteristics of its own … Rather, phobia appears to be closely related to hysteria, since the hysteric constitutes herself initially as the object suitable for plugging up the lack in the mOther" (ibid., p. 164). "Successful" phobia, then, seems to have an odd status as not having many defining characteristics of its own—in terms of the phobic's relation to desire, sexuality, fundamental fantasy, etc.,—but somehow constituting "the fertile moment of neurosis" (Lacan, 1958–1959, p. 503).

Certainly, in the clinic we see hysteric or obsessional neurotic individuals who have more or less prominent phobias which have either persisted since the castration complex or arisen afterwards. For example, an hysterical analysand whose first memory, from age four, was when her mother, who was suffering from cancer, fell (recall the role that the "fall-of-the-mother" played in Lacan's explication of Hans's phobia) on the floor and was rushed to the hospital where she died soon thereafter. Her father was on active duty in the military, and so he was mostly absent from her life for the next few years, leaving her in the care of her grandmother. The grandmother told her that she was much loved by her mother and her father, but she often felt uncertain about what she meant to her father. At age six, an older cousin forced her to watch the movie *IT*, in which the titular character can morph into the form most feared by a child in order to first immobilise her or him with fear and then consume her or him. Most frequently, IT appeared as a clown, and so the analysand developed a phobia of clowns that persisted into adulthood with such intensity that even a picture of a clown caused her heart to race. Notably, as a child, her mother's cancer had been explained to her as something that *ate* away at her mother's body. The elements of the devouring other are plain to see in this phobia, although in this case it helped bolster her sense of being desirable in the eyes of the other. One strategy of the neurotic to deal with the fact that the object *a* is connected to the Other's desire is to avoid approaching the object. As Lacan (1958–1959) put it in Seminar VI, "One way, as we have seen, is by creating a phobic object, a prohibited object. What must be prohibited? In the final analysis, a jouissance that is dangerous because it exposes the true abyss of desire to the subject" (p. 504).

The fetish object

In contrast, a subject who has a fetish can potentially have his structure or his orientation to lack, sexual difference, and the Other defined by the fetish object. That being said, having a fetish does not necessarily mean being perverse; neurotic individuals can and often do have fetishistic traits. Similarly to Lacan's (1958–1959) designation of phobia as "the simplest form of neurosis" (p. 503), Lacan gave a primary place to fetishism in the perversions. Lacan spoke of the "fundamental fetish in every perversion as an object perceived in the signifier's cut" (Lacan, 1957, p. 610), implying that the fetish object is present in every perversion. In Seminar IV, Lacan referred to fetishism as "the perversion of perversions" (Lacan, 1956–1957, p. 194). For all perversions, including fetishism, Lacan said that the primary problem has to do with "how the child, in his relation to the mother … identifies himself with the imaginary object of [her] desire" (ibid., pp. 197–198), the imaginary phallus. It is in this way that perversion, like childhood phobia, is the consequence of a partial failure of the paternal function, since the child becomes stuck in the position of the imaginary phallus without the intervention of the prohibition associated with the Name-of-the-Father.

In fetishism, as in all perversions, the relationship to the phallus plays a central role. Whereas for Freud the fetish stands in for the penis, for Lacan the fetish *"represents the phallus as absent, the symbolic phallus"* (ibid., p. 154, my italics). However, the symbolic phallus for the fetishist can only function via what Lacan calls the veil. In the ninth session of Seminar IV, Lacan provides the Schema of the Veil (ibid., p. 156), in which there is a curtain in the middle, with the subject on its left side, the object on its right side, and the nothing which lies beyond the object, hidden by it. The schema portrays the fetish object as an image projected onto the veil that hides the mOther's lack in being. The fetish hides "the nothing, which is also the symbol, or the phallus in as much as the woman doesn't have it" (ibid., p. 156). As I have argued elsewhere, the subject's desire is produced when object *a* is veiled or disguised, whereas the subject's anxiety is provoked when object *a* lacks the veil's adornment and is experienced in its nakedness as over-proximate (Swales, 2012, p. 113). If the curtain rises, the distinction greatly diminishes between the fetish as object-cause of desire and the phobic object as object-cause of jouissance (in the form of anxiety). The absence of the veil faces the fetishist with the Other's lack in being. The fetish is at root an image projected onto the veil at the level not of the field of vision, but instead the scopic field of the partial drives.

What constitutes the fetish object as, say, a shoe instead of a raincoat? Lacan noted that its inception is related to the moment "just before the moment when what is sought for in the mother, which is to say this phallus which she has and which she doesn't have, must be seen" (Lacan, 1956–1957, p. 157). The fertile moment functions as a screen memory, the *Deckerinnerung*, Lacan said, as it "is not simply an instant, it is an interruption in the story, a moment when it is stopped and frozen, and when, by the same token, it indicates the pursuit of its movement beyond the veil" (ibid.). While in the ninth session of Seminar IV this presence-absence is directly related to the symbolic phallus, which the so-called phallic mother both has and does not have, in the first session of the seminar Lacan said that the fetish "is related to the perception of the lack of a phallic organ in the female subject, and to the negation of that absence" (ibid., p. 23)—an observation which is repeated when he discusses little Hans's belief that his little sister's *Wiwi-macher* will grow, as if girls have little penises instead of qualitatively different genitalia. On this account, the fetish object is a signifier which both designates the ambiguity around sexual difference and the symbolic phallus.

The fetish object is constituted in response to the problem of the mother's desire. The fetish is isolated by the signifier, by a parent's enunciation of a prohibition. For instance, a common fetish object of a neurotic, such as the breast, does not come into play until the mother prohibits the child's access to her breast. This signifying cut forms the breast as an object *a* out of a previously undifferentiated ground.

To elaborate on the constituting effects the signifying cut has on the fetish, consider the case Freud (1927e) discussed in his article "Fetishism". The adult analysand had lived in England as a young child before moving to Germany. The analysand developed a fetish for women with "a shine on the nose" (*Glanz auf der naze*), resulting from the homonymic relation between "*Glanz*" (translated as "shine" in English) and "glance." The constituting screen memory was when the analysand, in a moment of sexual curiosity, tried to glance at his English nurse, and she told him his nose would be punished if he tried to look at her. And so *Glanz* and glance became linked to the nose, the forbidden object being the sexualised object of the scopic drive. The fetishist identified with the gaze, and this is what structured his relationship with the Other. Lacan said that via *Glanz auf der naze* we can "see here come into play and project itself at a point on the veil, the narrative chain, which may even contain a quite different phrase, and more still, a phrase in a forgotten language" (Lacan, 1956–1957, p. 158).

In Bruce Fink's case of W (2003), who had a fetish for black boots, we learn not only of the constituting moment of the fetish, but also how the fetish serves two main functions: propping up the paternal function and standing in for the ambiguity around sexual difference. Reading Fink's case considering what we have learned about fetishism from Seminar IV, we can trace one of the moments of the absence of the veil to W's memory of having been "horrified one day when he came home from school and saw his mother's dining room table pulled apart, "a gaping hole in the middle of it" (ibid., p. 58). [W] commented that he "couldn't handle it" (ibid.), he was so upset. The boot fetish was as a symptom overdetermined, but one of the key moments in its constitution was that on one occasion while the father was giving W's younger sister a "horsy ride" on his boot, he got very angry when she accidentally scratched his boot (ibid., p. 53). This memory may very well have formed W's association between the boot and female genitalia. As such, the boot as "presence-absence" (Lacan, 1956–1957, p. 157) could veil the lack in the Other. What is more, the boot came to stand in for the Name-of-the-Father—which had been substantially weakened when W was five years of age and his mother discovered that his father had never divorced one of his previous wives and that their marriage was consequently a sham. Why was "boot" the chosen signifier for the fetish, other than the memory with his little sister riding his father's boot? For one thing, the father's last name was associated with boots, and for another, when W was young, his mother read him a story about

> pirates who wore tall black boots, and she specifically pointed to their boots (it was the "boot book"). Part of the family lore was that they were direct descendants of Captain Kidd. She perhaps viewed these pirates as real men, unlike her husband, whom she considered to be too weak to fill the shoes (or boots) of her own strong father (whose boots W put on when he first masturbated). (Fink, 2003, p. 53)

Boots, then, were associated with strong fathers and the kind of men W's mother found to be desirable. The boot fetish was a way to insert a father figure between himself and his mother, staging that the father, and not W, was what the mother really wanted. The boot fetish thus functioned as a Name-of-the-Father, bolstering the paternal function so as to achieve a perverse structure but being insufficient for W to become neurotic.

Concluding thoughts

Lacan's early work has justifiably been criticised for phallocentrism. That being said, in Seminar IV Lacan's re-writing of the Oedipus complex via the imaginary phallus goes a long way toward de-emphasising the penis as a biological organ, which plays such a primary role in Freud's work. Nevertheless, at times in the seminar Lacan uses imaginary phallus in a way that seems equated with the penis. What is more, Lacan's comments that a required precondition for fetishistic perversion is that the male child perceives the female's lack of a penis and negates that absence. While on the one hand this could seem like a reductive theoretical move which as a consequence makes perversion a male prerogative, there is compelling clinical evidence of the disavowal of the female genitalia in cases of perversion. Freud's case of little Hans, Fink's case of W, Tostain's (1977) case of Jean, and my work with Jay (2012)—as well as my unpublished clinical experience working with perversely structured individuals—all testify to the importance of disavowal of the female genitalia. From this perspective, reference to the penis as a biological organ is necessary even if it might seem theoretically unsophisticated. And of course, it is the symbolic significance of the absence of the penis and the presence of something unnamable that is what counts. Successfully encountering sexual difference in the castration complex depends upon the process of nomination of the two types of genitalia.

The fact that both the fetish and the phobic objects can frequently be part of the life of neurotic subjects speaks to their crucial function of veiling the object *a*. In that vein, in Seminar VI Lacan (1958–1959) commented that the "fetish is in fact the fur, edge, fringe, or frill, the thing that hides, and nothing is better designated to serve the function of signifier of the Other's desire" (p. 564). Indeed, clinical work continues to testify to the challenge that each subject has in finding a way to deal with the Other's desire. In that regard, a fetish for being shat on, for the anal object, can be just as sophisticated, just as earth-shattering, and just as life-sustaining as a phobia of IT.

References

Fink, B. (1997). *A Clinical Introduction to Lacanian Psychoanalysis Theory and Technique*. Cambridge & London: Harvard University Press.

Fink, B. (2003). The Use of Lacanian Psychoanalysis in a Case of Fetishism. *Clinical Case Studies*, 2(1): 50–69.

Freud, S. (1909b). Analysis of a Phobia in a Five-Year-Old Boy. *S.E.*, 10: 3–149. London: Hogarth Press.

Freud, S. (1927e). Fetishism. *S.E.*, 21: 147–159. London: Hogarth Press.

Lacan, J. (1956–1957). *Le Séminaire. Livre IV: La relation d'objet*. Paris: Le Seuil, 1994.

Lacan, J. (1957). The Direction of the Treatment and the Principles of its Power. In: *Écrits: The First Complete Edition in English* (pp. 489–542). B. Fink (Trans.). London & New York: W.W. Norton & Company, 2006.

Lacan, J. (1958). The Signification of the Phallus. In: *Écrits: The First Complete Edition in English* (pp. 575–585). B. Fink (Trans.). London & New York: W.W Norton & Co, 2006

Lacan, J. (1958–1959). *Le séminaire livre VI: Le désir et son interprétation, 1958–1959*. Paris: Éditions de La Martinière et Le Champ Freudien, 2013.

Lacan, J. (1959). On a Question Prior to Any Possible Treatment of Psychosis. In: *Écrits: The First Complete Edition in English* (pp. 445–488). B. Fink (Trans.). London & New York: W.W. Norton & Company, 2006.

Lacan, J. (1960). The Subversion of the Subject and the Dialectic of Desire in the Freudian Unconscious. In: *Écrits: The First Complete Edition in English* (pp. 671–702). B. Fink (Trans.). New York and London: W.W. Norton & Company, 2006.

Lacan, J. (1962–1963). *The Seminar, Book X, Anxiety*. J.-A. Miller (Ed.) and A.R. Price (Trans.). Cambridge, UK and Malden, MA: Polity Press, 2014.

Lacan, J. (1966). Position of the unconscious. In: *Écrits: The First Complete Edition in English* (pp. 703–721). B. Fink (Trans.). London & New York: W.W Norton & Company, 2006.

Mathelin-Vanier, C. (2008). Fears and phobias in child analysis. *Journal of Infant, Child, and Adolescent Psychotherapy*, 7(3): 176–184.

Swales, S. (2012). *Perversion: A Lacanian Psychoanalytic Approach to the Subject*. New York & London: Routledge.

Tostain, R. (1977). Fetishization of a Phobic Object. . In S. Schneiderman (Trans.), *How Lacan's Ideas are Used in Clinical Practice* (pp. 247–260). New Jersey & London: Jason Aronson Press.

PART 2
Lack

5

PRIVATION

A logical step between castration and frustration

Rolf Flor

Jacques Lacan (1964) wrote that castration is "the altogether new mainspring that Freud introduced into desire" (p. 723). But what is castration for Lacan? And what does it mean for it to be a mainspring in relation to desire? One memorable and oft quoted characterisation of castration is the penultimate sentence of "The Subversion of the Subject and the Dialectic of Desire in the Freudian Unconscious": "Castration means that jouissance has to be refused in order to be attained on the inverse scale of the Law of desire." (Lacan, 1960, p. 689). An effort to unpack this gnomic sentence could lead us through a large swath of Lacanian metapsychology covering several years of his teaching (for a systematic explication of this compressed sentence see Van Haute, 2001, pp. 271–283). Suffice it to say that Lacan began to develop the distinctions assumed in this sentence—between need, demand, desire, and jouissance —as early as his fifth public seminar on the formations of the unconscious Lacan (1957–1958, p. 58ff).

His explication of castration did not start there. In his fourth seminar from the year before, on the "Object Relation" (Lacan, 1956–1957a), Lacan elucidated aspects of castration in terms that one could call "Oedipal" or even "developmental", i.e., as part of the parent-child relationship. At this point he is interested in presenting his understanding of castration in a way that is intended to contest the specific erosion he finds in psychoanalytic theory post-Freud. Part of this erosion harkens back to Melanie Klein's assertion that pre-Oedipal frustration in the mother-child relationship is defining for Oedipal development (Klein, 1928, p. 202). Largely through her impetus, the theoretical focus of Oedipal dynamics turned from castration to frustration, a shift that accelerated during the subsequent twenty-five years. Frustration, as Lacan noted in the year before this seminar, has become the very "*leitmotiv* of the prolific mothers of analytic literature in English" (Lacan, 1955–1956, p. 235), which he protested "abandons the very inspiration behind the work of Freud" (ibid.). This is in keeping with Lacan's overall approach throughout his first seminars, where he repeatedly directs his auditors back to Freud and cautions about deviations in the theoretical developments of Freud's followers.

As part of his "return to the meaning of Freud" (Lacan, 1955a, p. 335), Lacan works to shift the focus back from frustration to castration. Lacan does this in his fourth seminar by introducing a new notion, the concept of "privation". This essay will examine the role played by privation in the mother-child relationship, a kind of lack which Lacan thinks is essential to a properly Freudian understanding of both castration and frustration. It will survey Lacan's argument that if we can situate these "kinds" of lack (privation, castration, frustration) with regard to what he calls our registers of experience, we return to a properly Freudian understanding of castration, specifically *symbolic* castration. By introducing his notion of privation, this Oedipal version of the logic of lack, Lacan will not only lay the foundation for the equally pivotal notion of demand in his metapsychology, he will show that castration is about both the castration of the subject *and* the castration of the mother.

The Imaginary versus the Symbolic

The public teaching in which Lacan calls for a return to Freud begins with the introduction to "three quite distinct registers that are essential registers of human reality: the Symbolic, the Imaginary, and the Real" (Lacan, 1953, p. 4). I will say more about all three of these later, but at this time it is helpful to make a few schematic comments about how and why Lacan contrasts the Imaginary and the Symbolic.

The Imaginary is the register of experience Lacan (1949) associates with the ego and with a propensity for infants to create a sense of wholeness or completeness via images of an other (pp. 74–81). Not knowing what it is for itself, the subject "speculates" with this semblable, it imagines itself via an other. This happens through a variety of image experiences: I am what is seen by the other; or, I am like what I see. At a certain moment in childhood—somewhere between six and eighteen months—a critical mass of these experiences precipitates a change for the subject,

> caught up in the lure of spatial identifications, (who can now) turn out fantasies that proceed from a fragmented image of the body to what I call an "orthopedic" form of its totality—and the finally donned armor of an alienating identity that will mark his entire development with its rigid structure.
>
> *(ibid., p. 78).*

This rigid structure, the ego, is a unifying function acquired through the introjection of a total image of the body (Lacan, 1949, p. 76). The construction of the Imaginary carries with it ontological insecurity; to find myself via a specular ego comes without guarantee. Even worse, the ego formed by imaginary identifications is an illusion, itself (Lacan argues in his very first seminar) constructed like a symptom (Lacan, 1953–1954, p. 16). Whatever else I may be, I am not, for example, my brother, even if it is via an image of this other that I become something for myself. "I can in no way expect to attain my accomplishment and my unity from the recognition of an other who is caught up with me in a relation of mirage" (Lacan, 1955–1956, p. 241).

Some of Freud's followers called for a maturing or strengthening of the ego (Anna Freud, Heinz Hartmann, Ernst Kris); they looked for an "adaptation to reality [via an] alliance of the healthy part of the ego ... by its agreement with the point of view [of the analyst]" (Lacan, 1955a, p. 127). Lacan will dismiss any strategy of maturing or strengthening the ego. "Freud's experience forces him to remodel the structure of the human subject by decentering it in relation to the ego" (Lacan, 1954–1955, p. 116). If anything, Lacan will recommend the opposite, a dissolution of the identifications that form the ego needs to be pursued, because "the ego represents the center of all resistances to the treatment of symptoms" (Lacan, 1948, p. 96).

He directs us instead to attend to what he calls the Symbolic. Speech, language, words, signifiers: these comprise the material with which we treat symptoms and they belong to this "other" register of experience. Lacan claims that, for Freud, something "decentered" (Lacan, 1956, p. 241) from the ego—the *speaking* subject—is the principal focus for psychoanalysis. Speech is the only tool psychoanalysts use in the consulting room to combat human troubles; words are the very "crux of technique" (ibid., p. 202). The unconscious is, he says, structured analogously to the realm of signifiers as outlined in Saussurean linguistics; and the speaking subject finds itself inserted from the start in a lawfully organised order of signification. Lacan's overarching stance can be described thus: Freudian psychoanalysis *hinges* on the Symbolic.

He supports his argument with a careful reading of Freud's formative works—"The Interpretation of Dreams" (Freud, 1900a), "The Psychopathology of Everyday Life" (Freud, 1901b), and "Jokes and the Relation to the Unconscious" (Freud, 1905c). In the semesters during which he was holding his third seminar, Lacan gave a short talk for the general public entitled "An Address: Freud in the Century" that summarises his understanding of these texts (Lacan, 1955–1956, pp. 231–247). He finds in these seminal texts the many ways that Freud shows that psychoanalysis must take account of the functions of speech and the field of language. His positions on castration in his fourth seminar are a response to what he saw as "deviations" (Lacan, 1955b, p. 273), post-Freudian models of psychoanalysis that either misplace the tools of language or centre their therapeutic goals on shoring up the ego.

Contra Bouvet

An example of *both* critiques is his repeated challenge of influential French psychoanalyst Maurice Bouvet (Lacan, 1956–1957a, session of 21 November 1956; session of 28 November 1956; Lacan, 1958, p. 505). Working from the British school made famous by Klein, Winnicott, and Balint, as well as the ego psychology promoted by Hartmann, Kris and Lowenstein, Bouvet theorised that the frustrations inevitable in pre-Oedipal relationships could be understood as important analysable source material and that we could push back with patients in analysis to the age *before* speech to infantile object relations (Bouvet, 1956, pp. 51–52). This connects Bouvet's work with Klein and object relations theory. Bouvet explored internalised objects from infantile development since, for him, neurosis developed during those pre-linguistic years as a result of "immature" object relations. Of interest to Bouvet were identifications from the oral and anal phases of pre-genital development in which the relationship with the mother is central because of her typical function in nursing and toilet-training. However, Bouvet was also in line with ego psychology in important ways. He argued that attachments gone awry during infancy require psychoanalysts to move the ego of their patients towards "mature object relations"; patients need to develop "from pre-genital to genital relations" (Lacan, 1958, p. 506). Ultimately, for Bouvet, the only appropriate goal of psychosexual development was enjoyable heterosexual relations, any other relations being pathological (Evans, 2017, p. 1).

Bouvet's position has several core commitments which draw from both object relations theory and ego psychology: that the ego and the speaking subject are one and the same thing; that there is one natural process of maturation from partial to whole object relations, which ends for the healthy ego with "untroubled" genital relations; and that the (healthy) ego of the psychoanalyst provides the yardstick of successful maturation. Lacan has been arguing for some time against the first commitment. With regard to the second, the least bit of experience as an analyst in the consulting room shows that, notwithstanding any moralising hopes, the harmonious maturity presumed to underlie genital love-making is a chimera (Lacan, 1960, p. 41). Finally, he downright ridicules the notion that a measure of neuroticism (how stuck someone was in pre-Oedipal relations) is to be taken from the "obviously healthy" psychoanalyst's perspective (ibid, pp. 449, 506).

However, the question of maturation is a line of argument that must be taken more seriously because it is fathomable given Freud's "Three Essays on the Theory of Sexuality" (Freud 1905d), an early work on psychosexual development which seems to suggest just such a process. Nevertheless, for Lacan this is also ultimately wrong-headed; specifically, it fails to take account of the transformative edits Freud made to the "Three Essays" over the decades that followed its publication. Lacan (1956-1957a) contends (p. 50) any notion of development must be *thought together with* the other above-mentioned early works emphasising signifiers which shows us why the ego and the speaking subject are not the same thing. Moreover, the post-Freudian notion of a whole object (something Freud never spoke about) is challenged by Freud's positions on narcissism and the ego. The latter, works like "On Narcissism" (Freud, 1914c), "Group Psychology and the Analysis of the Ego" (Freud, 1921c), and "The Ego and the Id" (Freud, 1923b), should steer us away from a celebration of imaginary constructs.

Lacan makes clear his standpoint in his comment with regard to Bouvet that "if one confines oneself to an imaginary relation between objects there remains nothing but the dimension of distance to order it" (Lacan, 1960, p. 508). There is every reason *not* to limit oneself to the experience of the Imaginary once one has taken the proper measure of the Symbolic. The child finds itself in a symbolic environment. Names are introduced. One plays hide and seek games with them using words. Injunctions are pronounced. In other words, the child is spoken to almost from the get-go. Freud's formative texts shows ways in which psychoanalysis *must* take account of the functions of speech and the field of language. "[P]sychoanalytic action develops in and through verbal communication, that is, in a dialectical grasping of meaning. Thus it presupposes a subject who manifests himself verbally in addressing another subject" (Lacan, 1948, p83). This terrain of the Symbolic, the dimension in which this addressing of an other takes place, is what Lacan calls "the Other". It is with regard to the Other that we must develop our understanding of castration.

Symbolic castration and its retroaction

In the opening moments of his fourth seminar—fully entitled "The Object Relation and Freudian Structures"—Lacan (1956-1957a) reminds his listeners of his commitment to this speaking subject alluded to in the latter part of his title, by presenting his L-schema (p. 2). This schema graphically represents the dialectical speech relationship between the subject and the Other, as well as the conflictual relationship between the Imaginary and the Symbolic. It illustrates the seed of his alternative: to suspend the subject's certainties (their ego identifications) until "their final mirages have been consumed" (Lacan, 1960, p. 209) by pursuing instead the speech relationship between the speaking subject and the Other.

In this seminar he specifically turns to the moment of origin for the speaking subject, the moment when the subject first begins to accept the existence of the radically Other dimension of signification itself, a process that continues into the following year's seminar on the formations of the unconscious. He ties this moment of origin to a particular notion of castration.

Lacan acknowledges that Freud did indeed explore the *pre*-linguistic, infantile, pre-Oedipal foundations of human development. However, Freud emphasised that strong forces from later life shape that development retroactively, making the status of infantile material aporetic. Lacan identifies castration as a force of this type because for Lacan castration is not about surrendering some part of one's body, rather it is to experience the loss of imagining oneself completely, i.e., without the intrusion of the symbolic environment. Castration, for Lacan, is symbolic castration; we will need to return to this in more detail below, but for now, suffice it to say that castration is the assent to absence which enables symbolising in the first place.

Since it permits the child to find its way with the signifier, and signifiers are the tools of psychoanalytic work, castration means that any symptom associated with pre-Oedipal frustration can only be worked through from an Oedipal dimension. Lacan (1956-1957a) protested "analysts today in fact reorganise analytic experience by beginning with the level of frustration, and neglect the concept of castration, which was nevertheless Freud's original discovery" (p. 52). How specifically does castration relate to the mother-infant relationship? The discovery that Lacan will find in his fourth seminar and hold onto into his later work is that castration is first discovered during the (imaginary) mother-infant relationship by the child *in the mother.*

This shows that when Lacan theorised the pre-Oedipal mother-infant relationship he was in fact himself indebted to the work of Melanie Klein.

> Only Melanie Klein, studying children on the verge of language, dared to project subjective experience into that earlier period.... Through Klein we have become aware of the function of the imaginary primordial enclosure formed by the imago of the mother's body.
>
> *(Lacan, 1960, p. 93)*

However, as we would expect, Lacan also counseled that we cannot stop at the level of the Imaginary:

> [What] allowed Freud to track down the treasure in [psychoanalysis], treasure that made his followers rich, is the symbolic determination to which the imaginary function is subordinated and which in Freud's work is always powerfully recalled.
>
> *(Ibid, p. 388)*

The Real object

To take the next step in Lacan's logic of lack it will be necessary to introduce Lacan's third register or category: the Real. At least for the purposes of this paper, which is limited to Lacan's early seminars, we can start with the first two things Lacan (1956-1957a) tells us about the Real: "the Real has more than one meaning and (whatever else it may be) the Real is at the boundary of our experience" (p. 26). Lacan knows he is not saying much about this; but indeed that seems to be the point. The Real is what remains somehow just beyond our ability to imagine or express.

Throughout his early seminars he remains coy about saying exactly what the Real is; in 1956 Lacan will suggest that the German words *wirklich* (for Real), *wirklichkeit* (reality), and *wirkung* (effect) may help us glean what he is calling the Real (ibid, p. 28). As a process of approximating the notion, with these linguistic references we can distinguish the more quotidian notion "reality" as being what we express with signifiers, from the "Real" *as that which we can feel the effects of but just can't get our words around.* With this point, Lacan can finally put front and centre his issue for the object in regard to the so-called object relation:

> We are thus led to the fundamental question with which we must begin because to it we must return, and it is the question with which we shall end. The whole ambiguity of the question concerning the object and its management in analysis comes down to this—is the object Real or not.
>
> *(Ibid, p. 25)*

But what object are we talking about? Is the object an element of reality, in the ordinary sense of the word, or is it "real"?

Lacan's answer will centre on two extraordinary propositions which he sees as the Freudian core on the topic of the "object": from the moment the subject begins to speak we know that the subject has a relation with an object *that is lost*; and the always-already lost object *is* the phallus (ibid, p. 7). The object according to Lacan *is* real, "real" in Lacan's sense, and its *wirkung* is precisely what makes castration happen.

Lacan elaborates this lost phallus by introducing an experience with not one but three objects: the imaginary, the symbolic and the real phallus. None of these usages of the term phallus should be equated with the penis. An imaginary phallus can be an image or a model of a penis. However, for the subject *every* embodiment of what was lost through castration would also be an imaginary phallus. A penis *can* be *but does not have to be* an embodiment of what was lost. Certainly, for the mother, who has never had one, a child could hypothesise the existence of an imaginary phallus. A real phallus is *also* not a penis. What makes it "real" is the impossibility of simply representing it; it is the ineffable experience of presence (or loss) without representation. Nor is the symbolic phallus a penis. Such a phallus is something that has "been introduced into the place of the signifier as such" (Lacan, 1956, p. 53) and in that way has become a kind of signification. Typically one may think of a signified as something that exists first and is then given a signifier. But for the advent of signification, we could say, the signifier creates and erases the signified. The Symbolic is the register in which lack proper can first appear because the word is "a presence made of absence" (Lacan, 1960, p. 228), in other words, a "Real" made palpable through some embodiment of loss.

Operations and agents of lack

Lacan explains that to know what these losses are is to know how they function, and for that two more components must be added. Objects of lack (the imaginary, the symbolic and the real phallus) have "operations of lack" (Lacan, 1956–1957a, p. 42)—this is how Lacan refers to distinguishable experiences of the infant—namely castration, privation, and frustration. Then also we must incorporate the infant's perspective of the *other* that apparently causes lack. Lacan refers to the other that brings about lack as the "agent". Hence Lacan's theory of phallic lack is a knotting of the three registers (Symbolic, Imaginary, Real) with three components (object, lack, and agent). He presents this in his seminar in table form.

Frustration is the lack associated with the experience of an injury, a harm, a damage done. The agent imposing this injury is symbolic in that their coming and going is essential to the idea of signifying structure. She is the "symbolic mother, the first element of reality symbolized by the child, in that she can be absent or present" (Lacan, 1956–1957a, p. 422). The object is the real phallus in the sense of an indescribable "something"; a powerful other, a mother, or another in her stead, may come and go. For a reader versed in Lacan, this notion of a "symbolic mother" may be striking since one often associates the Symbolic with the father

AGENT	LACK OF OBJECT	OBJECT
Real Father	Castration *Symbolic Debt*	Imaginary Phallus
Symbolic Mother	Frustration *Imaginary Injury*	Real Breast/Penis
Imaginary Father	Privation *Real Hole*	Symbolic Phallus

FIGURE 5.1 Table of lack
(Adapted from Lacan, 1956-1957b, p. 269)

and the mother with the Imaginary/Real. His point seems to be that the infant experiences this mother, this first Other, as the one who introduces an effraction of the Symbolic. The infant attempts to fathom the lack associated with the mother (Lacan, 1956, p. 32). The source of this effraction is that the infant questions the oscillation of some quantum of anxiety. Why does she come and go? Does she lack something herself? Am I what she lacks? And, perhaps most importantly, is it possible to find our way back to the time before or beyond anxiety? Lacan's answer will be "no" for two reasons: first, psychoanalytic experience shows that what is found will always be marked as repetition, which demonstrates that it is not what was lost. What was lost is "found and embraced elsewhere than it was sought" (Lacan, 1956–1957a, p. 6). But the more important reason is the second: what the mother brings to the infant-mother relationship is pivotal. *The mother herself will have undergone castration.* Lacan (1960) refers to this as the "function of mothering in the genesis of the object" (p. 511). She brings with her to the child's experience a seed of perpetual lack in the form of *her own* imaginary phallus.

Hence Lacan (1956-1957a) can say that the imaginary phallus has "a certain complementary function with regard to something which appears as a hole, indeed as an abyss in reality" (p. 15). The imaginary phallus is *any* embodiment for the subject of what was lost. The abyss is "complementary" in that it applies to the mother as well. Because the mother brings her lack with her, the first object relation for the child is not child-to-mother but rather *child-to-mother-to-phallus (qua lack)*. For Lacan, this is the primal object relation: an anxious arrangement for the child in which both lack and other are present for *both* participants.

Thus, in this matrix—a word of apt origin—begins the process of castration. The complementary function allows that the child might frame the concern symbolically: "The other lacks or it does not. I am what she lacks or I am not what she lacks". The child considers an imaginary object (imaginary for the mother, because it would be the embodiment for the mother of what was lost) where the agent imposing this injury would be real (because it remains ineffable in the experience of the infant.) The fact that it is an imaginary phallus implies that it can be detached from the notion of a real penis, symbolically allowing the child to stand in as a phallus *for the mother*. Hence the child can consider at least that it may be exactly what the mother lacks. Lacan draws here on Winnicott's notion of the transitional object (Winnicott, 1953), itself an extension of Klein's object of the mother, to develop the idea of the endless movement of the signifier. Lacan says in one of his *écrits:*

> [W]hen I discussed object-relation themes one year in my seminar, I showed the value of a conception in which child observation is nourished by the most accurate reconsideration of the function of mothering in the genesis of the object: I mean the notion of the transitional object introduced by D. W. Winnicott.
>
> *(Lacan, 1960, p. 511)*

The phallus, Lacan says, is "an instrument for masking and guarding against the fundamental ground of anxiety which characterises, at different stages of his development, the subject's relation to his world" (Lacan, 1956–1957a, p. 15). Lacan will say that in its ultimate incarnation the phallus is the instrument that enables the child to promote itself into a speaking subject, the very condition of psychoanalysis, because the symbolic phallus will come to "signify" signification itself (Lacan, 1960, p. 579). But his phrase "stages of development" implies that there is somehow a precursor for this ultimate role of the phallus. What are the intermediate steps that enable the child-mother-lack to transform into a speaking subject? Or as Lacan (1956-1957a) asks, "What is the turning point at which the mother-child relation opens towards elements that will introduce what we have called a dialectic" (session of 19 December 1956, p. 69)?

Privation is pivotal

For this, Lacan will need to bring in the kind of lack we have not yet touched upon, privation. He summarises our trajectory so far:

> Never, in our concrete experience of analytic theory, shall we be able to do without a notion of object lack as being central. This is not a negative, but the very spring of the subject's relation to the world.
>
> From its origin, analysis, the analysis of neurosis, began with the notion of castration, a notion so paradoxical that one can say it has still not been completely worked out.
>
> We think we are still speaking about it as they spoke of it in Freud's time. This is totally erroneous. We are speaking of it less and less, and we are wrong. What we speak about much more is frustration. There is still a third term of which we are beginning to speak, or more precisely, we shall see how

> necessary it was to introduce this notion, by what route and what imperative, and that is the notion of privation.
>
> *(Lacan, 1956–1957a, session of 28 November 1956, p. 31)*

So far we have seen that effraction of the Symbolic, in the form of the presence/absence of the mother seems to frustrate the child, leaving it with an imaginary injury. If the mother lacks, or better, if the child can consider an economy in which the mother's lack allows for substitutions ("Maybe I am what she lacks; maybe I am not what she lacks?"), the child could bridge these losses with a logical construction: there is a real hole here. This real hole, the sense of privation, brings with it a kind of reflexivity. Something ineffable is missing. The symbolic nature of the agent that frustrates can be imagined: there is now an Other at the center of this injury. The imaginary nature of the object can be mobilised symbolically: the lack that the mother brings, her *own castration insofar as it is experienced by the child*, allows the child to imagine itself as what may or, more importantly, may not make the mother whole.

With privation, the symbolic mother becomes a real "power"; what had been merely objects of satisfaction or dissatisfaction become "objects of gift deriving from this power" (Lacan, 1956–1957a, p. 69). So the imagined object becomes a symbolic object, an object of exchange. As Lacan will say in the following year, "privation is completely real, even though it only bears upon a symbolic object" (Lacan, 1957–1958, session of 13 March 1958, p. 261). Privation is in that way a very particular lack, a logically constructed one that initiates the separation of the inchoate mother-child relationship and will permit the child to move the imaginary injury to a symbolic debt.

With this notion of privation and power, Lacan will start to move the theoretical exposition away from objects and the Oedipal dynamic. The pivotal roles of privation and power lead him to explore the notion of demand upon which the advent of the subject will depend. This will be given as a distinct, but related, logic of lack in terms of need, demand, and desire (Lacan, 1960, p. 580). In this, demand (instead of privation) will provide the pivot that allows Lacan to describe the logic of lack. The advantage of starting from demand means that he starts with something that is expressed *in signifiers*. We ask for things. Things are asked of us. In other words, demand is a term that carries the mark of language which has always specified for Lacan the Freudian unconscious.

> [The specifics of this logic] beginning with demand … eluded in the notion of frustration (a notion Freud never used) … bear on something other than the satisfaction it calls for. It is a demand for a presence or an absence. This is what the primordial relationship with the mother manifests, replete as it is with an Other who must be situated *shy* of the needs that the other can fulfill.
>
> *(Ibid, p. 579)*

In both versions of the logic of lack what remains true is that the phallus will be the privileged signifier, the first mark of that signification. From there we cannot find our way back to frustrations in the analytic material without the impact of that mark. There is no frustration without castration, and no castration without privation. But in the logic of lack which Lacan will henceforth develop, that of demand and desire, it will be possible to focus on the dialectic between the two in the life of the speaking subject beyond its Oedipal roots.

References

Bouvet, M. (1956). La clinique psychoanalytique: La relation d'objet. In: *La psychoanalyze d'aujourd'hui* (pp. 41–121). Paris: PUF.

Evans, J. (2017, September 11). Commentary on Maurice Bouvet's description of Object Relations Theory (Seminar IV). Lacanian Works. Retrieved from: http://www.lacanianworks.net/?p=12130.

Freud, S. (1900a). *The Interpretation of Dreams. S.E.*, 4–5. London: Hogarth Press.

Freud, S. (1901b). *The Psychopathology of Everyday Life. S.E.*, 6. London: Hogarth Press.

Freud, S. (1905c). *Jokes and the Relation to the Unconscious. S.E.*, 8. London: Hogarth Press.

Freud, S. (1905d). Three Essays on the Theory of Sexuality. *S.E.*, 7: 123–230. London: Hogarth Press.

Freud, S. (1914c). On Narcissism: An Introduction. *S.E.*, 14: 67–102. London: Hogarth Press.

Freud, S. (1921c). Group Psychology and the Analysis of the Ego. *S. E.*, 18: 65–144. London: Hogarth Press.

Freud, S. (1923b). The Ego and the Id. *S.E.*, 19: 3–69. London: Hogarth Press. Klein, M. (1928). Early Stages of the Oedipus Conflict. In: *Contributions to Psycho-analysis 1921–1945* (pp. 202–226). London: Hogarth Press.

Lacan, J. (1948). Aggressiveness in Psychoanalysis. In: *Écrits: The First Complete Edition in English* (pp. 82–101). B. Fink (Trans.). New York: W.W. Norton & Company, 2006.

Lacan, J. (1949). The Mirror Stage as Formative of the I Function as Revealed in Psychoanalytic Experience. In: *Écrits: The First Complete Edition in English* (pp. 75–81). B. Fink (Trans.). New York: W.W. Norton & Company, 2006.

Lacan, J. (1953). The Symbolic, the Imaginary, and the Real. In: *On the Names of the Father* (pp. 1–52). B. Fink (Trans.). London: Polity Press.

Lacan, J. (1953–1954). *The Seminar of Jacques Lacan Book I: Freud's Papers on Technique*. J. Forrestor (Trans.) New York: W.W. Norton & Company, 1988.

Lacan, J. (1954–1955). *The Seminar of Jacques Lacan Book II: The Ego in Freud's Theory and in the Technique of Psychoanalysis*. S. Tomaselli (Trans.). New York: W.W. Norton & Company, 1988.

Lacan, J. (1955a). The Freudian Thing, or the Meaning of the Return to Freud in Psychoanalysis. In: *Écrits: The First Complete Edition in English* (pp. 334–363). B. Fink (Trans.). New York: W.W. Norton & Company, 2006.

Lacan, J. (1955b). Variations on the Standard Treatment. In: *Écrits: The First Complete Edition in English* (pp. 269–302). (B. Fink, Trans.). New York: W.W. Norton & Company, 2006.

Lacan, J. (1955–1956). *The Seminar of Jacques Lacan Book III: The Psychoses*. J. -A. Miller (Ed.) & R. Grigg (Trans.). New York: W. W. Norton & Company, 1993.

Lacan, J. (1956). The Function and Field of Speech and Language in Psychoanalysis. In: *Écrits: The First Complete Edition in English* (pp. 197–268). B. Fink (Trans.). New York: W.W. Norton & Company, 2006.

Lacan, J. (1956–1957a). *The Seminar of Jacques Lacan Book IV: The Object Relation, 1956–1957.* J.-A. Miller (Ed.), L.V.A. Roche (Trans.). Unpublished Manuscript.

Lacan, J. (1956–1957b). *Le Séminaire, livre IV: La relation d'objet.* Paris: Seuil, 1994. Lacan, J. (1957–1958). *Formations of the Unconscious: The Seminar of Jacques Lacan Book V.* J.-A. Miller (Ed.) & R. Grigg (Trans.). Cambridge: Polity Press, 2017.

Lacan, J. (1958). The Direction of the Treatment and the Pinciples of Its Power. In: *Écrits: The First Complete Edition in English* (pp. 489–542). (B. Fink, Trans.). New York: W.W. Norton & Company, 2006.

Lacan, J. (1960). The Subversion of the Subject and the Dialectic of Desire. In: *Écrits: The First Complete Edition in English* (pp. 671–702). (B. Fink, Trans.). New York: W.W. Norton & Company, 2006.

Lacan, J. (1964). On Freud's "Trieb" and the Psychoanalyst's Desire. In: *Écrits: The First Complete Edition in English* (pp. 722–725). (B. Fink, Trans.). New York: W.W. Norton & Company, 2006.

Van Haute, P. (2001). *Against Adaptation: Lacan's Subversion of the Subject.* P. C. Vankerk (Trans.). New York: Other Press.

Winnicott, D. (1953). Transitional Objects and Transitional Phenomena. *International Journal of Psychoanalysis*, 34: 89–97.

6

ASEXUALITY, ABSENCE, AND THE DIALECTIC OF SUBSTITUTION

Kevin Murphy

One obvious challenge in approaching the concept of asexuality is how to understand its manifest absence of sexual desire. Despite its central position, this absence is referenced only obliquely in the widely accepted definition of asexuality provided by the Asexual Visibility & Education Network (AVEN): "An asexual is a person who does not experience sexual attraction" (AVEN, 2001). Researchers in this field also generally eschew an engagement with the concept, preferring instead to focus on predictors of asexual identity (Prause & Graham, 2007), on social and sexual behaviours (Brotto et al., 2010; Carrigan, 2011), and on mapping its statistical prevalence (Aicken, Mercer & Cassell, 2013; Poston & Baumle, 2010). Research that *does* privilege it focuses on neurological or physiological factors (Bogaert, 2006) to explain the absence of sexual desire. Furthermore, within the asexual community there are divergent approaches. On the AVEN website, for example, there is the view that the "cause" of asexuality and, by default, the absence of sexual desire, needs no enquiry; it is enough for asexuals to experience it for its legitimacy to be established. On the other hand, there is also an essentialist viewpoint that acknowledges asexuality, and the primacy of absence of sexual desire, as a "natural" condition that one is born with. This ambivalence regarding absence of sexual desire indicates an unease that may derive from an inadequate theoretical foundation from which to interrogate it. It also exposes asexuality to those who seek to pathologise it. If sexual attraction, understood as a manifestation of sexual desire, is the psychological core of sexuality (Bogaert, 2012, p. 23), then its absence would, presumably, undermine asexuality's claim to being a legitimate and unique "sexual" orientation (Brotto & Yule, 2017, p. 620). In the context of this equivocal dialectic, Lacan's Seminar IV offers considerable scope to approach the absence of sexual desire by employing his insights regarding the concept of lack in the formation of the human subject. Extending his thinking in this area allows for a theoretical consideration of asexuality in relation to absence and offers a possible aetiology of this emerging orientation. Asexuality is contemporary culture's newest and most enigmatic mode of sexuality, one that appears to offer a particular form of enjoyment deriving from the very absence it represents.

Lacan (1956–1957) situates lack as central to subject formation and rather than being a negative it is, instead, the "very spring of the subject's relation to the world" (p. 31). In this regard, he emphasises how sexuality occurs in the earliest experience of the breast as the lacking object of frustration when refused or absent for the child. It is not the object itself which plays the essential role in this. For Lacan, the significance of the breast as object derives from "the activity" or interplay between child and feeding Other. This oral function as activity, including as it does a pleasurable dimension, takes on an eroticised function on the plane of desire. In Lacan's terminology it enters into the "dialectic of substitution in the demand for love" (ibid., p. 211). He moves forward from this with a discussion of anorexia in which he considers how absence itself can become eroticised. He reconsiders the subject who is "not eating" as the subject who is instead "eating nothing" (ibid.). This "eating nothing", he argues, is something other than a negation of activity because the child uses this "absence savoured as such" (ibid.) in the face of the mother on whom the child depends. As he puts it: "Thanks to this nothing he makes her depend on him" (ibid., p. 214). If the relation to the nothing in anorexia enters a "dialectic of substitution for satisfaction" (ibid., p. 210), thus bringing about an absence that can be savoured, then absence becomes eroticised. From this perspective, it is possible to glean a theoretical insight into what might be taking place in asexuality. Rather than "not desiring", the asexual might be actively "desiring nothing" in a dialectic that allows for an engagement with the Other while at the same time avoiding a dependence for the satisfaction of need which the real of bodily jouissance would entail.

The object annulled as symbolic

Lacan makes the point that the main purpose of anorexic refusal is about the object, the symbolic object of the subject-Other dialectic which appears, as he says clearly, under the sign of the nothing (Lacan, 1956–1957, p. 214). He also identifies the mechanism which brings this refusal about. "It is with regard to the object annulled as symbolic that the child puts his dependency in check, precisely by nourishing himself on nothing" (ibid.). The mechanism of annulment that he introduces here offers considerable scope in approaching the relation of asexuality to absence. Using Freud's term, *Versagung,* Lacan speaks of it as, "the concept of annulation, in the sense that one speaks of annulling a treaty or of a retreat from an engagement" (ibid., p. 206). From this perspective, frustration is not just the refusal of an object of satisfaction but is, rather, frustration as the refusal of a gift, in this case the gift of the breast as object. According to Lacan:

> [T]he gift arises from a beyond of the object relation, since it supposes behind it the whole order of exchange into which the child has entered, and it can

> only arise from that beyond with a character which constitutes it as properly symbolic.
>
> *(Ibid., p. 208)*

Here the oral object is the gift, whereas in his subsequent work he continues the Freudian tradition (Freud, 1917c) in which the gift is associated with the anal object. In *Television*, for example, Lacan (1963) describes the oral object as the breast which the "astonished" child realises belongs to the mother (Seminar of November 20 1963, p. 85). The anal object, by contrast, is the gift, "the present offered in anxiety" (ibid., p. 85). In *Seminar IV*, however, it is the breast that is the gift and Lacan (1956–1957) says the refusal of the gift involves for the child the experience of a frustration that is only thinkable as the refusal by the mother of the gift as symbol of love (p. 207). At this point in Lacan's account "the nothing" enters as "the gift that is not constituted by the act which has previously annulled or revoked it" (ibid., p. 208). In other words, the child is presented with "the nothing" representing the absence of the mother's reply to its call for the gift, a call which only makes itself heard when the object of satisfaction is *not* there (ibid.). When it *is* there the object appears as the *sign* of the gift and, as the object of satisfaction, is the "nothing" (ibid.). He will go on to say that against this "background of revocation" (ibid.), the gift as sign of love is given or not given in reply to the call. This "symbolic game" (ibid.) has a fundamentally disappointing character but is, nevertheless, the manner in which satisfaction takes on its meaning. He says:

> [A]ll satisfaction called up in frustration comes in against the background of the fundamentally disappointing character of the symbolic order. The satisfaction here is only a substitute, a compensation. The child crushes what is disappointing in the symbolic play in the oral seizure of the real object of satisfaction, the breast in this instance. What puts him to sleep in this satisfaction is precisely his disappointment, his frustration, the refusal that he has experienced.
>
> *(Ibid., p. 209).*

Laplanche and Pontalis (1973) point out that *Versagung* as frustration includes an active sense and define the word as a "condition of the subject who is denied, *or who denies himself*, the satisfaction of an instinctual demand" (p. 175, emphasis mine). The authors add that while the translation as "frustration" implies the subject is "passively" frustrated, *Versagung*, "in no way lays down *who* does the refusing" (ibid.). Lacan's observation of the child crushing what is disappointing is coterminous with this conception of *Versagung*.

A jouissance of renunciation

If the asexual experiences no sexual attraction for another person and, according to research, does so without subjective distress (Prause & Graham, 2007, p. 350), does this desexualised position offer a unique and hitherto unrecorded form of jouissance? To quote Freud (1916–1917), albeit from a different context, does it offer "a mode of satisfaction which alone the subject desires" (p. 345)? In other words, can Lacan's teaching with regard to the annulled object provide a perspective on a jouissance that ultimately derives from this crushing of what is disappointing? This is of distinct relevance in terms of understanding how the asexual unconsciously situates him or herself in relation to the object of sexual satisfaction. In Seminar IV Lacan is working with what are, essentially, oral-stage effects and this prompts an important question: what happens at the moment when the satisfaction of need comes into play and is substituted for a symbolic satisfaction? The fact of substitution means there is a transformation of the real object (the breast) into, as he puts it, a sign of the demand for love or a symbolic request. This is how, for Lacan, orality comes into being and, as an instinctual form of hunger, it is the bearer of libido. It has entered the dialectic of substitution and in doing so has become an eroticised activity: "It is libido in the strict sense, and sexual libido" (Lacan, 1956–1957, p. 210). Lacan's premise concerning *Versagung,* of the child crushing what is disappointing in the symbolic, holds out the possibility of an unconscious, prototypical refusal of the eroticisation of the first real object. In *Seminar VI, Desire and Its Interpretation*, Lacan elaborates on how the speaking subject is marked by the structural difficulties expressed in the phantasy of the barred S with the o object. This is because what he terms "the code of demand", or "vocabulary", passes through a certain number of relationships *via* food, excrement and so on (Lacan, 1958–1959, session of 7 January 1959, p. 8). These relationships involve the same process of substitution by way of an interchangeable object that he defines as food for the oral relationship and excrement for the anal relationship. If, therefore, the "code of demand" or "vocabulary" can encompass the *Versagung* as Lacan speaks about it, then the stamp of a renunciation or annulling of the object would appear to be distinctly possible, carrying through from the first relation to the breast as object in the dialectic of substitution. When it comes to the genital relationship, in turn, Lacan says that it is by a "kind of imprint, or prolongation" of the relation to demand established in the oral and anal relationships that its "symptomatic incidences" come to appear in a disguised fashion *via* the signifier phallus (ibid.). He explains it thus:

> For a very good and simple reason, that the phallus is well and truly not this interchangeable object, that it only becomes it by its passage to the rank of signifier, and that everything that is involved in a complete genital maturation reposes on the fact that everything that, in the subject, should present itself as being here the completion of his desire is indeed to put matters clearly, something which cannot be demanded
>
> *(Ibid., p. 9).*

If, beginning with the oral stage, a *Versagung* as refusal brings about an unconscious and prototypical renunciation of eroticisation, as Lacan has been positing it, then this allows for a number of possibilities. As a result of the "prolongation" of this "code of demand" passing through oral, anal and into the genital relation, the symbolic phallus can potentially emerge annulled in order to protect the subject from the omnipotence of the first Other's desire. It can also potentially keep the subject protected from the desire of subsequent others. The phallus as an annulled signifier becomes stripped of some or all of its signifying effects. However, it continues to operate as a space holder in the signifying chain much as the zero in mathematics. At the root of this *Versagung* is the relation to the mother as first Other and within this dialectic Lacan says the mother constitutes, "a virtual field of symbolic annihilation [*néantisation*], from which all objects henceforth will each in turn draw their symbolic value" (Lacan, 1956–1957, p. 211).

The "nothing" in relation to desire

In speaking about the anorexic child "eating nothing" Lacan is also distinguishing anorexia as something other than a negation of activity. This is an important distinction. It is not a drive that is negated or repressed, but a drive that gains satisfaction from "absence savoured as such" (Lacan, 1956–1957, p. 211). In his paper one year after Seminar IV, "The Direction of the Treatment and the Principles of its Power", he examines, *inter alia*, Ernst Kris's "fresh brains" case. Here, again, he is considering the idea of a desire for nothing. For Lacan, Kris's case study is about absence rather than about the presence of the idea of being a plagiarist. What he draws out from it is the very notion that this patient's fear of plagiarism functions as a form of "stealing nothing" (Lacan, 1958, p. 502). However, unlike his desire for a plate of fresh brains after his analytic session, it is not an oral drive but is instead an "anorexia" of the "mental realm" (ibid.). In this regard it is similar to, but not the same as, asexuality in that it concerns "the desire on which the idea lives" (ibid.). The "idea" in both cases amounts to a desire for the nothing, but, particularly in the case of asexuality, it signals a desire for no sexual desire. Now absence *becomes* the desire and while asexuality is not anorexia it is similar to the extent that something of the Other is refused so that desire can be protected. Writing about anorexia, Gherovici (2014) describes it as a refusal in order to preserve an "appetite for nothing" (p. 49). In what we might think of as the asexual phantasy, the o object operates *as* the nothing, as cause of desire for no sexual desire, and in its paradoxical way desire is supported. Lacan returns to the idea of refusal in *Seminar XIV, The Logic of Phantasy,* when he considers refusal of the oral object as a way "to save oneself from being engulfed by the maternal partner" (Lacan, 1966–1967, session of 10 May 1967, p. 4). In Seminar IV, the unavoidable reality or *Wirklichkeit,* for the child is that of the omnipotence of the (m)Other, *qua* real being and "primordially all-powerful" figure (Lacan, 1956–1957, pp. 211–212). It is with regard to the object, under the sign of nothing, that "resistance against omnipotence in the relation of dependence is elaborated" (ibid., p. 214). He continues this theme in *Seminar VI, Desire and its Interpretation,* and says that in the primitive presence of the opaque and obscure desire of the Other, the subject is without recourse. The subject experiences *Hilflosigkeit,* helplessness, and this is the foundation of the traumatic experience (Lacan, 1958–1959, session of 12 November 1958, p. 13). The cause of this trauma of helplessness, Lacan says, cannot be defined in any other way than simply "the desire of the other" (ibid., session of 10 June 1959, p. 3). The trauma associated with the desire of the Other, therefore, allows for an understanding of the asexual experience of no sexual desire for another person, as outlined in the AVEN definition.

Asexuality is not simply a refusal, however. Rather, asexuality is an experience of the subject as voided of sexual desire which, I am proposing, begins in the first experiences of the child in the relation to the first Other. An encounter that every subject experiences with regard to the primordial Other produces a unique and contingent effect for the asexual subject. This, I propose, results in a desexualisation of desire, phantasy and jouissance in relation to the Other which, in essence, is the manifest sexual orientation of asexuality. What Lacan's Seminar IV is pinpointing is the moment at which the increase in drive tension is experienced as unpleasurable for the child. If desire structures the drives, and if an increase in drive tension *is* unpleasurable then, as he posits in "The Subversion of the Subject and the Dialectic of Desire", desire will adjust to a phantasy aimed at avoiding this (Lacan, 1960, p. 691). An early question posed by Freud (1896b) is stated thus: "In my opinion, there must be an independent source for the release of unpleasure in sexual life: once that source is present, it can activate sensations of disgust, lend force to morality, and so on" (p. 222). As Verhaeghe (1998) puts it: the drive tension at the core of human sexuality contains potentially the same effect for the subject as external trauma. He says: "Drive in itself, independent of any externally determined trauma, has a potentially traumatising effect, to which the psyche has to come up with an answer, that is, with a psychological elaboration" (p. 96). When the primordial place of structural trauma in relation to the first Other is considered, it becomes possible to see where sensations of disgust and the release of unpleasure in sexual life might come from. While the latter sensations are associated with hysteria, I am proposing that asexuality represents a form in which the classical sexual symptom takes on a *sinthomatic* character. It is outside the scope of the current essay but the *sinthome,* as elaborated in Lacan's later teaching, is the specific act of artifice whereby the invention or creation of a fourth ring ties the Borromean knot of Real, Symbolic and Imaginary together (Lacan, 1975–1976, session of 11 May 1976, p. 131). This allows for the possibility that some subjects, under the signifier "asexual", can unconsciously choose a desire for no sexual desire. However, the unpleasure of sexual life is still based on an originally unwelcoming Real experienced through an increase in drive tension and is implicitly determined by trauma caused by the first encounter with this Real. The psychological elaboration of this trauma for sexual subjects who reach so-called genital maturity is to seek discharge for the unpleasurable rise in tension through a repetitive engagement in a sexual act which for Lacan has symptomatic "sediments" (Lacan, 1966–1967, sessions of 22 February 1967, p. 7., and 10 May 1967, p. 10). In the repetition of the sexual act, the sexually desiring subject reproduces the initial relation to the Other, which was potentially traumatic and is, Lacan says, the very relation which maintains the o object (ibid, Session of 1 March 1967, p .9). For the asexual subject, on the other hand, the rise in drive tension is unpleasurable and causes anxiety (Brotto et al., 2010, p. 607) and so psychological elaboration is achieved through what might be called a "Nirvana principle" (Freud, 1920g, pp. 55–56) response to reduce that tension to zero, to borrow the term Freud borrowed from Barbara Low. According to Laplanche and Pontalis (1973) "the Nirvana principle must be understood as something more than a law of constancy or of homeostasis: it is, rather, the radical tendency to reduce excitation to zero-point" (p. 273). At the same time, they say the word "Nirvana" evokes a profound link between pleasure and annihilation: a link that always remained problematic for Freud. They note that the term Nirvana in Buddhism connotes the "extinction" of human desire (ibid, p. 272). Asexuality, in this context then, might be considered a contingent response to the traumatic initial encounter with the omnipotent Other's desire in which desire as the desire of the Other is radically annulled.

What is the asexual phantasy?

Many self-defined asexuals participate in relationships with others, despite the caveat of no sexual attraction (Carrigan, 2011, p. 469). In some cases these are romantic relationships where love, affection and even occasional sexual interactions do take place. If heterosexual and homosexual subjects structure their relations to the Other *via* phantasy, that is, as a defence against castration, what then is the asexual phantasy? One approach to this question would be to consider again the "nothing" which asexuals say they experience in the place of sexual desire. If, as Lacan (1962–1963) says, phantasy is the support of desire (session of 16 January 1963, p. 1), then a key element in the phantasy is the o object. Furthermore, the link between the nothing and the o object is clearly made when he includes it as an o object in "The Subversion of the Subject and the Dialectic of Desire". The "unthinkable" list that he produces there reads "the phoneme, the gaze, the voice … and the nothing" (Lacan, 1960, p. 693). In fact, in *Seminar XI* he extends his thinking in this regard when he says that at the oral level the o object is "the nothing", in that the real object from which the child is weaned has been lost and is "no longer anything for him" (Lacan, 1964, pp. 103–104). Boucher (2005), referring to Lacan's 1960 "list", suggests that by adding "the nothing" to the phoneme, the gaze, and the voice, Lacan appears to indicate that "the nothing" underpins these o objects. As he puts it: "the nothing is not merely another item, but the very 'substance' of which 'the phoneme, the gaze, the voice' are specifications" (Boucher, 2005, p. 85). If so, then the o object has a place in the fundamental phantasy that emanates not from the extimate materiality of the subject-Other dialectic in the way the penetrating voice or gaze does, or the breast, or the phallus with its links to the penis, or the phoneme's material roots in language. It is instead linked to the foundation of the very subject, not only as *want-to-be*, or lacking, but as the absence in language which the speaking subject seeks to fill, thus creating himself. In his ninth seminar on Identification (Lacan, 1961–1962, session of 28 March 1962, pp. 153-154), some three years after his consideration of Kris's "fresh brains" case, Lacan looks to Kant's "four nothings" and selects the *nihil negativum* as the object to represent the nothing, the empty object without a concept. With it he is seeking to situate a "partial" (Le Gaufey, 2008, pp. 33-34) that is free of a specular unity to the object, one that can become a space holder, empty of content and yet capable of fundamentally transformative effects, particularly in relation to desire.

If o objects are representatives of the partial drives, indicators of limits, remainders of loss, and markers of a cut that comes between unity and the subject, then the nothing, too, is a marker of a cut. But in this case the cut is between presence and absence, the empty space where something was once present but has been lost, where an absence exists to hold out the promise of a presence to be refound in the symbolic beyond of the object. In the case of asexuality, it is an absence that also allows the subject a defence against desire. If this proposition holds then asexuality has an o object which is not tied to the Real of the body or related to need or demand, rather it is an object that is located in a realm beyond sexuality and sexual satisfaction. Lacan (1964) emphasises this concept a number of times in *Seminar XI* where, again speaking about the oral drive, he says that no object of any need can satisfy the drive (p. 167). A little later in the same seminar he argues that the o object is not the "origin" (ibid, p. 180) of the oral drive, it is not the "original food" (ibid). The o object, he says, "is introduced from the fact that no food will ever satisfy the oral drive, except by circumventing the eternally lacking object" (ibid.).

This o object would then represent a lack inherent within every human subject but would allow the asexual, to varying degrees of personally chosen engagement, carve out a desire for him or herself that would answer the "*Che vuoi?*" of the Other and satisfy the subject's desire for recognition of being. In this way, nothing physical remains unsatisfied because desire has shifted from the axis of bodily need and demand to the ontological ground of being. In terms of the matheme of phantasy it could be written as the barred subject in relation to the o object-annulled or, provisionally, S ◊ a° where the a° represents the object cause of no sexual desire. This, in turn, allows for a jouissance derived, like eating the nothing in anorexia, from desiring the nothing in asexuality. Seen in this light, asexuality becomes an active, driven form of sexuality that emanates from a dialectic, albeit one which annuls the phallus as signifier and the o object as cause of sexual desire. In *Seminar IV* Lacan (1956–1957) argues that libido has active effects in every instance, even in the passive position, because activity is necessary in order to adopt the passive position (p. 41). His work in this seminar also allows for a sketching of what is akin to a short-circuiting of the work of analysis. Instead of free association *via* the dyadic transferential encounter aiming at a traversal of the fundamental phantasy, the asexual phantasy ensures that the desire of the Other is countermanded. Fink speaks about an analogous concept when he considers the subject becoming "cause of itself" (Fink, 1995, p. 69). He says this also occurs as a result of the subject traversing the fundamental phantasy. This movement "subjectifies" the *cause* of the subject's existence (formerly the Other's desire through the o object) which, he says, comes to be characterised by a kind of pure desiring without an object, or what he terms "desirousness" (ibid.). I would argue that this view similarly posits a form of desire which includes the "nothing" and in which there is no grounding of the subject's existence in the Other's desire. The symbolic is embraced but its phallic content is annulled and so there is a sublimation of the drives into the order of the signifier aimed at a non-phallicised object. It could also be argued that Lacan's concept of the *sinthome*, as outlined in Seminar XXIII, is operating on similar terrain. Through a process of suppletion, rather than substitution, it employs nomination and inventive creation to make up for a real absence of the Name-of-the-Father as agent of castration. In this way it allows the subject encounter its own desire despite the condition of absence.

Preserving a necessary gap

The o object has the same purpose in asexuality as it has for the sexually desiring subject, namely to support a desire against what Lacan (1958–1959) defines in Seminar VI as "aphanisis", the disappearance of the subject rather than the disappearance of desire (session of 10 June 1959, p. 2). It supports the subject at the moment he faints, vanishes, fails before the lack of the signifier which corresponds to his place at the level of the Other. This clearly reprises something of the original experience in which *Hilflosigkeit* was first encountered, only now there is an o object to support the subject, one that is ambiguous, that derives from the subject but is in the field of the Other and, as remainder, is where a jouissance takes refuge that does not fall under the pleasure principle (Lacan, 1966–1967, session of 7 June 1967, pp. 7–8). In the case of asexuality, the o object supports a desire for no sexual desire while establishing the subject in a relation of lack. Lacan illustrates the place of the o object as the intersection between the connecting Euler circles representing subject and Other and says that "intersection defines the o-object for us" (ibid, session of 16 November 1966, pp. 6–7). The concept of intersection also defines the o object's position in asexuality's relation to the Other since asexuals form non-sexual relationships. The fundamental relation that it preserves, however, is a relation based on a necessary gap that is maintained between subject and Other. As proposed above, this derives from the earliest experiences of the subject in relation to the Other which set in train a repetitive restaging of a desire for no sexual desire. In this contingent manner, asexuality becomes a curious proof of Lacan's (1972–1973) statement that there is no such thing as a sexual relationship (p. 12). Sexual subjects, on the other hand, deal with the lack *via* phantasy in which the o object veils it by the repetitive restaging of a symptomatic sexuality, thereby revisiting the original encounter. For the asexual, however, the o object fulfils a very different function by providing a jouissance through the presence of the nothing as the o object. There is no revisiting the original encounter *via* the sexual act. Because of a contingent choice in response to structural *Hilflosigkeit*, the asexual unconsciously resolves lack by emptying the drives of their phallic connotation and draining jouissance of its sexual component.

The primary state of being, before language, before the word becomes the death of the thing, represents a unity between subject and Other that the subject perpetually wishes to refind. Or as Ragland (2010) puts it: "We might describe the join between desire and language as the desire to replace the lack-in-being ($) created by the primordial loss of an object that first caused an infant to desire its return via the reminiscence of a trace of it" (p. 71). In the endeavour to refind it, a surplus jouissance is created, by way of compensation for an imaginary and real original lack, one that is embodied in the o object. Žižek (1999) describes Coca-Cola as the perfect embodiment of the o object, a drink removed of all that is needed to sustain the body, "transcending any use-value", functioning as the pure surplus of enjoyment over standard satisfactions (p. 1). It is, quite literally, a "nothing" from which surplus jouissance is extracted. In similar terms, the asexual could be said to utilise this dynamic interchange between presence and absence to sustain desire through a "leaning on nothing" (Gueguen, 2009, p. 7). Seen in this context, asexuality can be said to represent a consciously experienced absence of desire driven by an unconscious *desire for absence* where the absence represents what Finn (2011), in an archaeological context, has described as a "potency in the not-thereness" (p. 1). Lacan's Seminar IV offers the theoretical coordinates with which to begin a mapping of the particularity of this desire.

References

Aicken, C.R.H., Mercer, C.H., & CassellJ.A. (2013). Who Reports Absence of Sexual Attraction in Britain? Evidence from National Probability Surveys. *Psychology & Sexuality*, 4(2): 121–135.

Asexual Visibility & Education Network (AVEN). (2001). Retrieved from: http://www.asexuality.org.

Bogaert, A.F. (2006). Toward a Conceptual Understanding of Asexuality. *Review of General Psychology*, 10: 241–250.

Bogaert, A.F. (2012). *Understanding Asexuality*. Maryland: Rowman & Littlefield.

Boucher, G. (2005). One Hand Clapping: The Phoneme and The Nothing. *Filozofski Vestnik*, 26(2): 83–93.

Brotto, L.A., Knudson, G., Inskip, J., Rhodes, K., & Erskine, Y. (2010). Asexuality: A Mixed-Methods Approach. *Archives of Sexual Behaviour*, 39(3): 599–618.

Brotto, L. A., & Yule, M. A. (2017). Asexuality: Sexual Orientation, Paraphilia, Sexual Dysfunction, or None of the Above? *Archives of Sexual Behaviour*, 46(3): 619–627.

Carrigan, M. (2011). There's More to Life than Sex? Difference and Commonality within the Asexual Community. *Sexualities*, 14(4): 462–478.

Fink, B. (1995). *The Lacanian Subject: Between Language and Jouissance*. New Jersey: Princeton University Press.

Finn, C. (2011). Absence and Evidence. Retrieved from: https://www.edge.org/response-detail/10824.

Freud, S. (1896b). Extracts from the Fliess Papers: The Neuroses of Defence (A Christmas Fairy Tale). *S.E.*, 1: 220. London: Hogarth Press.

Freud, S. (1916–1917). *Introductory Lectures on Psycho-Analysis, S.E.*, 15–16. London: Hogarth Press.

Freud, S. (1917c). On Transformations of Instinct as Exemplified in Anal Erotism. *S. E.*, 17: 127–134. London: Hogarth Press.

Freud, S. (1920g). Beyond the Pleasure Principle. *S. E.*, 18: 1–64. London: Hogarth Press.

Gherovici, P. (2014). *Where Have the Hysterics Gone?: Lacan's Reinvention of Hysteria. English Studies in Canada*, 40(1): 47–70.

Gueguen, P. -G. (2009). The Plunge of the Symptom in Hypermodernity. *Lacanian Compass: Psychoanalytic Newsletter of Lacanian Orientation*. 1(14): 5–12.

Lacan, J. (1956–1957). *The Seminar of Jacques Lacan, Book IV, The Object Relation*. J. Stone (Trans.). Unpublished.

Lacan, J. (1958). The Direction of the Treatment and the Principles of its Power. In: *Écrits: The First Complete Edition in English* (pp. 489–542). B. Fink (Trans.). London & New York: W.W. Norton & Company, 2006.

Lacan, J. (1958–1959). *Desire and Its Interpretation, Book VI*. C. Gallagher (Trans.). Unpublished.

LacanJ. (1960). The Subversion of the Subject and the Dialectic of Desire. In: *Écrits: The First Complete Edition in English* (pp. 671–702). B. Fink (Trans.). London & New York: W.W. Norton & Company, 2006.

Lacan, J. (1961–1962). *Identification, Book IX*. C. Gallagher (Trans.). Unpublished.

Lacan, J. (1962–1963). *Anxiety, Book X*. C. Gallagher (Trans.). Unpublished.

Lacan, J. (1963). *Television: A Challenge to the Psychoanalytic Establishment*. New York: W.W. Norton & Company, 1990.

Lacan, J. (1964). *The Four Fundamental Concepts of Psychoanalysis, Book XI*. A. Sheridan (Trans.). London: Penguin, 1994.

Lacan, J. (1966–1967). *The Logic of Phantasy, Book XIV*. C. Gallagher (Trans.). Unpublished.

Lacan, J. (1972-1973). *Encore: The Seminar of Jacques Lacan XX: On Feminine Sexuality, The Limits of Love and Knowledge, 1972–1973*. B. Fink (Trans.). New York & London: W.W. Norton & Company, 1999.

Lacan, J. (1975–1976). *The Sinthome, Book XXIII*. J.-A. Miller (Ed.) & A.R. Price (Trans.). Cambridge, UK: Polity Press, 2016.

Laplanche, J.B., & Pontalis, J. (1973). *The Language of Psycho-Analysis*. D. Nicholson-Smith (Trans.). London: Karnac.

Le Gaufey, G. (2008). Towards a Critical Reading of the Formulae of Sexuation. C. Gallagher (Trans.). *The Letter*, 39: 19–69. Retrieved from: http://www.lacaninireland.com/web/wpcontent/uploads/2010/06/TOWARDS-A-CRITICAL-READING-2506.pdf.

Prause, N. & Graham, C.A. (2007). Asexuality: Classification and Characterization. *Archives of Sexual Research*, 36: 341–356.

Poston, D.L. Jr. & Baumle, A.K. (2010). Patterns of Asexuality in the United States. *Demographic Research*, 23(18): 509–530.

Ragland, E. (2010). The Discourse of Science, the Imaginary Axis and a Concept of the Differential, From the Perspective of Lacan's Psychoanalytic Topological Logic. *(Re)-turn: A Journal of Lacanian Studies, 5*, Spring: 63–100. Retrieved from: http://return.jls.missouri.edu/Lacan/archive.html.

Verhaeghe, P. (1998). Trauma and Hysteria within Freud and Lacan. In: *The Letter: Lacanian Perspectives on Psychoanalysis*, 14, Autumn: 87–106.

Žižek, S. (1999). The Superego and The Act: A Lecture by Slavoj Zizek, August 1999. The European Graduate School. Retrieved from: https://belfioreword.files.wordpress.com/2011/11/the-superego-and-the-act.doc.

7

MUCH ADO ABOUT MORE THAN NOTHING

Thoughts on "difficult" cases and Lacan's Seminar IV

Manya Steinkoler

Lacanian psychoanalysis aims to go beyond the fantasy that is the unconscious support of the neurotic symptom. This does not mean that the symptom is cured, or disappears, but that analytic work can, in many cases, empty it of meaning. In neurosis, analysis moves from the symptom to the Real. In psychosis, analysis moves from the Real to the Symbolic. In both instances, analysis is directed towards the object as cause rather than aim, a constitutive separation that grounds the speaking being in discourse. In "Radiophonie", Lacan tells us that the analyst incarnates and produces the object: she does this by making lack appear whenever there is a demand, that "incorporeal function" made, carved, instantiated by "mathematics and typology" (Lacan, 1970, p. 55). This empty place of lack is the cause of desire. But what of those cases that aren't so simply categorised as neurosis or psychosis? Or cases where we are not quite sure how to diagnose? What is the aim of the cure then?

Many readers of this essay are familiar with traditional Lacanian coordinates of clinical work, and no doubt many are more familiar with the well-known position of the analyst as *objet a*. And yet. Increasingly, in clinical supervision, we hear of the impasses and ensuing fatigue with regards to what Americans call "borderline" cases, or what their French Lacanian supervisors make it a point to categorise as *either* psychotic or hysteric. These more problematic cases do not fit so easily into the two trajectories that opened this essay. Acting out, mad jouissance, nonsensical claims, uncanny repetition, and seemingly incessant demand don't always "civilise" themselves by way of the transference and in many cases, time seems to stand still. Is it possible for Lacanian theory, and in particular the developments in Seminar IV, to help us think about such patients? More than think about them, can we make useful clinical interventions, making cuts into the jouissance standoff that one often finds in such cases? If so, how?

In Seminar IV, Lacan's theorisation of lack as phallic allows us to theorise such cases with regard to the mother, the phallus, and the elaboration of modalities of lack. In this seminar, arguing counter to what was more and more popular at the time, Lacan specifically emphasises that analytic technique is not about "frustrating the patient" (Lacan, 1956-1957, p. 37). In Lacan's critical formulation, a challenge to object relations theory, an object is an object insofar as it lacks not insofar as it "satisfies" or answers a demand.

By linking early theorisations with later elaborations in Lacan's work, I will show how, rather than being altogether "different" in the so-called "late Lacan", these early concepts actually develop and become more nuanced, allowing us to work more efficiently with what are often the clinical impasses of difficult cases. In this regard, following Lacan's work in Seminar IV, I use the categories of perversion and phobia to elaborate on the so-called "borderline" making use of the theoretical elaborations developed in this crucial early seminar.

Lacan's fourth seminar, *La relation d'objet* is an interrogation not only of what will later on become the *objet a*, i.e., a lack that is both something and nothing, but is an example of Lacan's sustained theorisation of lack, an elaboration of a *via negativa* that characterises the symbolic order. The preceding third seminar concerned the Name-of-the-Father and already characterised the Symbolic as a kind of metaphoric grounding, a distance that makes "reality" possible. *La relation d'objet* (Seminar IV) is the seminar that will allow us to also understand why this metaphoric grounding is more difficult for some patients, and perhaps even hypothesise why the "borderline" is most often featured on the American clinical menu as a national speciality.

Most Americans think of Lacan as a theorist of the father, the Name-of-the-Father, the concept of the phallus, and of course, of the signifier. For many American clinicians, he is accused of being "phallically" impossible to read, despite being concerned with language. In Seminar IV, it is the inclination towards the mother that takes precedence, indeed that is central, to understanding the object as a form of lack or negativity. Lacan's mother is not a "good enough mother" or some 1970s watered down Winnicottian notion of "good enough" or "nurturing mother-child dyad" (Winnicot, 1971, p. 149). Instead, Lacan underlines the way the mother takes her child as an object precisely insofar as the mother is also a woman. In the seminar, Lacan lays out three fundamental terms that concern the early relation with the mother: mother, phallus, and baby. The phallus here is the imaginary phallus. The child aims to be this phallus for the mother and he discovers the "*mère inassouvie*" (unsatisfied mother 179), (Lacan, 1956–1957, p. 179). Importantly, the initial oral dialectic, initiates the symbolic register in terms of the lack that it instantiates. Here, in this lesson in particular (27 February, 1957), we see that the signifier is of another heterogeneous order, and this is what the mother answers with *as well as* with her being; there is thus something heterogeneous to being that cannot be accounted for in the answer of the mother, but that the mother initiates and as such, helps invent. If the mother is the virtual field that is "nothinged" by the invention of the Symbolic, then we could say with Lacan that all objects are there, making up this "nothinged" field. Lacan calls this "*la deception fondamentale*" (Lacan, 1956–1957, p. 81) where the child realises he is not the sole object of the mother, and the "register of the call" on the level of a "vocalise" (ibid., p. 67) instantiates a primary, albeit fragmented Symbolic (ibid., p. 81). He separates the mother then from simply being "a primitive object" (ibid., p. 68). In this sense, the seminar participates not only in a Lacanian trajectory of theorising lack, but also of thinking through the feminine position and feminine sexuality that he will take up in *Seminar XX, Encore* (Lacan, 1972–1973).

This "making nothing" doesn't always work, especially in an American context where "nothing comes of nothing" and "nothing succeeds like success" and where the ego is "nothing to be sneezed at". When discussing a difficult case in supervision, a senior analyst rejoined, "Ah! *Those*! We've all had one of *those*!" What does it mean "to have one of those"? What nosographical group do *those* patients belong to? Knowing I was going to write on this seminar, I sent an email asking colleagues from different formations, trained in diverse theoretical orientations to tell me whether they had "one of those patients" and what such a designation meant to them. I asked permission to publish their responses, promising not to name names of the clinicians who gave them to me. They responded by sharing private aliases they gave these patients, invented often out of exasperation or despair, and included the following sobriquets: "The Bald Soprano", "The Queen of the Borderlines", "Marie Antoinette", "The Rabbit (in *Fatal Attraction*)", "Veda Pierce" (Mildred's spoiled daughter in Curtis's Noir film, *Mildred Pierce*), "Ophelia", "Soldier of the Impossible", "Chairman Mouth" (denoting the imperial oral character of the patient), "Better than Ordinary Psychosis", "Chimp Funeral" (see the beginning of Wilder's *Sunset Boulevard*), "The Count", and "Law and Order Special Victims Unit". The penchant for the theatrical should not go unnoticed.

The aggression and humour in these appellations underline a wish to symbolise an aggression and impossibility heard in the patients' speech, the very character neurosis or "actual neurosis" that Lacanian analysis aims to dialecticise via the trajectory of the subject, the name designating something of the insistent jouissance at stake. In this regard, Lacan, when discussing the early object relation and the pathos of the mother and the Real, uses the phrase from Macbeth's "Tomorrow, tomorrow and tomorrow" monologue that follows the suicide of Lady Macbeth: "the sound and the fury", as it pertains to the Real (Lacan, 1956–1957, p. 65). We recall the end of that phrase that Lacan curiously omits, "*signifying nothing*". Consider fixation, or repetition that does not find repose in a word, or the power of the "not to be able not to be" (Lacan, 1971–1972, p. 14) that "signifies nothing" from which the patient suffers. The patient signifies "nothing" since, paradoxically, this insistent jouissance can never become nothing.

It is useful to recall that during the period Lacan is giving Seminar IV (1956–57), he is also penning "The Situation of the Psychoanalyst in 1956" included in his *Écrits*. In that essay, he bemoans the move away from Freud's discovery of the unconscious as well as the concomitant stagnation of the field of psychoanalysis. Seminar IV takes the state of psychoanalysis to task in order to disrupt stagnation via a sustained critique of the phallus as lack, and of the foundations of the Symbolic in terms of a structuralist critique of the unconscious. Lacan maintains that analytic theory and practice cannot be dissociated. He reminds us that the famous "object relation" is not found in Freud's texts except as a relation to a lost object (Lacan, 1956–1957, p. 15). He reads Freud and sees that what is at stake is instead a lost object, an object to be re-found in the *wiedersufindung,* and he further critiques the idea of an "object that would harmonise man with his world" (ibid., p. 16) underlining that there is a tension in the object relation not theorised in object relations theory. What is sought is not sought in the same way as what will be found (ibid., p. 15). He calls it a "search for an outgrown satisfaction", adding that, "reality is in fundamental opposition to what is sought by the drive" (ibid., p. 53).

Such claims are particularly germane to the American context both at the time Lacan gave the seminar as well as today. It is a context where an ersatz meritocracy, a fetishising of financial gain, and obedience to social norms—particularly success and a belonging we might characterise as imaginary—have enormous ideological power and weight. This even includes the "norms" imposed on young clinicians in becoming analysts. For example, one needs a documented and supervised "case" which translates into a certain number of hours with a patient "on the couch" to qualify to take the multiple choice licensing test to "be an analyst".

By Seminar IV, Lacan had already developed the "mirror stage" (Lacan, 1949) where the conflictual nature of the dual relation was underlined, elaborating the aggressive nature of the pre-genital drives as both destructive and unconditional. Lacan is responding here to the theoretically specious and ideologically-influenced tendency of psychoanalysis at the time to privilege frustration in both clinical work and theoretical elaboration. Frustration had even come to concern how symptoms were understood. Lacan states in no uncertain terms that frustration is in the domain of "revindication" (Lacan, 1956–1957, p. 37). According to Lacan, this had the result of obfuscating, and worse, damaging the clinical efficaciousness of psychoanalysis. For Lacan, frustration was one of the forms of the lack of the object. In frustration, the lack is imaginary, the object is real and the agent is symbolic. In frustration we have to concern ourselves with the demand that is inexhaustible. Lacan thus reminds us that Freud does not speak of frustration, or at least the word frustration is a poor translation of *Versagung,* which means denial or refusal (Lacan, 1956). Freud's term *Versagung* suggests something more like a promise of a taking away of a promise (refusal, denial), and comes from the word *sagen*, or saying, something at the level of the Symbolic. Already in Freud, we see the move from the object to the signifier, illustrative of Lacan's work at this time. Lacan explains that frustration nourishes the wish for satisfaction and adds that an object is an object insofar as it is lacking, insofar as it lacks. Freud's *nebenmensch complex* in the *Project for a Scientific Psychology* harkens to an originary loss that is developed in Lacan's notion in Seminar VII of *Das Ding*. Lacan posits *Das Ding* as "beyond the original Good." He tells that this "beyond" is why "The Good is also a bad object … but is not distinguished as bad" and cannot be handled (Lacan, 1959–

1960; p. 73). It only exists for a subject via the fantasm. We could call *Das Ding* a loss that makes a real hole, and for Lacan, psychic structure stems from this hole.

We might characterise the difficult cases, the impossible ones we name with sobriquets, as taking a stand against the hole. One of my patients who had been previously hospitalised following her father's death put it quite succinctly:

> I used to think I was just running around happily like a cartoon character. Then I realised I ran off the cliff. I am sure I had done that many times before—but I never noticed there was no ground beneath my feet. After my father died, I noticed, and I fell and I haven't gotten up since. Why should I?

Or another, a sex worker and only child from an Evangelical family, put it like this: "You think I don't know what God is? I know very well what God is! God is what covers a hole. Who wouldn't rather turn trick than go to church?" A patient with severe obsessionality that has marked his entire life stated quite clearly, "My last therapist tried to get me to give up my obsessions. He thought I should just, you know, agree to the empty nothingness of existence. Didn't he realise I agree to it every time I count?"

Such theorisation of an originary void is key to Lacan's seminar, crucial to understanding the invention of lack as phallic as a result of a destitution of the mother, or a making of the mother into language. Seminar IV allows for the most elaborated discussion of the invention of lack via separation from the mother and includes Lacan's discussion of Freud's cases of little Hans and the Young Homosexual Woman. The object is hallucinated against a background of a threatening reality of a void that is constitutive of subjectivity. Freud explains that this initial loss creates the subject who loses his being and runs after it (Freud, 1914g, p. 151). Freud understood: there is a loss at the beginning that is inaugural for subjectivity that puts the machine in action, a machine that tries to make good on the initial loss. What Lacan calls the object is, therefore, retroactively made out of this initial loss. This is clearly distinct from any notion of a satisfying object and underlines that while the subject might be aiming at satisfaction, the analysis is not. These notions fly in the face of the idea of harmony and the end of the cure as a "happy ending". Many of the patients above are all well aware of the hole. They have their own how-to-make-do: deadening melancholia, prostitution, and paralysing obsessionality.

In neurosis, this lost object galvanises the invention of the ideal. Lacan explains that the ideal aims at a "normalisation of the subject"; it keeps her on the path that necessitates lack and repression. In the case of the pervert, this is compromised due to the "syncope with jouissance" and the fetish functions as a protection against the anxiety of the hole. In perversion, Lacan explains that there is "a syncope of the subject that allows an access to a beyond", but his point is that these moments are always symbolically ordained, adding that the pervert's idea of utopia does not arise from nowhere. His recourse to plenitude invites the fetishist position wherein there is an identification with the object. Lacan reads Freud's case of the Young

Homosexual as identifying with the object (Lacan, 1956–57, p. 133); whereas, Freud reads this as a regression to narcissism (Freud, 1920a, p. 158, fn. 1). In "those" difficult patients, existential impasse concerns a knowledge of the hole that is defended against with the ego, phallically. Indeed, often prior treatment "builds up" the ego and the subject imagines that the ego alone is the defence against the hole.

Lacan calls the "oral character of the imaginary relation" (Lacan, 1956–1957, p. 28) that which alludes to the primary void where we find the object, or better put, the lost object, or eventually, the *objet a* in clinical work. Here Lacan discovers a fantasy of phallic incorporation and plenitude. The melancholic patient punctuates her narrative with what seems a chorus of her epic song, "my mother is a cannibal". Following the death of her father, she has "reinvented" herself as filthy, smelling, and clinically depressed so that her mother "will not eat her". This is where Marie Antoinette, The Queen and The Count balk at the impotent analyst, underlining a recalcitrance towards the Symbolic well depicted by a bulimic patient who laughed at her neologism: "Custard's last stand", adding that like her bulimia, "it is a last stand that never ends". The impasse testified to by these patients concerns the very dual relation that analysis could easily fall into, especially in America, and one that Lacanian psychoanalysis critiques and takes to task. In fact, the term frustration must be heard in its coincidence with capitalist reality as it invokes the notion that there has been an imaginary wrong, the very notion that fuels much of the contemporary politics of revindication (one that is a willing partner, a "Me Too", a perfect inverse to the perverse, sadistic, megalomaniacal, and tyrannical tweets of the Commander in Chief).

For Lacan, this Real encountered is always in its place and "sticks to the holes of one's shoes" (Lacan, 1956–1957, p. 39). We might associate this remark with one he made later in his career in "L'Etourdit" that "dancing is only possible" when the "discourses hold sway" (Lacan, 2009, p. 76). The Real makes the holding sway of the discourses, and as a result, dancing, impossible; something sticks to holes in the shoes that impedes movement. "I would move", says my melancholic patient, "but I am just too heavy". Indeed, in the difficult cases, nothing seems to move and one feels that the Real is all the more present. In Seminar IV, Lacan explains that when the mother does not respond to the symbolic call, she becomes Real as is evident in psychosis. It is why Lacan (1971–1972) can say in *Ou Pire* that, "foreclosure is not discordance" (p. 22). However, we can note the presence of the Real in regression in neurosis and as a threat in perversion as well.

Noting the link with the Real, in Seminar IV, Lacan tracks the way the mother lacks the phallus; she is destituted, or deprived of something. Rather than see the object as portending any kind of plenitude, he reads the *Fort Da* game, following Freud, as a manner of constituting the initial coordinates of the symbolic order (Lacan, 1956–1957, pp. 41–57). Presence exists on a foundation of absence. In neurosis and in perversion, the moment the child is dependent upon this power given to the mother, the mother becomes Symbolic.

It is via the use of Freud's cases that Lacan can wonder what kind of consistency can be given to lack. He notes that the lack is an element external to the structure that conditions or defines the structure as such. Lacan had been using the three registers—Imaginary, Symbolic and Real—since 1953 (Lacan, 1953). He invents *objet a* in 1960 by way of an important equivocation between the *objet a* and the other, or small *a*, the original letter designating "the other" (*l'autre*) (Lacan, 1962–1963). *Objet a* is made from something of the relation to the other. Following his early work, in *Encore* he explains that the essence of the object is *ratage*, a failure (Lacan, 1972–1973, p. 50). Seminar IV lays out the origins of this trajectory. The *objet a* is drive-related, non-specular, and partial. The *objet a* is an important clinical concept because it can enable a body, somebody, any-body to exist by way of separation. The object is what remains of the signifying operation by which the coming to being of a subject is produced as a subject of the unconscious, as a subject divided by jouissance. The image of the body proper, or of one's own body is on the same line of the object as of the subject. The more the subject and the body (ego) are disconnected, the more the *objet a* has body.

Both Freud and Lacan found the origins of the Symbolic in the *Fort Da*, a game of presence and absence. It is a game that has an aspect of satisfaction that engages another register of compensation. Any object (including the demand for analysis or for sessions) takes on meaning and even satisfaction in terms of this other register. In this regard, when Lacan speaks of the direction of the cure (Lacan, 1956) we should take this literally, it aims at the subject of the unconscious.

The mother's organ: Jouissance

The primordial mother is all-powerful; it is where the child has a sense that there is such a thing as "all powerful". One is reminded of the Kleinian notion that the primordial mother contains everything. Thus is the Kleinian depressive position related to the Lacanian all-powerful mother. The mirror stage affords the child a feeling of mastery, accompanied by primordial splitting as well, as a kind of proto-symbolic. Importantly, the only power of the child against this all-powerful mother without the Name-of-the-Father is to say no. Such nay-saying, however, does not lead to independence, but dependence in the form of negativism, elaborating itself in terms of the object on the side of nothing or what we might call perversion. The point is that the mother depends on the child for her omnipotence. What psychoanalysis calls "regression" occurs when the real object and the activity deployed to seize upon it, or get it back, become substituted for symbolic exigency. This is the clinic of "those" patients. And we could call this business as usual in the US where "satisfaction" is always "guaranteed" by the Big Other. More than one of my patients has said in some form or another: "What I need is a guarantee. If there was a guarantee, then I would be able to accomplish something". We recall that in "L'Etourdit", Lacan says that

> [I]t is rather that the more it is snapped up (*happé*) by the *a posteriori* of the discourses that await it (happiness as it is called in the U.S.A.) the more does the organ have things to carry (*se porter*) from them.
>
> *(Lacan, 2009, p. 60)*

He explains that discourse touches on the relation with the phallus. It is thus that according to Lacan, culture can create and exacerbate mental illness.

The imaginary phallus is introduced via the dialectic of frustration and hopefully resolved at the level of Oedipus. Often it is here that we encounter what some would call "the perversions" that concern the phallus and how it is that the child realises that her mother is missing something. In *Seminar IV*, Lacan underlines that the fetish has a protective function. It controls the devouring desire of the mother (Lacan, 1956–1957, p. 152). In phobia as well, the symptom is installed to protect against anxiety, serving as a kind of stand-in for the Name-of-the-Father. They are defences when the desire of the Other becomes too devouring and insatiable, and one's shoes stick to the floor and one is unable to move, let alone dance. Lacan shows that in the pre-Oedipal, in this exchange with the mother, there is a phallic something in front of which the veil is situated. The fetish figures the lack onto the veil and thereby tries to rejoin with the lost object. The subject identifies with what is behind the veil, i.e., to the object insofar as it is lacking something—the phallic mother. This is the clinic of the "more than nothing" and it is not limited to moments in childhood.

Whaling and harnessing: Case notes

A forty-seven-year-old male had suffered, and continued to suffer, an austere, intrusive, and demanding mother who put him in ballet school most of his childhood against his will. As an adult, having inherited an enormous family fortune, he bought harness race horses and raced them regularly. This was his way of diverting the maternal burden from his own body onto the body of the racehorse. It allowed him also to spend his parents' fortune on "nothing", but importantly not the same "nothing" as speech in analysis, which he felt indignant to have to pay for. The horse was an apostrophe to the void over which the object is formed, a kind of answer. How to be at the height of the maternal phallus? To have a horse that wins. Lacan explains that the fetish is between the mother and the baby. The fetish is a solution to what the mother wants on an imaginary plane (Lacan, 1956–1957, p. 156). At his first session, he showed me a photograph of himself and his winning harness horse some years back, Beast of Burden. "What is a harness horse?" I asked the patient. "You know, like a buggy". "A harness", he added, "like what you strap a baby into, only on the harness strapped to the horse there is nothing in it". I stopped the session there.

A patient came to analysis at the age twenty-three. She had been in regular treatment since the age of five when she vomited on her father and refused to attend school afterwards, developing a fear of vomiting that inhibited her entire functioning. This fear was alive and well when she first stepped through my office door, poised and eager to tell me all about it. A lifetime of various forms of therapy, analysis, and religious counselling had done nothing to diminish its power. I told her that she could work with me but that she would have to speak about something other than her fear of vomiting. She said she found this very strange because it is the only thing that had ever bothered her, bothering her so much she was unable to travel, and as a child, often unable to go to school lest she vomit, a fate she feared more than death, she said. She wondered what else there was to talk about. The primal scene, which changed a bit from time to time, involved a memory of being nearly five years old and coming down the stairs to find her mother absent and her father sitting on the sofa reading. She said she felt ill and thought she might throw up which she immediately did on her father's lap. Her father panicked and, not knowing how to react, waited for her mother to return from her morning jog. They took their daughter to the hospital after the mother yelled at the father for being incompetent and not knowing anything about how to be a father. The patient's first session centred around her envy of her best friend, chosen because she was able to projectile vomit at will through grade school and high school. A few weeks into the work, unable to "talk about the fear of vomiting all the time"—a fate that enraged her I might add—she had a dream that reminded her of her recurring childhood nightmare that had terrified her almost as much as the paralysing fear of vomiting. She is at the seashore with her parents where a baby whale has washed up and is stranded on the shore. She runs to the whale to take care of it and save it. She throws water on it with her toy pail to keep it alive and to her horror, the uncanny opposite takes place! Despite her desperate attempts to keep it alive, the whale begins to shrink until it is in her arms like a baby, and then, continuing to shrink, in the palm of her hand, a "dried out piece of beef jerky", or "pure desiccated flesh". Terrified, she wakes up.

Lacan's work on phobia in Seminar IV allows us to see this dream in a context distinct from the one that her childhood therapists were thinking about it. What is the whale but the maternal phallus that was the patient herself? What is the vomit but the splashing of the baby whale with her pail of water? In the dream, the exact opposite of what she wants to happen happens. The whale is not restored to the water and her mother but is dried out and desiccated—the Symbolic is "made" via the phobic action itself, a solution for an imaginary object to restore a world where there is phallic signification where the father did not intervene as an agent of castration.

Perhaps with "these" patients, while not psychotic, we nevertheless seem to help invent the Symbolic—or better, instantiate it by way of the work. For some of them, analysis itself can become the way this is done. Even if they come to complain that it doesn't work and it's all "good for nothing", they come to our offices to register this complaint with us. Some will even become analysts when "more than nothing" can become "nothing more". And some, like a melancholic patient mentioned earlier, will fall upon a question, as if at a rainbow, asking: "Is there an end to nothing?"

References

Freud, S.(1895) Project for a Scientific Psychology. *S.E.*, 1: 283–387. London: Hogarth Press.

Freud, S. (1914g). Remembering, Repeating and Working-Through (Further Recommendations on the Technique of Psycho-Analysis, II). *S.E.*, 12: 145–156. London: Hogarth Press.

Freud, S. (1920a). The Psychogenesis of a Case of Homosexuality in a Woman. *S.E.*, 18: 145–172. London: Hogarth Press.

Lacan, J. (1949) La Stade de Miroir: Communication faite au XVIè Congrès international de psychanalyse, à Zürich. In: *Écrits*. Paris: Editions Seuil, 1966.

Lacan, J. (1953). The Function and Field of Speech and Language in Psychoanalysis. In: *Écrits: The First Complete Edition in English* (pp. 197–268). B. Fink (Trans.). London & New York: W.W Norton & Company, 2006.

Lacan, J.(1956–1957). *Le Séminaire Livre IV: La Relation d'objet*. Paris: Le Seuil, 1994.

Lacan, J. (1959–1960). *The Ethics of Psychoanalysis 1959–1960: The Seminar of Jacques Lacan Book VII*. J.-A. Miller (Ed.) & D. Porter (Trans.). New York: W.W. Norton & Company, 1992.

Lacan, J. (1962–1963). *Seminar X: Anxiety, 1962-63*. Paris: Editions Seuil, 2004.

Lacan, J. (1956). Situation de psychanalyse en 1956. In:*Écrits*. Paris: Editions Seuil, 1966.

Lacan, J. (1970). Radiophonie. J. Stone, (Trans). *Scilicet* 2/3: 55–99. Paris: Editions Seuil.

Lacan, J. (1971–1972). *Le Séminaire Livre XIX. Ou Pire*. Retrieved from: http://www.lacaninireland.com.

Lacan, J. (1972–1973). *Le Séminaire Livre XX: Encore*. Paris: Le Seuil, 1975.

Lacan, J. (2009). L'Étourdit. *The Letter: Irish Journal for Lacanian Psychoanalysis*, 41: 31–80. Dublin: The School of Psychotherapy.

Winnicott, D.W. (1971). *Playing and Reality*. London: Tavistock Publications.

PART 3
Phallus

8

THE PHALLUS OF THE FIFTIES

Those years of "tranquil possession"

Olga Cox Cameron

"It is the fault of the pronouns" (Beckett, 1959, p. 408) opines the speaker in the last volume of Beckett's great trilogy. Readers of Lacan face a different grammatical conundrum in the fate of the phallus as it moves from the status of noun to that of adjective over the course of the twenty-five seminars. As Guy Le Gaufey has pointed out, in the first ten years of Lacan's teaching the phallus as noun appears more than 1500 times. This drops to about 200 over the next ten years, and further subsides to not more than forty in the final six years (Le Gaufey, 2009, p. 127). The initial surge is at its most insistent in the seminars under consideration in this book, *Seminar IV, The Relation to the Object,* and *Seminar V, Formations of the Unconscious*. The teaching of these years represents the heyday of the phallus, held aloft and sustained on Lacan's part by some brilliant, if questionable, intellectual prosthetics.

Why would we look closely at seminars which stake out positions later modified, and in some cases, abandoned by Lacan? Surely the subsidence of the phallus as charted by Le Gaufey indicates that Lacan's own later insights will provide a more than adequate critique of these earlier stances. In this regard one could do worse than trace the slippage of the *Nom du père* along a path of uncertainty leading to the Beckettian position of *les non-dupes errent*. However a number of the major theoretical tenets established in Seminars IV and V continue to skew psychoanalytic thinking today, notably the extraordinary substitution of the multiple by the one with respect to the phallus and the Name-of-the-Father. If, as Alain Badiou (2001) says, "the multiple is the law of being" (p. 25), it could be argued that whereas a position of openness to the multiple is visible in Seminar I, and is gradually re-established from Seminar VI onward, in Seminars IV and V, the proliferating medleys of imaginary formations are all subsumed under the term "imaginary phallus". In analogous fashion, the mesh of the symbolic order, the world of pact and law held together by the play of signifiers, is gradually compressed into a totalitarian structure maintained in existence by a single signifier, the Name-of-the-Father. This astonishing reductionism is brilliantly achieved, and strongly insisted on, by means of what Lacan, in the seminar on Identification, calls the "Aristotelian" logic of patriarchy (Lacan, 1961–1962. p. 93). This logic continues to prevail in psychoanalytic thinking.

In terms of general Lacanian scholarship it is always worth asking; how does Lacan build a given theory, and having built it, when and how does he begin to undermine the edifice he has created? I would suggest that halfway through Seminar V, almost directly after the coping stone has been placed on the impressively theorised Oedipus complex, it is possible to discern faint tremors heralding a seismic shift in the underpinning of this enormous edifice. Not that Lacan wanted to altogether dismantle the edifice he had erected, but the lure of the Imaginary, visible in all his finest writing ever since his article in *Minotaure* on the Papin sisters, starts to make itself felt with increasing magnetism.

Seminars IV and V represent the apogee of masculinism in Lacanian theory. Despite notable revisions regarding this bias he never quite succeeded in flying the nets of masculinist fantasy. That said, given that the world we live in is still imbued with masculinism, and given too that for many heterosexual men, the trajectory sketched out by Lacan rings absolutely true, Seminars IV and V remain important and relevant. It is not possible to remotely do justice to the sheer volume of text involved, so since an inadequate commentary is inevitable I will limit myself to three angles of approach; the manner in which the androcentric bias of the symbolic order, acknowledged in Seminar II, is tautologically justified as structural by way of this same bias; the vorticial pressure on both the phallus and the Name-of-the-Father to subsume multiplicity into totalitarian hegemony; and thirdly, the manner in which the theory set forth in these seminars seems paradoxically to give rise to its own undoing. Surprisingly, in the wake of such a major statement of the primacy of the Symbolic, Lacan, more and more over the next few years, will veer towards the power and passion of the Imaginary.

An androcentric symbolic order

"Girls don't want to be the hero, they want to be had by the hero" (Scherfig, 2016). In a recent film, *Their Finest*, set in the 1940s, a film director thus curbs the imaginative suggestions of a female scriptwriter, adding as a throwaway rider the terms of employment "Of course we won't be able to pay you as much as the chaps" (ibid.). Being and having. The film director is closer to Freud's sexual computation of these two essential verbs than to Lacan's, but the fall-out for women looks much the same. The obviousness of these statements to the speaker is what draws the attention today. In a similar manner the case Lacan makes in Seminars IV and V is impressive, and to a degree unassailable, since both the symbolic order and the Oedipus complex which will be shown to underpin it, are specified as androcentric, permitting him not only to reiterate but to expand Freud's phallocentrism.

A year or so before he embarked on the vast theorisation of the Oedipus complex in the seminars under consideration, Lacan unhesitatingly specified the symbolic order as androcentric and patriarchal. In *Seminar II* he makes it clear that it is only because of an androcentric bias that the penis takes on this imaginary value (Lacan, 1954–1955, p. 272), a situation which he posits in 1955 as "not without remedy" (ibid., p. 262). Lacan in these early years writes very persuasively of the power of this symbolic order. As he says in *Seminar III*, it is "what yields us the entire world system ... that which appears to be open to the neutrality of the world of human knowledge", as opposed to the Imaginary "which seems to be the very domain of the eroticization of the object" (Lacan, 1955–1956, p. 177). The incommensurability of this symbolic system with the natural order is an observable fact. In the course of these years it is invoked in excess of thirty times as part of the prosthetics of the phallocentrism being established. It is unequivocally stated in *Seminar III*;

> It is in so far as the function of man and woman is symbolized, it is in so far as it is literally uprooted from the domain of the imaginary and situated in the domain of the symbolic, that any normal sexual position is realized. Genital realization is submitted to symbolization as an essential requirement that the man be virilized, that the woman truly accept her feminine function.
>
> *(Ibid.)*

He emphasises its ineluctability in *Seminar IV*. "It is in a human world organized by this symbolic order that the child appears, and this is what he must confront" (Lacan, 1956–1957, lesson twenty-three, 26 June 1957, p. 472). Certain conditions exist in this world which as he says:

> allow the subject to preserve a sufficient presence, not only in the real world but also in the symbolic world, that is to say so that he can tolerate himself in the real world organized as it is with its weft of the symbolic.
>
> *(Ibid., lesson twenty-one, 5 June 1957, p. 429)*

These conditions pre-date the subject. "For as long as there have been signifiers that function, the psychic system of subjects has been organized by these signifiers" (ibid., lesson three, 5 December 1956, p. 47). In the 1950s, at the height of the post-World War II reinstallation of patriarchy, it is perhaps understandable that Lacan would see 4000 years of androcentrism as an immutable state of affairs. Furthermore, if, as he persuasively insists, the symbolic order is what literally gives us our world, it will be very difficult to think outside of this frame. Lucien Fèbvre's magisterial study of Rabelais in *The Problem of Unbelief in the 16th Century* is a vivid demonstration of this apparent impasse; an impasse created and maintained via a tautological torsion brought about by the parameters of the frame itself. The inevitable scotomisations and competing antagonisms involved are visible from outside the frame but of course much less so from within.

The symbolic order then is established as ineluctable and ineluctably androcentric. "It is the particularities of the symbolic order as I have underlined in passing that give its prevalence for example to that element of the imaginary which is called the phallus" (ibid., lesson twelve, 6 March 1957, p. 228). The consequence of this for women, he says, is that "one of the sexes is obliged to take the image of the other as the basis of its identification" (Lacan, 1955–1956, p. 176). In fairness, Lacan does not spell this out without fully recognising the aporias to which it gives rise. Mapping it out for the first time in Seminar II, he points to "the impasse into which the woman is pushed by her specific function in the symbolic order" (Lacan, 1954–1955, p. 262), acknowledging that there is "something insurmountable, let us say unacceptable, in the fact of being placed in the position of an object (to be had by the hero) in the symbolic order" (ibid., p. 262). In *Seminar IV*, speaking of Freud's 1923 paper "Infantile Genital Organization", where Freud poses the primacy of phallic organisation as a principle, Lacan, echoing Freud, points out that making the possession or non-possession of the phallus into the principal differential element is actually founded on a mistake, in particular, ignorance of the female sexual organ (Lacan, 1956–1957, lesson six, 9 January 1957, p. 102). This exactly exemplifies the patriarchal framing of the symbolic order in question here.

How is difference to be computed? Is one looking at an apple and a non-apple or at an apple and a pear? If the task in hand is to count the apples, then what I see will correspond to the first distinction, if to categorise the fruits in front of me to the second. So two things can be equally present but only one "counts" as seen. A wonderful anecdote recounted by my American husband comes to mind. In 1818 in a town in Massachusetts the wives of the town burghers, incensed by something or other, called a women's meeting. To their consternation a black maid showed up asking the unanswerable question "Ain't I a woman?" Every day, babies in the womb with differing and very distinctive sexual organs are examined, but as recently as 2013 the "objective" findings of this examination were described in a psychoanalytic journal not as the presence of two different organs, but in terms of presence and absence;

> Through nuchal translucency testing for example, the scientific machinery registers in advance the presence of the "wee-wee maker" in the fetus. There being or not "a wee-wee maker" thus discriminates the man from the woman on a certain evidence (there is or there is not).
>
> *(Recalcati, 2013, p. 73).*

This is a completely accurate instance of the workings of the symbolic order, seemingly so self-evident that its underpinning scotomisation is not at all evident. What extraordinary occlusion permits someone looking at a vulva, even the remarkably large vulva of an unborn baby girl to see not something but nothing, not presence but absence? The above is a perfect example of what patriarchy "sees" and this "seeing" is reflected with crystalline and repeated clarity in Freud's writings. One recalls for example his commentary on a dream where the phrase, "there's something missing", describes – I quote Freud, not his patient – "the principal feature of the female genitalia" (Freud, 1900a, p. 333). The "blindness of the seeing eye" to use Freud's own phrase (Freud, 1895d, p. 117).

Lacan, in fairness, repeats very regularly throughout Seminars IV and V that in the Real, with respect to female sexual organs there is nothing missing. But rather oddly for someone who, less than a decade earlier in his article on *The Family Complexes in the Formation of the Individual*, had emphasised the imago of the maternal womb as indelible (Lacan, 1938, p. 20) and its symbolisation visible in burial practices as well as in dwelling houses and caverns, (ibid., p. 22), he now asserts that only the penis is amenable to symbolisation because it can be seen, which thereby transforms it into the phallus; "Besides it isn't the penis, it's the phallus, that is to say something whose symbolic usage can be seen, because it is erected. There can be no possible symbolic usage for what is not seen, for what is hidden" (Lacan, 1954–1955, p. 272). A year later he takes this statement a little further, explaining that "where there is no symbolic material there is an obstacle, a defect in the way of bringing about the identification that is essential for the subject's sexuality to be realised" (Lacan, 1955–1956, p. 176). Lacan's view here is that;

> this defect comes from the fact that on one point the symbolic lacks the material – for it does require material. The female sex is characterized by an absence, a hole which means that it happens to be less desirable than is the male sex for what he has that is provocative.
>
> *(Ibid.)*

He also says "I should say that strictly speaking there is no symbolization of woman's sex as such because the imaginary only furnishes an absence where elsewhere there is a highly prevalent symbol" (ibid.).

Whose Imaginary? And what fuels this denegation? Towards the end of Seminar VI Lacan refers to "what is symbolically the most intolerable thing in our experience, namely the form which responds to it in the place of the female sexual organs" (Lacan, 1958–1959, lesson twenty-three, 3 June 1959, p. 295). For whom is this intolerable? Hard not to line up this thinking with Freud's never borrowed/already returned pot! One is reminded too of Lacan's stellar reading of Freud's Irma dream in Seminar II, where the horror evoked appears to be very much Lacan's and is not to be found in Freud's dry phraseology. Lacan describes Freud examining Irma's throat as the first break in the dream leading to;

> the apparition of the terrifying anxiety-provoking image, to this real Medusa's head, to the revelation of this something which is properly speaking unnameable, the back of this throat, the complex unlocatable form which also makes it into the primitive object par excellence, the abyss of the female sexual organ from which all life emerges.
>
> *(Lacan, 1954–1955, p. 164)*

The paradoxical result of this (possibly phobic) scotomisation is that the female sexual organ is, Lacan says in Seminar IV, "never symbolically located as something which might have a meaning. It is always essentially problematic" (Lacan, 1956–1957, lesson eight, 23 January 1957, p. 158). The question "what counts?" which pervades *Seminar IX, Identification* (Lacan, 1961–1962), is vividly exemplified here.

But while the phallus is indeed indubitably a "highly prevalent symbol" can Lacan really have thought that no equivalent female symbols existed? It is perhaps understandable that he might not have heard of *sheelagh na gigs*, the carvings of fertility goddesses with huge vulvas and deeply incised vaginas, most commonly found in Ireland but also well disseminated throughout Western and Eastern Europe and certainly known to Mircea Eliade in France. More surprising is his apparent non-knowledge of the Paleolithic "Venus" carvings, the oldest of which dates from 35,000 years ago, figurines often deployed as apotropaic devices on gates, the vulva symbolised as the primordial gateway into life. Can he really not have known any of this?

Nonetheless, while focussed on endorsing Freud's phallocentrism, Lacan is unable to prevent himself from describing it as literally "stupefying". However, he opts for compliance; "well one must start with what is stupefying" (Lacan, 1956–1957, lesson eleven, 27 February 1957, p. 219). The result is that like Freud, he can only see the woman as existing for the other, in effect the masculine partner. Colette Soler points out that *all* of the formulations Lacan provided to specify the place of woman make her a partner of the masculine subject: 1) being the phallus, that is the representative of what man is missing; 2) being the object that serves as cause of his desire; and 3) being the symptom on which his jouissance is fixated (Soler, 2002, p. 102). As Soler adds "the result is that everything that can be said about women is said from the point of view of the Other, their own being remaining … foreclosed from discourse" (ibid., p. 102).

So the necessity for an androcentric symbolic order will be examined through the prism of androcentrism itself. When Lacan provides a compelling justification for patriarchy he is simply restating its own premisses.

From the multiple to the one

While the shortfall occasioned by this androcentric framing is the focus here, it is important to recognise that notwithstanding their masculinism, many of the theoretical elaborations to which this gives rise are so rich, so complex, so insightful, and so brilliant that they have tended to carry the day and have made it difficult to separate out some of their questionable underpinnings. In particular his starting point in Seminar IV, the concept of the imaginary phallus represents a tremendous widening and deepening of the existential drama undergone in the Freudian Oedipus. This concept, unknown to Freud, fits like a glove into two major tenets of Freud's phallocentrism, *penisneid* and fetishism, and widens out for Lacan into enormously evocative questions about desire: how shocking is it to realise that the Other on whom I depend is herself lacking? What does the other see in me? Can I be what the other desires? Or might it be something other than me? And the most momentous question of all: how is the transition to be effected from the impossible exigencies of the Imaginary to the relative stability of a symbolically validated identity which bears "the mark which modifies desire"? (Lacan, 1957–1958, lesson seventeen, 26 March 1958, p. 225). In effect, this last question will be answered via an interplay of penis, phallus, and Name-of-the-Father largely endorsed by, and therefore presumably commensurate with, male experience. The imaginary phallus also very impressively steps into the breach over and over with respect to all of these questions. Perhaps too impressively, obscuring the fact that some of them are unanswerable or would best be answered with an X. Unlike certain Lacanian algorithms such as o-object, barred S, etc., the word phallus enters our vocabulary freighted with centuries of semantic ballast which cannot but render questionable its all-encompassing range of reference. When Lacan, a few years later, justifies the "algebraic equation" that is the o-object, he describes it as "something very straightforward that's designed to make something very complicated manageable" (Lacan, 2014, p. 65). The semantic history of the phallus renders it unsuitable for this task. As he himself says in *Encore,* language "brings with it considerable inertia compared to mathemes" (Lacan 1972–1973, p. 110). So the polyvalence accorded to the imaginary phallus in these seminars means that it colonises territories far outside its proper range of reference.

One standard example; female power, undoubtedly a force in human affairs is "phallic", a distortion which continues in psychoanalytic writing. Anything a woman could possibly want, a life, a career, a child, will devolve from a single avatar, the phallus. Anything she might want to be, will similarly be unimaginable outside of this monolithic silhouette.

Initially in Seminar IV, the phallus appears as something that disrupts the mother/child dyad, but, as stated above, it rapidly becomes the single answer to a series of crucial and complex questions. The phallus is insistently evoked each time these reiterated questions surface. Far less frequently Lacan recognises simply that "what is loved in a being is beyond what he is" (Lacan, 1956–1957, lesson eight, 23 January 1957, p. 158). The baby in fact occupies a place in the mother's desire and unconscious fantasy which will forever be inaccessible to both of them. Similarly for every subject his/her "lived incompleteness" (ibid., lesson ten, 6 February 1957, p. 201) will attach itself to specific signifiers not always reducible to a universal avatar. Lacan very effectively fuses Freud's primordially lost object with the imaginary phallus in these seminars. One year later he will develop this strand of his thinking with great power and poignancy via his introduction of the o-object. Guy Le Gaufey has pointed to the similarity in Lacan's writing of the notations o and o-object as evidence that the second had its origins in the first (Le Gaufey, 2009, p. 27). In Seminar V, something of the same rapprochement is visible with respect to the phallus, when in lesson eight he specifies the relation of the ego to the specular image as "more than" the homologue of what he describes as "this phallus as fundamental function to which the subject imaginarily identifies himself" (Lacan, 1957–1958, lesson eight, 8 January 1958, p. 112), specifying "it is in a way in a mirror that the subject identifies himself with what is the object of desire of the mother, and this is … the primitive phallic phase" (ibid., lesson ten, 22 January 1958, p. 137). Despite the ever widening claims for the circumference of the phallus, it nonetheless comes as somewhat of a surprise to the unwary reader when in lesson thirteen of Seminar V it becomes the single signifier upholding the whole world of meaning; "The signifier of the signified is in general the phallus" (ibid., 12 February 1958, p. 173), a leap into the ludicrous repeated some months later in his Munich paper "The Signification of the Phallus" where it is "the signifier intended to designate as a whole the effects of the signified" (Lacan, 1958, p. 285).

While Lacan himself certainly went on to think somewhat differently, the effects of this leap are still visible in psychoanalytic writing, which on this topic sometimes looks as if authored by

> the lunatic of one idea
> in a world of ideas, who would have all the people
> live work suffer and die in that idea
> in a world of ideas
>
> *(Stevens, 2006, p. 285)*

And indeed its effects have been felt beyond psychoanalysis via a perhaps now outmoded semiotic shift whereby "the phallus" absorbed into itself a whole range of meanings, hitherto moored to entirely different concepts. As Marina Warner pointed out in 1985, prior to Lacan's setting up of the phallus as the organising principle which maintains the Symbolic Order itself in existence, binary thinking, with its simple and complex processes of discrimination, was presumed to be a property of thought itself.

> The phallus today has absorbed into itself these meanings, but only today. Thought processes themselves, especially during the Aristotelian Christian centuries, were considered to achieve fine discriminations between one thing and another; Aquinas' *Summa*, constructed in question and answer form, represents a perfect model of a binary mode.
>
> *(Warner, 1985, p. 160)*

Today – and in some psychoanalytic circles unquestioningly – the phallus has been gifted with this ability to uphold binarism. Its function is that of ordering, selecting, separating, and unifying. (A naïve thinker might come up with a quite different set of "phallic" adjectives – thrusting, surging, insisting, even, perhaps, drooping, but no; these do not figure in the usual descriptions of "the phallic function".) As well as the above, a recent superficial trawl through psychoanalytic literature provided the following results. The universalising and totalising drive of Western epistemology is now characterised as phallic, as is the circuit of production and consumption. It functions as the bar between signifier and signified. It is of course *the* signifier of lack, rather than one of several possible and plausible such signifiers. It functions as a synonym for the verb "sexualised" ("sexualised that is phallicised"; Verhaeghe, 2002, p. 114). It is named as S1, the master signifier. The statement that the conditions of desire are unconscious for each of us can apparently be much more effectively conveyed by saying that the phallus always functions as veiled. Bizarrely, given the claims Lacan makes for it in these seminars as that which grounds all meaning, it also manages to be the sole signifier whose very meaning is its failure to signify – that which ruins the very possibility of affirmation or negation (Copjec, 1995, p. 215).

Although we laughed at it thirty years ago, the barb circulating in our training group about the symbolic order being peopled by a solitary regal inhabitant, the phallus, still commands a degree of recognition.

How did this happen? And when? And what is the relation between the phallus and the other signifier which fulfils this all-encompassing function with respect to the symbolic order, the Name-of-the-Father? At the beginning of Lacan's teaching, in Seminar I, the symbolic order is a mesh. The pact which links subjects is founded on laws and contracts (Lacan 1953–1954, p. 230) and is extraordinarily intricate, marked as it is by the property of crisscrossing

> "every easily isolable linguistic symbol is not only at one with the totality but is cut across and constituted by a series of overflowings, of oppositional overdeterminations which place it at one and the same time in several registers"(ibid., pp. 53–54).

The transference which maintains the enigmatic authority of this mesh-like structure is ordinarily not locatable. History demonstrates that the social fabric alters its shape but does not easily tear apart. It appears to be held together by a necessary, though unsubstantiated, belief in meaning as such as opposed to its absence. Lévi-Strauss called this the zero institution, something devoid of any positive determinative function (Lévi-Strauss, 1963, pp. 131–163). Žižek, commenting on this zero institution, sees its only function as the purely negative one of signalling "the presence and actuality of social institution as such, in opposition to its absence, that is in opposition to social chaos" (Žižek, 2002, p. 62).

While Lacan, throughout Seminars II, III, and IV continues to use the phrase "the play of signifiers" in describing the symbolic order, the number of signifiers involved begins to shrink from Seminar III onward.

The assertion that there exist "basic signifiers without which the order of human meaning would be unable to establish itself and that all sorts of cultural myths embody these signifiers" (Lacan, 1955–1956, p. 200) becomes soldered to the Oedipus complex in a manner which is both a tremendous tribute to Freud and a tremendous recentring of the relevance of psychoanalysis to modernity. These primordial signifiers, the mesh that sustains the symbolic order, are, in Lacan's view, very few in number; "the significant points of purchase that uphold the little world of the solitary little men in the modern crowd, are very few in number" (ibid., p. 203). In fact at this point it is no longer the metaphor of the intricate criss-crossing of a mesh-like structure that is in question, but the rather homelier metaphor of a three-legged stool. "Not every stool has four legs. There are some that have only three. Here though there is no question of their lacking any, otherwise things go very badly indeed" (ibid.). But a degree of plurality is still what is in question; "as the signifier is never solitary, the lack of one signifier necessarily brings the subject to the point of calling the set of signifiers into question" (ibid.). What needs to be established is a signifying element which is irreducible to any type of imaginary conditioning, he says (ibid, p. 316). And while the Name-of-the-Father as he theorises it will work well here, Lacan at this time eschews the encroaching exclusivity of the next two years: "I'm not saying that the Name of the Father is the only one of which we can say this" (ibid.).

Two years later, returning to the topic of psychosis in Seminar V, it has indeed become the one and only signifier to fulfil this role. In lesson eight, commenting on a presentation by Gisela Pankow, a distinguished clinician in the field of the psychoses, Lacan propounds the necessity for "a word which will stabilise the whole signifying system, which will ground signification itself" (Lacan, 1957–1958, lesson eight, 8 January 1958, p. 102) and proposes one word only for this task. "There is something that authorises the text of the law … namely the name of the father, that gives support to the law, that grounds the law" (ibid., p. 103). This idea gathers momentum in the early months of 1958, so five weeks after the above statement it is expressed in even stronger terms: "in a way within the signifying system, the name of the father has the function of the whole signifying system, the one who signifies, who authorises the signifying system to exist, who establishes its law" (ibid., lesson thirteen, 12 February 1958, p. 173). The not always clearly marked interplay between phallus and Name-of-the-Father had been specified as metaphorical a little earlier. The desired outcome of the Oedipus complex, "this relation to the power of the law … corresponds to, metaphorically echoes, the relation to the phantastical object which is the phallus" (ibid., lesson eleven, 29 January 1958, p. 152). But Lacan is not entirely at ease with how this transmutation comes about. In lesson ten he tries to articulate step by step "the thing that in it is not altogether clear, nor altogether clearly symbolised … this 'genesis' which ensures that the position of the father in the symbol is fundamental for the position of the phallus in the imaginary plane" (ibid., lesson ten, 6 February 1959, p. 131). This doubt persists and will surface again in the seminar on Identification. Here in 1958, the groundwork for the reduction to this one metaphor is laid by relegating the mother to the Imaginary – "the imaginary pure and simple, namely the mother" (ibid., lesson twelve, 5 February 1958, p. 163) – and therefore in need of subsumption by a superior symbolic power. So what of the penis then? Not to be tucked away in the folds of metaphor it would seem. Entry into the symbolic order cannot happen "without the male sexual organ playing a role of the first importance" (ibid., lesson eleven, 29 January 1958, p. 141). It, and not the phallus or the Name of the Father, is the pivot, although referencing this statement five minutes later, this pivot is now the phallus (ibid., p. 142). This non-separability is evident throughout these seminars. The Name-of-the-Father is also inextricably linked to the penis since it corresponds to the "title deeds" ensuring that "in the most successful cases" the subject can assume "in all tranquillity ... the fact of having a penis" (ibid., p. 147). So it would seem that what we have here is a kind of three in one, with all psychic reality converging on one metaphoric transmutation.

The whole thrust of Seminar V up to a certain point has been this phenomenally comprehensive installation of the paternal metaphor as the lynchpin of a world where sexuality is humanised and desire has a liveable space in which to function. However it is only in totalitarian regimes that one signifier can take on this task by basing itself on a founding exclusion, and invariably this gesture provokes protest. Furthermore, metaphor tends to search out multiplicities. It is closer to the *mi-dit* of the later Lacan than to the implausible tyranny of that "which authorises the signifying system to exist" and it is to Lacan's credit that the successful trajectory traced under the auspices of this solitary signifier cannot but appear ridiculous.

Tranquillity disrupted

Anyone engaging with the enormous corpus of Lacan's work will recognise the aptness of the Moebius strip as metaphor for the experience of reading. Transitions occur and the same vocabulary is imbued with new meaning brought about by serpentine and not easily discernible moves from one surface to another. Lacan himself does not facilitate the wish to create lines of demarcation, often blurring innovative edges by retrospective gestures of inclusion. So we are fortunate in being able to recognise an entirely new strand in Lacan's thinking making its first appearance in Seminar V. Having very convincingly outlined the trajectory of the successful Oedipus with the installation of the paternal metaphor, Lacan cannot but see that the emerging subject, with the title deeds to the penis stuffed tranquilly in his pocket, is, if not a bit of a prick, at least overly cocksure; "insofar as he is virile a man is always more or less his own metaphor. This is even what attaches to the term virility a certain shadow of ridicule" (Lacan, 1957–1958, lesson ten, 22 January 1958, p. 140). So if a real man is a prick, what would a real woman be after this alienating process whereby she has been "obliged to take the image of the other sex as the basis of her identification" (Lacan, 1955–1956, p. 176)? Astray in the head says Lacan in Seminar V; "real women always have something a bit astray (*égarée*) about them" (Lacan, 1957–1958, lesson ten, 22 January 1959, p. 140). Well, well! These observations which might seem to shaft the impressive theoretical edifice he has just erected do not in fact signal any overt change of direction in the general thrust of Seminar V. They are nonetheless worth noting. But the attentive reader will also register the appearance for the first time in lesson thirteen of an altogether new vocabulary, a vocabulary edging towards poetry, and that will infuse that great seminar of the Imaginary, Seminar VI, one year later.

The Moebian shift from one surface to another is remarkable. By the middle of Seminar V the Oedipus complex had subsumed the exigencies of the Imaginary from the domain of the impossible into that of the feasible. A year later Lacan will reverse this orientation and open up an altogether new dimension to psychoanalytic theory. This dimension is tragedy. It will be explored and made explicit over the next two years to the point that the final section of Seminar VII will bear the title "The Tragic dimension of Psychoanalytic Experience". The more sombre dramatic vocabulary in which Lacan will explicate this theme is heard first in lesson thirteen of Seminar V, and, not surprisingly, in the context of phantasy. In Seminar IV, Lacan had just once referred to "that passage through annihilation we call the Oedipus complex" (Lacan, 1956–1957, lesson twenty-one, 5 June 1957, p. 429). Here for the first time in Seminar V, the phrase "the pain of being" – a pivotal concept in Seminar VI – appears; "this pain of being is something really fundamental to him as being linked to the very existence of the living being" (Lacan, 1957–1958, lesson thirteen 12 February 1958, p. 178). Annihilation is spelled out similarly to Seminar VI as something that "reduces to nothing the subject as desiring" (ibid., p. 171), tending to abolish him, and the phrase "*ne phunai*" ("better not to be"), taken from Sophocles' *Oedipus at Colonus*, attributed correctly in earlier seminars to the Chorus, now for the first time is (wrongly) cited as the final curse on existence of Oedipus himself, a misquote which will be hugely expanded on in Seminars VI, VII, and VIII. Also in this lesson, the St. Augustine story which had featured in Lacan's work since the 1940s reappears with a new tragic resonance. From the seminar on Desire to that on Anxiety it will be invoked as the specimen story for the founding catastrophe which marks the birth of the Imaginary. Furthermore, still in the remarkable lesson which is lesson thirteen, after this lengthy and brilliant exposition of a process of subjectification installed as resting on the phallus and the Name-of-the-Father, Lacan (1957–1958) re-states it in much less constricted terms;

> [H]uman beings are as such all under the rod, that is to be a human being who has entered into the world of desire, it is well and truly in the first place to suffer from this something which exists beyond – that we should call it the father has no longer any importance here, it does not matter, it is the law.
>
> *(Lesson thirteen, 12 February 1958, pp. 175–176).*

And four weeks after the appearance of this new direction, in lesson seventeen a hitherto unheard of notation is written on the board. The Big Other is barred, marked as failing, a notation of enormous import, to be developed at length over the following years.

In Seminar VI he will call Ophelia the bud and blossom of life, alternatively referring to her as the phallus and "at the place of the o-object".(Lacan, 1958–1959, p. 215) A year later Antigone rivets onlookers with her *éclat.* It is probably idle to wonder if Lacan was at all close at that time to recognising that there are avatars other than the phallus, but including the latter, for the surge of life and its brief flowering. One thinks of Proust's *jeunes filles en fleur*, but the adolescent boy or the child, as well as countless other images, can also occupy this place.

The tranquil certainties of Seminar V will be left far behind as Lacan turns his attention to the "subjective elision" attendant on the coming into being of the subject (Lacan, 1958–1959, lesson twelve, 11 February 1959, p. 150).

While it is fair to say that in the following years he in no way modifies his phallocentric stance to pursue the power and pathos that subtend the dramas of the Imaginary, his new focus on the verb "to be" begins to undercut the masculinist opposition of the verbs "to be" and "to have". What will be in question in Seminar VI is "a subjective assumption inflected between being and having" (ibid.).

But the phallus of the fifties cast a long, long shadow, making it necessary for girls who wanted to *be* the hero rather than be *had* by him to look outside of psychoanalytic theory for the necessary *derring do.*

References

Badiou, A. (2001). *Ethics: An Essay of Understanding Evil.* London: Verso.

Beckett, S. (1959). *Molloy, Malone Dies, The Unnamable.* London: Calder and Boyars.

Copjec, J. (1995). *Read my Desire.* London: Cambridge: MIT Press.

Freud, S. (1895d). *Studies on Hysteria. S.E.*, 2. London: Hogarth Press.

Freud, S. (1900a). *The Interpretation of Dreams. S.E.*, 4–5. London: Hogarth Press.

Lacan, J. (1938) Les complexes familiaux dans la formation de l'individu. In: *Autres Écrits.* Paris: Seuil, 2001. Unpublished English translation by C. Gallagher as: Family Complexes in the Formation of the Individual. Retrieved from: www.lacaninireland.com.

Lacan, J. (1953–1954). *The Seminar of Jacques Lacan, Book 1:Freud's Papers on Technique.* Cambridge: Cambridge University Press, 1988.

Lacan, J. (1954–1955). *The seminar of Jacques Lacan, Book II: The Ego in Freud's Theory and in the Technique of Analysis.* Cambridge: Cambridge University Press, 1988.

Lacan, J. (1955–1956). *The Seminar of Jacques Lacan, Book III: The Psychoses.* London: Routledge, 1993.

Lacan, J. (1956–1957). *The Seminar of Jacques Lacan, Book IV: The Relation to the Object.* L.V. A. Roche (Trans.). Unpublished.

Lacan, J. (1957–1958). *The Seminar of Jacques Lacan, Book V: The Formations of the Unconscious.* C. Gallagher (Trans.). Retrieved from: http://www.lacaninireland.com/web/wp-content/uploads/2010/.

Lacan, J. (1958). The Signification of the Phallus. In: *Écrits: A Selection* (pp. 281–291). A. Sheridan (Trans.). London: Tavistock Publications, 1977.

Lacan, J. (1958–1959). *The Seminar of Jacques Lacan, Book VI: Desire and its Interpretation.* C. Gallagher (Trans.). Retrieved from: http://www.lacaninireland.com/web/wp-content/uploads/2010/06/Book-06-Desire-and-its-interpretation.pdf.

Lacan, J. (1961–1962). *The Seminar of Jacques Lacan, Book IX: Identification.* C. Gallagher (Trans.). Unpublished.

Lacan, J. (1962–1963). *The Seminar of Jacques Lacan, Book X: Anxiety.* A. Johnson (Trans.). Cambridge: Polity Press, 2010.

Lacan, J. (1972–1973). *Seminar of Jacques Lacan, Book XX: On Feminine Sexuality: The Limits of Love and Knowledge, 1972–1973.* B. Fink (Trans.). New York & London: W.W. Norton & Company, 1999.

Le Gaufey, G. (2009). *C'est a quel sujet?*Paris: Epel.

Recalcati, M. (2013). Love and Feminine Jouissance. *Lacunae*, 2(2): 71–97.

Scherfig, L.(Director). (2016). *Their Finest* [Film]. UK: Pinewood Pictures.

Soler, C. (2002). What does the Unconscious know about Women? In: S. Barnard & B. Fink (Eds.), *Reading Seminar XX* (pp. 99–108). Albany: State University of New York Press.

Stevens, W. (2006). *Collected Poems.* London: Faber & Faber.

Strauss, L. (1963). *Cultural Anthropology*. New York: Basic Books.
Verhaeghe, P. (2002). Lacan's Answer to the Classical Mind/Body Deadlock. (pp. 109–140). Albany: State University of New York Press.
Warner, M. (1985). *Monuments and Maidens*. London: Picador.
Žižek, S. (2002). The Real of Sexual Difference. In: S. Barnard & B. Fink (Eds.), *Reading Seminar XX* (pp. 57–75). Albany: State University of New York Press.

9

THE PHALLUS

Crossroads or impasse? Queering desire via Seminar V

Sarah Meehan O'Callaghan

The topic of the phallus in Lacanian theory has always proved contentious, as demonstrated in Jan Campbell's *Arguing with the Phallus*. Debates still rage over its patriarchal and conservative connotations, such as the privileging of the male organ as symbol of power and the historical exclusion or devaluing of female sexuality from the theoretical paradigm of psychoanalytic theory. As Campbell (2000) argues, "however deconstructive Lacanianism is in terms of a humanist, transcendental ego, it fails to dislodge the mastery of the ego because it privileges on a totalising level the symbolic, linguistic phallus" (p. 132). The phallus is also targeted with supporting a heterosexist ideal, where heterosexuality is deemed to be the most desired and "normal" state of being. Nonetheless, a close inspection of the phallus in Lacan's fifth seminar, *Formations of the Unconscious* (Lacan, 1957–1958), opens up pathways to thinking of desire and sexuality from a non-normative, non-binary or queer perspective. In this seminar, Lacan is already problematising heterosexuality and theories privileging genital maturation as the desired-for outcome of analysis or a life trajectory. As Lacan asks, "this heterosexual relation between human beings, is it something so simple?" (ibid., lesson XXI, 7 May 1958, p. 337). In later seminars, such as *Encore* (Lacan, 1972–1973), this idea will be developed into the "non-rapport of the sexual relation", with a precursor to this idea at the end of his sixth seminar, *Desire and its Interpretation* (Lacan, 1958–1959). This breach, or non-rapport, between the sexes is envisaged through the introduction of the phallus as "signifier of desire" (Lacan, 1972–1973, p. 339). In this, a movement occurs from the imaginary realm of identification pertaining to the ego and to that of desire as unconscious.

This chapter offers a reading of the phallus in Seminar V that will emphasise its innovative direction in moving beyond traditional debates of male/female sexual and gender identity as were occurring at the time, while not disputing its chauvinistic and patriarchal overtones such as virility/ potency (as discussed in Meehan

O'Callaghan, 2016). In fact I would say, as Hector Kollias (2012) has shown, that the phallus is an inherently queer concept which has been neglected as a topic of queer research. I am here referring to the ideas of Queer theory, or Queer theories, that interrogate subjectivities and configurations of identity that do not conform to, or reflect, proscribed normative ideals, such as, what Butler (1993) calls "compulsory heterosexuality" (p. 18). Traditionally Queer theory has attempted to subvert the status quo and challenge the concept of normativity in relation to sexuality and sexual acts, including binary or dualistic assumptions inherent to models of identity, such as heterosexual, gay and lesbian subject positions, as Eve Sedgwick captures in her statement:

> [Q]ueer is a continuing moment, movement, motive – recurrent, eddying, troublant. The word "queer" itself means across – it comes from the Indo-European root – twerkw, which also yields the German quer (transverse), Latin torquere (to twist).
>
> *(Sedgwick, 2005, p. 8)*

While Queer theory has highlighted the diversity of sexuality and the political and societal consequences of the exclusion of non-normative sexualities, from a Lacanian perspective it has its limitations. As Tim Dean (2003) notes, Queer theory's utopianism in attempting to engage a freedom from the oppression of heteronormative society, leads at times to the privileging of the imaginary dimension of identity over the unconscious. Therefore, I do not want to suggest that Lacan was a Queer theorist in this respect, but rather that, ironically, the phallus, though targeted as an agent of the binary conception of male-female relations, is actually a signifier which leads to their undoing.

In Seminar V, Lacan begins to challenge the parameters of normal/normativity that encircle heterosexuality. This challenges its privileged position within the cultural imaginary as a state of aspired-for satisfaction and as an ideal outcome of therapeutic practice. The parameters of normativity, as echoed in the debates at the time, are evidenced by the expositions and critiques in chapter V of Karen Horney's *On The Genesis of the Castration Complex in Women* (1924) and Helen Deutsch's *Significance of Masochism in the Mental Life of Women* (1930). The interplay between these female analysts demonstrates pertinent issues relevant to female sexuality at the time. Horney advocated that the sensations of the vagina, as opposed to the clitoris, were more central to infantile female sexuality than had been previously believed. Hence the vagina served a more active role than the passive one often assigned to it (Horney, 1930). Deutsch on the other hand, did not attribute the same sensibility to the vagina, taking a more phallic view of the female genitalia, such that after the "phallic phase" the clitoris becomes forbidden as a source of pleasure and the female is bereft of an avenue for jouissance. Deutsch (1930) contends that this loss of the clitoris as an active pleasure "phallic" zone is then compensated for with the desire for a child (p. 7). Female masochism is associated with a natural instinct to child bearing, and frigidity is a component factor of this passivity. From this point of view the ability to bear a child satisfies the masochistic instinct in the female and compensates for the passive position. We shall see how Lacan responds to these female clinicians later in this chapter and what this implies for conceptualisations of sexuality during the 1950s and today. Although I am using the terms sexuality and desire in tandem so far, this chapter will challenge this coupling, and, utilising insights from Seminar V, will demonstrate how desire, while intersecting with sexuality, is not reductive to it. This decoupling will be useful in thinking about sexuality in our modern times and the proliferation of identity categories emerging within the sexual societal paradigm. These identity categories suggest that identity can be aligned with desire, whether that is gay, straight, queer, bisexual, asexual, etc. Lacan asks in this seminar, why there is not a proliferation of identities – "Why not the greatest plurality of identifications? – as many identifications as unsatisfied demands? – as many identifications as there are Others, supposing themselves in the subject's presence as responding or not to the demand?" (Lacan, 1957–1958, lesson XIX, 23 April 1958, p. 312).We see here that the realm of demand is linked with that of identification. Lacan shows that it is in the refusal of demand within the Oedipal dialectic, and with the ensuing frustration/disappointment that identification may form. We can thus consider the plurality of identity categories in today's times within the framework outlined here of demand/desire. This implies that an imaginary stability of subjectivity is demanded via the mechanisms of identification at the expense of living with the uncertainty of unconscious desire, a desire that has no specific object of satisfaction but operates to "enjoy" as desire. This enjoyment or masochistic quality of desire is akin to jouissance and causes suffering for the subject. Hence, while I contend that the phallus can be read as a queer or non-binary signifier, and consequently unconscious desire as something non-essential, and not specifically heterosexual, we need to be careful not to descend into that queer utopia where, as Rob Weatherill articulates, "to blow apart 'identity' and replace it with 'fluidity', destroys what even Žižek (2009) refers to as 'the ultimate difference, the "transcendental" difference that grounds human identity itself'" (Weatherill, 2017, p. 331). This transcendental difference grounding human identity is the function of the phallus as signifier. It is what Lacan refers to in Seminar V as the "alterity … through which being (*l'être*) divides from its own existence" (Lacan, 1957–1958, lesson XIX, 5 March 1958, p. 228).

The phallus as crossroads signifier: *Signifiant carrefour*

Lacan has defined the phallus as a crossroads signifier; a point of tangency or connectivity in a juncture where differing paths coincide. We shall see how this positioning of tangency relates to the process of identification as explained by Lacan in Seminar V, and how it serves as a function in the concept of the Name-of-the-Father or *le Nom du Père*. The phallus is at the crossroads of desire, identification and the transformative identificatory dialectic of the Oedipus complex. As a crossroads signifier the phallus is conceived as an organisational defile through which desire is both transformed and nominated: as Lacan says on many occasions the phallus is "the signifier of desire" (Lacan, 1957–1958, lesson XXI, 7 May 1958, p. 344). If we leave aside for one moment the problems with this designation of "the signifier" in the singular, we can approach how the phallus is deemed to function within the Oedipal matrix of mother, father and child. As Lacan says:

> [T]here's always something ternary in it – even in the most primitive relation, that of the child and the mother: the phallus, as object of the desire of the mother, which sets up an uncrossable barrier to the satisfaction of the desire of the child – which is to be, himself, the exclusive object of the desire of the mother.
>
> *(Ibid., lesson XV, 12 March 1958, p. 255)*

This ternary aspect of the phallus will be important in tracing the non-binary resonances inherent to its function as crossroads signifier of desire and sexuality, and will allow us to consider desire as something connected with identification but also pointing beyond. In Seminar V Lacan gives a formula for the process of identification and the implications for desire:

> Finally, an exchange is produced – what had been the object of the libidinal relation becomes something else, is transformed into a signifying function for the subject – and the desire pertaining to it passes to another plane, the plane of desire established with the third term. In this operation, this other desire comes to substitute itself for the first desire – which is repressed, and fundamentally transformed.
>
> *(Ibid., lesson XVI, 19th March 1958, p. 263)*

This is a hugely dense formula, condensing as it does, a reference to, and movement beyond, Freud's conceptualisation of the ego-ideal in relation to identification, loss and narcissistic structure. In "The Ego and the Id", Freud theorises the connection between object cathexis and identification and the ego-ideal. The ego-ideal retains the traces of the lost libidinal object, which occurs in melancholia. Identification in this sense constitutes a compensatory process where, as Freud (1923b) puts it, the object "is forcing itself, so to speak, upon the id as a love-object" (p. 30). Freud admits that this transition from object cathexis to identification is complex and uncertain, and aligns it with sublimation – where the energy of the drive is redirected to a different destination, transforming the original object. Lacan's reworking of these terms and the addition of the phallus as signifier formulates the operational mechanisms of the transition from object to signifier (Lacan, 1957–1958, p. 263). Lacan aligns the ego-ideal with that of the subject (the unconscious) and the process of secondary identification (secondary narcissism in Freud). The ego-ideal marks the transition of the loved object's descent into the Symbolic and retains the traces of this object. Therefore it is not so much an introjection of a good or bad object, but rather a phenomenon demonstrating how the traces of identification (the insignias of the Other) mark the unconscious of the subject. As Lacan describes: "this point of identification where the subject takes on the insignias of what she's identified with – which plays the role, the function, of ego-ideal" (ibid., p. 263).

The formula for identification as outlined above illustrates the dynamics of the paternal metaphor, one term comes to substitute for another and as a result transforms the original libidinal object into a signifier (ibid.). As Chiesa (2007) points out, in understanding the role of the phallus in the paternal metaphor it is important not to collapse it with the Name-of-the Father. The phallus is an element in this metaphor, not the metaphor itself. It is the signifier of the X of the mother's desire, which the Name-of-the-Father comes to substitute for. We could say that the Name-of-the-Father is the operational function of the metaphor and the phallus is the signifier within that operation. The phallus remains more on the side of metonymy, and a function of the endless and shifting movement of desire as it forms and conjugates within linguistic perimeters. "Desire is the metonymy of being in the subject; the phallus… is the signifying element subtracted from the chain of the word" (Lacan, 1958–1959, lesson 1, 12 November 1958, p. 17). It must be said that if Lacan had stuck to the use of X to signify the mother's desire there would be much less controversy around this term. X is a term used in mathematics to signify a random variable, something we cannot know in advance or outcome predict such as, for example, what it is that sustains the mother's desire. The use of X for the mother's desire denotes an outcome that is subject to chance and not prescribed. The phallus on the other hand, while not being reducible to any particular signified, retains the resonances of the penis. However, and this is perhaps what Lacan intended, to give a name to the signifier X is to align it with a signified, to illustrate that it also functions as a signified as well as a signifier. "What's at work is the x, the signified. And the signified of the mother's coming and going is the phallus" (ibid., lesson IX, 15 January 1958, p. 156).

To recap, we have several intersecting theoretical paths, or points of connectivity, with the phallus as crossroads signifier; that of the ego-ideal, desire, identification and metaphor. The phallus is that which links these agents in the developmental movement of Oedipal negotiation. This crossroads is the juncture of the Oedipal complex, an alchemic moment where the child's libidinal objects are transformed via pathways of loss and disappointment into the realm of the symbolic: what was an object becomes a signifier, and moves from the level of demand to desire. As Chiesa (2007) explains, Lacan is attempting to find the crossroads between the Imaginary and the Symbolic, something that functions to explain the dynamics of how "love is transformed into identification" (Lacan, 1957–1958, lesson XVI, 19 March 1958, p. 261). This bridge between the Imaginary and Symbolic is conceptualised partly through understanding the father's role in the Oedipus complex as a component of a linguistic operation. In fact, Lacan refers to the father here as a metaphor: the "father is a signifier substituted for another signifier" (ibid., lesson IX, 15 January 1958, p. 155). In this sense the Oedipus complex becomes an operation potentially more fungible than essentialist, more normative than normal. Lacan is attempting to separate the function of the father within the Oedipus complex from the father as a concrete individual; the individual father may not be "normal" or conventional, yet the paternal function still maintains a normative role: "To speak of his deficiency in the family is not to speak of his deficiency in the complex" (ibid., p. 150). This theoretical distinction between the paternal function and the actual father, or the normative versus normal, allows for envisaging possibilities of family setups that do not conform to the heterosexist ideal.

For Freud, a successful outcome of the Oedipus complex differed for each sex. For the boy, an optimal outcome resulted in an intensification of identification with the father with affection for the mother, and for the girl, an intensification of identification with the mother. These identifications establish the boy as masculine and the girl as feminine. Freud (1923b) termed this outcome of the Oedipus complex "the more normal" (p. 32).

In Seminar V, Lacan problematises the concept of normal. In establishing the Oedipus complex as normative, Lacan introduces the distance between what is and what should be. Lacan adds another term to the process of identifications inherent to the Oedipus complex – that of the phallus. This introduces a movement from the biological and essentialist ideas of masculinity and femininity to what he will later develop in the graph of sexuation as the *dit*-mension of the sexes (Lacan, 1972–1973, p. 21) Sexuality and gender identity becomes untethered from thinking of it as a drive toward a so-called normative object to considering it as something that is impacted by language. Already, in 1958, Lacan questions essentialist understandings of gender, referring to masculine and feminine assumptions:

> [T]he Oedipus complex has a normative function; not simply in the moral structure of the subject, or in his relations with reality, but in the assumption of his or her sex – which, as you know, has an irreducible ambiguity about it.
> *(Lacan, 1957–1958, p. 147)*

Lacan clearly distinguishes here between genitalisation and the assumption of sex, which corresponds with gender. The Oedipus complex is the dialectic through which gender is "assumed", subjectively moving gender beyond an alignment with biology.

Beyond penis envy: From demand to desire

At various stages in Seminar V Lacan attempts to clarify that the phallus is not the penis:

> The phallus is not a form – it's not an objectal form, as a form that remains captivating … the phallus isn't a fantasy, or an image, or an object, even a

> partial or internal one – it's a signifier. That it's a signifier – well, this alone allows us to conceive and articulate the diverse functions it takes on, at different levels of the inter-sexual encounter.
>
> *(Lacan, 1957–1958, lesson XXI, 7 May 1958, p. 339)*

However, despite reiterating on many occasions that the phallus is a signifier, Lacan stumbles at times into collapsing or packing too much meaning into this signifier, such as saying that the phallus "represents the rise of vital power", designating it as a symbol of potency (ibid., lesson XXVI, 18 June 1958, p. 419). These resonances inherent in Lacan's conceptualisation of the phallus leads to imagining the phallus as something tangible, symbolic, an object whose meaning can be deciphered with the right interpretation, and hence to confusions in situating its position within the Lacanian theoretical framework. To view the phallus as an object of meaning is to attempt to define it, to align a particular signified in its path. However, to attempt to define the phallus is to run into a fundamental impossibility built into its very position within the signifying chain of language. As Hector Kollias (2012) says: "[T]he most blatant way to fuck with the phallus is to give it a name – how can the impotent signifier of that which resists signification have a name?" (p. 14). The phallus functions as "signifier of desire" (Lacan, 1957–1958, lesson XXI, 7 May 1958, p. 336) and also of what is barred in desire, which is the very imbrication of language within desire itself. At this juncture, Lacan is developing a theory of desire that pertains to the subject of the unconscious, rather than aligning it with the ego and the imaginary realm of identification where demand prevails. The implications for this movement beyond the penis as object are vital for the positioning of the analyst in the psychoanalytic "cure". Lacan warns against interpreting the phallus as an object to be demanded in the context of the clinical setting and gives various examples of how the phallus operates as a signifier both from the literary context and the clinic. It is the phallus as signifier that prevents identification and desire coalescing in the normative trajectory of gender and object aim, as Lacan postulates "perhaps it isn't the same thing – desiring to possess the phallus and desiring to be a man" (ibid., lesson XXV, 11 June 1958, p. 407).

While desire is intimately connected with identification, it is also not reduced to it. This is an important theoretical move, particularly at this time when cases of homosexuality were often referred to as cases of inversion; the scenario where same-sex attraction resulted from the assertion that inwardly (or psychically) the gender of an individual was assumed to be one of the opposite sex. Inversion theory "straightened" out same-sex desire and aligned sexual orientation with gender identity. So according to this theory, two homosexual females in a coupling could be assumed to fall on opposite sides of the gender spectrum, one female presumed to be identified as an internal male, having assumed qualities or traits of masculinity, and the other presumed to be inherently female. Apart from theories of inversion, other explanations of homosexuality featuring sexual desire and gender identification also figured, exemplified by Karen Horney's (1924) critique of female homosexuality and the castration complex. Horney elaborates on what she feels is the crux of the castration complex for women, and as is typical of her emphasis on cultural factors, she explains emotional or psychological difficulties arising for the female as an offshoot of the cultural valuation of the penis, and not as something inherently biological. Women envy some of the "perks" of having a penis, such as peeing standing up and the outward manifestation of the organ. This formulation of "penis envy" is illustrated by the recent version of the film *Jumanji* (Kasden, 2017), where one of the female characters embodies a male body and relishes experiencing the physicality of the penis. For Horney, the physical visibility of the male organ vs. the "hidden" component of female genitals lead her to formulate a theory concerning the differences of the sexes which explains why "a woman wears a low neck, while a man wears a dress coat" (Horney, 1924, p. 53). Due to the frustrated desire of not being able to exhibit her sexual organ, a displacement occurs where the female desires to exhibit her whole body (ibid.). She argues that identification with the father results from the disappointments of penis envy, and this identification may lead to female homosexuality: this is another way of saying that female to female homosexual desire is not natural or essential but rather neurotic. Lacan's critique of Horney's account of female homosexuality reveals that he does not collapse an unconscious male identification with female homosexuality. As he says, these theories do not take account of the penis or phallus as imaginary. To this effect, the phallus as concept inserts a wedge into object-relations theory; no longer are we dealing with a subject's direct relations to libidinal objects of the mother or father, but with this signifier of desire, we have the formulation that these relations concern a lack of an object. As Carol Owens (2017) has argued, the queer potential of Lacanian theory is diminished when "decontextualised and/or unreflexive usage of concepts such as lack and jouissance" emphasise a "tragic" account of lack and desire, associated with loss per se (p. 270). Hence the potential of Lacanian theory as a critique of non-normative sexuality has remained somewhat under explored. If desire is aligned with lack, this, as Lara Farina (2017) opines, categorises it as reactive as opposed to productive. So if we accept that desire is reactive to an absence, does this make it any less productive? Indeed why does it have to be productive? Is emphasising productivity not just another function of neoliberal discourse, bent on creating more of something, not less, in a movement of endless progression that denies the tragic quality of human existence? In Seminar V, Lacan begins to formulate the pathway toward the "tragedy of desire" that he will develop in *Seminar VI, Desire and its Interpretation* (Lacan, 1958-1959, Lesson 13, 4 March 1959, p. 161). Therefore, the phallus is the signifier of a tragic dimension of the subject and its import cannot be assessed without considering its correspondence with desire.

Desire

If the phallus is signifier of desire as Lacan reiterates frequently, what does this imply about desire? Is desire something that can be represented/signified or that which escapes representation? According to Lacan, desire is not something that can be fully spoken: "desire is articulated – insofar as it's linked to the presence of the signifier in man … Specifically because it's essentially a question of the link with the signifier, it's never fully articulatable" (Lacan, 1957–1958, lesson XVIII, 16 April 1958, p. 303). This statement implicates that desire is not encapsulated in phrases designating a desired-for object, although it has a part to play in the utterance itself. Desire is that which is always beyond demand, and yet also exists within demand. Desire is what is unknown in the Other and ourselves, and this unknown is what gives the enigmatic character to the gaze or the voice of another. It is that which distorts the fabric of reality, that aspect of ourselves that forms a crack in the contours of the Imaginary and the Symbolic. As soon as we speak and express a statement in language, our signifiers mask and indent desire. The phallus as signifier par excellence is what masks desire, in that it signifies the bar within desire itself, originating with the barring of the mother's desire. As Lacan points out, the phallus is not related to the prohibition of masturbation but to the castration of the mother primarily. It is the barring of the mother's desire (which is always something unknown) that renders us subjects of desire and subjects of jouissance. Thus, desire bears something of a masochistic quality, being closely aligned with suffering and "the pain of existence" – as Lacan says – "masochism at the foundation of the analytic exploration of desire; the subject grasping himself as suffering – he grasps his existence as living being in terms of suffering, that is to say, as being subject of desire" (ibid., lesson XVII, 26 March 1958, p. 290). We can see therefore that the line between desire and jouissance is a thin one, given that jouissance is something that a subject 'enjoys' and endures rather than masters. Lacan's later work will situate the subject of the unconscious as subject of jouissance. This is indicative of a theoretical shift that takes place in relation to the body relative to the unconscious (Verhaeghe, 2001). In 1958, desire is distinguished from that which can be demanded on the plane of egoic relations and, as Lacan shows on the evolving graph of desire, desire is always a signifying horizon of the signifying chain. It delineates the interval where the subject of the unconscious and fantasy will be situated. On the graph of desire, the phallus occupies a place which is just on the border of the signifying horizon, marking the limit where language and the unconscious overlap (Lacan, 1957–1958, lesson XXVII, 25 June 1958, p. 430). It is a signifier of lack, the signifier of the distance of the subject's demand from his desire, representing the movement between the egoic and imaginary dimensions of identification and the unconscious shifting underpinnings of desire. As Tim Dean (2003) claims, desire for Lacan is no longer a psychological category that is linked to the welding of identities, but as an effect of language and unconscious, it threatens the coherence of all identity categories (p. 272).

Today, identity categories appear to be endless, the letters on the LGBTQI acronym are expanding all the time allowing for more and more variations of sexual identity. While seeming to be categories that designate a fluidity of sexuality and that allow for agency regarding one's subjective position, these categories also perhaps attempt to corral the excesses of desire into an identificatory corner, so to speak. To find a category to which I belong explains and nominates my desire, it functions as a limit. This phenomenon is described by Alexandre Stevens (2007) as a communitarian demand, where sexual identities allow for collective belonging easing the anxiety of singularity. As he says "the problem of sex is presented in terms of the choice of identification, and that the subject is happy if his identification allows him to be part of a community" (p. 234). From the perspective of Seminar V, in considering identification as a mask, we can say that every identification leads to a dis-satisfaction, as Lacan stipulates "there are as many masks as dissatisfactions" (Lacan, 1957–1958, lesson XVIII, 16 April 1958, p. 305).

This link between identification and dissatisfaction can be seen within the psychiatric domain: an increasing array of diagnoses abound in the *Diagnostic and Statistical Manual of Mental Disorders* (DSM) leading to potential imaginary crystallisations forming within subjectivity. As Paul Verhaeghe (2008) points out, the method of the DSM is "go and name the things" (p. 31). Identification is also a means of categorisation, naming or specifying. One can identify with a "personality disorder" or "bi-polar disorder", temporarily palliating the anxiety underlying these states. Ultimately there is no identification that can satisfy the pulse of desire as it moves metonymically from object to object, remaining always on the edge of demand. And as we know, identification is always linked to loss and disappointment – the ego-ideal serving as a memorial to what was lost. As I have outlined here, the phallus is the marker of that loss, and Lacan will connect it with the *objet a* in *Seminar XI, The Four Fundamental Concepts of Psychoanalysis* (Lacan, 1964); that lost object that is separated from the body, but continues to haunt the subject in fantasy. By *Seminar XX, Encore,* the phallus becomes the signifier of non-signification, that which signifies, "the impossibility of the sexual relationship" (Lacan, 1972–1973, p. 15). This bar of non-signification between the sexes has major implications for thinking of the existence of homosexuality and heterosexuality within the unconscious. As Tim Dean (2000) deduces, "if there is no signifier for sexual difference, then as far as the unconscious is concerned, heterosexuality does not exist" (p. 86). The implications of this insight lead Dean to argue for a shift from understanding ourselves in light of sexuality, toward that of unconscious desire, where desire and sexuality are not coterminous, and desire emerges as the privileged concept of subjectivity. This desire, as Lacan explains, is not simply satisfied by the acquisition of an object but is what the subject "enjoys [and therefore] is an essential dimension of his *jouissance"* (Lacan, 1957–1958, lesson 17, 26 March 1958 p. 289). This enjoyment "is the eccentricity of desire in relation to every satisfaction … At the limit, what desire verges towards … in its pure and simple form – is this pain of existing" (Lacan, 1957–1958, lesson VI, 17 December 1958, p. 309).

The connection between desire and the pain of existing paves the way for his seminar of 1958–1959, *Seminar VI, Desire and its Interpretation.* Thus, as signifier of desire the phallus signifies the subversion of the subject vis-à-vis the unconscious.

References

Butler, J. (1993). *Bodies That Matter.* London: Routledge.

Campbell, J. (2000). *Arguing with the Phallus: Feminist, Queer and Postcolonial Theory.* London: Zed Books.

Chiesa, L. (2007). *Subjectivity and Otherness. A Philosophical Reading of Lacan.* USA: Massachusetts Institute of technology.

Dean, T. (2003). Lacan After Queer Theory. In: J.M. Rabaté (Ed), *The Cambridge Companion to Lacan*. Cambridge: Cambridge University Press.

Dean, T. (2000). *Beyond Sexuality*. London: University of Chicago Press.

Deutsch, H. (1930). Significance of Masochism in the Mental Life of Women. *International Journal of Psychoanalysis*, 11: 48–60.

Farina, L. (2017). Missing Something? Queer Desire. In: E. Watson & N. Giffney (Eds.), *Clinical Encounters in Sexuality: Psychoanalytic Practice and Queer Theory* (pp. 77–100). New York: Punctum.

Freud, S. (1923b). The Ego and the Id. *S.E.*, 19: 3–69. London: Hogarth Press.

Horney, K. (1924). On the Genesis of the Castration Complex in Women. *International Journal of Psychoanalysis*, 5: 50–65.

Kasden, J.(Director). (2017). *Jumanji: Welcome to the Jungle* [Film]. USA: Columbia Pictures.

Kollias, H. (2012, May 10). The Queer Phallus: Have It, Be It, Just Don't Fuck With It. Retrieved from: https://www.academia.edu/1771529/The_Queer_Phallus_Have_it_Be_it_just_Dont_Fuck_with_it [Accessed June 2016].

Lacan, J. (1957-1958). *The Formations of the Unconscious. Seminar V.* P.G.Young (Trans). Unpublished.

Lacan, J. (1958–1959). *Desire and its Interpretation: Seminar VI.* C. Gallagher (Trans.). Unpublished.

Lacan, J. (1972–1973). *Encore: The Seminar of Jacques Lacan, Book XX. On Feminine Sexuality: The Limits of Love and Knowledge, 1972–1973.* B. Fink (Trans.). New York: W.W. Norton & Co., 1999.

Lacan, J. (1964). *The Four Fundamental Concepts of Psychoanalysis: The Seminar of Jacques Lacan, Book XI.* A. Sheridan (Trans.) & J.-A. Miller (Ed.). London: Penguin, 1998.

Meehan O'Callaghan, S. (2016). Bending the Phallus: Considerations of Desire via Seminar V. *Lacunae International Journal for Lacanian Psychoanalysis*, 13: 115–129.

Owens, C. (2017). Queer Troubles for Psychoanalysis. In: E. Watson & N. Giffney (Eds.), *Clinical Encounters in Sexuality: Psychoanalytic Practice and Queer Theory* (pp. 261–273). New York: Punctum.

Sedgwick, E. (2005). *Tendencies*. UK: Routledge.

Stevens, A. (2007). Love and Sex Beyond Identifications. In V. Voruz & B. Wolf (Eds.). *The Later Lacan: An Introduction*. USA: State University of New York Press.

Verhaeghe, P. (2001). Subject and Body: Lacan's Struggle with the Real. In: P. Verhaeghe, *Beyond Gender: From Subject to Drive* (pp. 65–97). New York: Other Press.

Verhaeghe, P. (2008). *On Being Normal and Other Disorders: A Manual for Clinical Psychodiagnostics*. London: Karnac.

Weatherill, R. (2017). The Queer New Times. In: E. Watson & N. Giffney (Eds.), *Clinical Encounters in Sexuality: Psychoanalytic Practice and Queer Theory* (pp. 329–343). New York: Punctum.

10

TO BE OR NOT TO BE THE PHALLUS

Lacan, Genet and Wilde

Christine Gormley

In the middle of his fifth seminar, Lacan turns to comedy in an attempt to say something about the phallus. His comments on comedy appear within the broader context of a discussion of perversion, alongside his reading of Jean Genet's *Le Balcon*. Perversion is not considered in terms of a pre-Oedipal aetiology, nor as an uncompromised emergence of the drive in its "raw state" which might be attributed to a lack of, or deviance from, attempts to domesticate it. Rather, Lacan, after Freud, considers perversion to be just as subtle and complex as neurosis, showing "exactly the same structure of compromise and elusion, of the dialectic of repression, and the return of the repressed" (Lacan, 1957–1958, lesson 13, 12 February 1958, p. 1). Indeed, Lacan attempts to delimit the field of perversion by having it depend upon the position of the subject in relation to the phallus and the Name-of-the-Father. He is a long way away from describing the Oedipus complex as Freud's dream, but he nonetheless raises the question, "are there neuroses without Oedipus" (ibid., lesson 9, 15 January 1958, p. 3)? Genet's play *Le Balcon* was published the year prior to Seminar V, and undoubtedly had a considerable influence on Lacan. Much of his discussion about comedy in this seminar is borne out in this play or drawn directly from it. His comments occur alongside a reading of Joan Riviere's 1929 article "Womanliness as Masquerade" on the one hand, and the isolation of what Lacan considers to be a defining moment in the subjective history of André Gide, gleaned from Jean Delay's *The Youth of André Gide,* on the other. It is as good an example as any of the way Lacan worked; speaking about disparate topics side by side without explicitly drawing a link between them, leaving it to his audience to connect the dots.

Before looking at these texts, it is worth bearing in mind that many of the ideas Lacan attempts to work out here will soon be revised in light of one another, most notably his move towards the formula, already in Seminar VI, that the Other of the Other does not exist. For now, Lacan explicitly states that the Other of the

Other does exist. Other difficulties include the fact that the Real is at times conflated with reality or with what is "outside" the Symbolic, and the Name-of-the-Father reigns supreme as that which guarantees the successful resolution of the Oedipus complex, the ego-ideal being preserved for its dominion. Lacan states his thesis clearly in *Seminar V* when he says, "it's at the same place … that what forms here is, in one case, the ego ideal, and in another case, perversion" (Lacan, 1957–1958, lesson 14, 5 March 1958, p. 9). However, it is often unclear whether he is talking about the phallus as image or as signifier in this seminar, and while he is at pains to counteract the conflation of the phallus with the penis, he does not always escape this pitfall.

Lacan begins with "Womanliness as Masquerade". The article outlines a case, the defining feature of which, according to Riviere, is not unique to the woman in question. She tells us, "[W]omen who wish for masculinity may put on a mask of womanliness to avert anxiety and the retribution feared from men" (Riviere, 1929, p. 76). Read in terms of a dialectic of having/not having the phallus, she presents herself as lacking. It is a position which maintains a conservative respect for the phallus, and it is this position certain comedies set out to subvert. Lacan, still under the influence of Kojeve's reading of Hegel, uses this example to demonstrate that, "what's at stake in an analysis, in the comprehension of a subjective structure, is always something that shows us the subject engaged in a process of recognition, as such" (Lacan, 1957–1958, p. 5). But, he asks, recognition of what? Lacan variously calls this an unconscious need or desire for recognition which is situated on the plane of the signifier through which, he says, "being divides from its own existence" (ibid.). Consider the Bishop's words in *Le Balcon*:

> If I had wanted to become a bishop, I should have had to put all my energy not into being one, but into acting in the sort of way that would have led to my becoming one … – a function is only a function. It isn't a mode of being. But a bishop – that *is* a mode of being. It's a heavy responsibility. A burden. Mitres, lace, cloth of gold, costume jewellery … Stuff functions!
>
> *(Genet, 1991, p. 5)*

The Bishop is carried away in the middle of his monologue by an ecstatic portraiture of the insignia which go towards making up a bishop, however, these only concern him at the level of the image. Genet presents us with a character unwilling to pay the price of identification with the insignia of the Other: "I want to *be* a Bishop in solitude, in appearance only … And in order to destroy every vestige of function, I'm going to create a scandal – I'm going to violate you, you slut, you punk, you strumpet, you cunt!" (Genet, 1991, p. 6). Lacan is predominantly concerned with the mask throughout this seminar and his writing at the time, not so much as opposed to truth, but as on the same side of truth. He opens his article "The Youth of André Gide, or the Letter and Desire" from the same year with the dictum that truth is structured like a fiction, writing, "[I]t is nowhere but in this mask that the secret of desire is revealed to us" (Lacan, 1958, p. 637). Removal of this mask would not reveal a more authentic representation.

The same idea is prefigured by Riviere. She asks, "[H]ow do I define womanliness or draw the line between genuine womanliness and the masquerade? My suggestion is not that there is any such difference; whether radical or superficial, they are the same thing" (Riviere, 1929, p. 78). This is not of course a status specially reserved for women. As Lacan says, "Oedipal defiles aren't any less fabricated when men are in question" (Lacan, 1957–1958, lesson 15, 12 March 1958, p. 11). Throughout this seminar, Lacan links the outcome of the Oedipus complex for the masculine subject with ridicule (ibid., lesson 10, 22 January 1958, p. 17). The man is never virile except by an indefinite series of proxies. The ego-ideal, this point at which the subject arrives, and which, in the case of the boy, grants him the "title-deeds" (ibid., p. 15) of which he can make use when the time comes, is what allows this movement from being to having, the dialectic of which is Lacan's principal concern in relation to the phallus at this stage of his thought. Here, it is the identification with the insignia of the father, or the image as signifying, which sustains the subject, the father here meaning anyone who introduces this signifier, this process of metaphorisation, of naming the mOther's desire. What is important for Lacan here is the coalescence of desire with the mask, and it is here he locates the ego-ideal. He suggests that the ego-ideal and perversion are mutually exclusive, perversion resulting, not from the failure of the ego-ideal as such, but from its never having been installed in the first place.

In his study of the life of André Gide, Lacan recognises the phenomenon of splitting, which he criticises ego psychology for misrecognising as a weakness of the ego. Gide, he tells us, was in a totally unsituated position on account of his being a child who was not desired, the effect of which was an "infinite destructuration" (ibid., lesson 14, 5 March 1958, p. 7). For Lacan, the death of Gide's father was the death also of the language which could humanise desire, leaving Gide to be enveloped by his mother's desire, in a position of identifying with the imaginary phallus.

It is in Gide's passionate attachment to his correspondence with his wife, and his devastation at its loss, that Lacan sees something of the structure of comedy revealed. He compares it to the cry of Harpagnon in Molière's play *l'Avare*; the "comic cry par excellence" (ibid., p. 10) accompanying the loss of a certain object in which the desire of the subject is alienated. The laughter which greets this cry arises at once from the exposure of the mask, or anything of the order of imitation or mimicry according to Lacan, but it is also the laughter which greets "subjectivity caught off guard" (Lacan, 1958, p. 641). In other words, subjectivity captivated by the image; the image as signifying. In *Seminar V* Lacan suggests that any signifier which bars the subject which is *not* the Name-of-the-Father pertains to a perverse subjective structure. Linking the eruption of laughter to a liberation from the image, he says, "[O]n the one hand, something is liberated from the constraint of the image – and on the other hand the image continues its little stroll, all by itself" (Lacan, 1957–1958, lesson 7, 18 December 1957, p. 11). He evokes an image of a headless chicken who continues to run about after having its head cut off. This is as close as Lacan comes to linking comedy with the notion of the undead; here he reads it in terms of a tension between the Symbolic and the Imaginary. However, a lot more can be made of this headless chicken in light of subsequent theory. Why not read it in terms of the Real?

Alenka Zupančič's reading of Lacan is illuminating here. She engages the trajectory from desire to drive in his work in an attempt to theorise beyond the ontology of the One without collapsing into multiplicity. Pivotal to this movement is Lacan's theorisation of the category of the Real, which undergoes repeated revision throughout his work and appears in Seminar VII in the form of a primordial "beyond" of the symbolic order. It is this conception of the Real which Zupančič categorically rejects. Her body of work can be read as an elaboration of the consequences for ethics of failing to include the dimension of the Real as Lacan will later theorise it; not as an ontological category, but as something which disturbs ontology as such. The notion of the "undead" interests Zupančič on account of the fact that, "what is at stake here is not any kind of simple opposition between life and death, or vital forces and the 'dead' automatism of the symbolic, but is instead a paradoxical entity which traverses this divide" (Zupančič, 2012, p. 10). The interface between the body and language presents us with an ontological paradox because of the dimension which comes into play therein, making it impossible, try as Genet's bishop might, to speak of "being qua being" such that "the real is the bone in the throat of every ontology" (Zupančič, 2012, p. 10). The important point is that the Real is not conceived of as the remainder of or as that which resists symbolisation in such a way as to preserve a space for essentialism, but rather as that which complicates the binary: appearance versus reality. Lorenzo Chiesa also points to this shift:

> At this stage, Lacan has not yet completely overcome the (Sadean) idea that nature is One (differential, "fermenting") being that enjoys per se: this notion structurally contradicts all theoretical (and clinical) elaborations which presuppose the a priori of the barring of the Other and the logically concomitant reduction of nature to the not-one of the undead.
>
> *(Chiesa, 2007, p. 183)*

In Seminar V Lacan speaks about jouissance exclusively in the context of perversion and comedy. Of course Gide's loss is not comic, but for Lacan comedy is not the comic. He gives a precise definition of comedy. When it comes to the alienation of desire in the signifier the subject "can take hold of these very conditions – imposed on him, in his world – as if these conditions were made for him, as if he can satisfy himself with them" (Lacan, 1957–1958, lesson 14, 5 March 1958, p. 1). Furthermore, the comic character is one who profits from, and enjoys, this predicament. Lacan says that the univocal explanation of the function of comedy has to do with "the crucial character, for the subject and for his development, of *imaginary identification to the phallus*" (ibid., lesson 11, 29

January 1957, p. 16). This function being, we could argue, to stage this identification in such a way as to reveal its contingency. The Madame of Genet's brothel admonishes one of the prostitutes for wanting to poke fun at the fantasies they are hired to enact with the customers:

> IRMA: (*Very Harshly*) I certainly won't have any joking. A laugh, or even a smile, and the whole thing's on the floor. Where there's a smile, there's a doubt. The customers like their ceremonies solemn.*(Genet, 1991, p. 24)*

In contrast to comedy, tragedy represents the effect of the signifier as rendering the subject divided such that something remains impossible for them, to the extent that, "the chain that ties man to the signifying law, on the plane of the family, is not the same as that on the plane of the community" (Lacan, 1957–1958, lesson 14, 5 March 1958, p. 10). This is one of the criteria by which Zupančič differentiates tragedy from comedy; tragedy, she argues, configures – from the standpoint of demand – the fundamental discrepancy between demand and satisfaction within the ambit of the dialectic of desire, the constitutive non-satisfaction of which is its ultimate horizon (Zupančič, 2008, p. 131). Comedy on the other hand, articulates this discrepancy from the point of satisfaction which appears as jouissance, or as surplus-satisfaction. Satisfaction overtakes demand in comedy in a way that is not, as Freud (1927d) has it in his essay "Humour", in the service of the pleasure principle. Zupančič writes:

> Not only do we (or the comic characters) not get what we asked for, on top of it (and not instead of it) we get something we haven't asked for at all ... It is the discrepancy of something *en plus* that leads the way and drives the comedy.
>
> *(Zupančič, 2008, p. 132)*

What is surprising is that the demand finds an unexpected satisfaction which is always elsewhere than where it is expected. This is the meaning she gives to Lacan's statement in *Seminar V* when he says, "*Witz* restores its *jouissance* to the essentially unsatisfied demand" (Lacan, 1957–1958, lesson 7, 18 December 1957, p. 1).

Zupančič champions the eighteenth century dramatist Pierre de Marivaux, and in her reading of *The Game of Love and Chance* she recognises a specific formula which breaks down the binary opposition of truth and appearance. She writes, "one could almost formulate Marivaux's motto as follows: '[E]verything is deceptive, only the mask never lies'" (Zupančič, 2008, p. 103). In this play of mistaken identities, the protagonists, Lisette and Dorante, engaged to be married, both pretend to be their own servants in order to spy on one another only to inadvertently fall in love while performing their respective roles. Lisette's brother Mario remarks, "[T]hey must be brought to speak to one another often in these disguises" (Marivaux, 1988. p. 194). Marivaux's thinly drawn characters are sufficient to serve this fundamental axiom in what amounts to what Zupančič calls a pre-established disharmony "on account of which things attain their true goal only by following the wrong path" (Zupančič, 2008, p. 107).

This axiom appears in Oscar Wilde's *The Importance of Being Earnest.* Replete with exaggeration and word-play, litotes, parapraxes, paradoxes, oxymorons and Wilde's famous epigrams, the play is a comedy which satirises the English aristocracy as the paradigmatic arena of the masquerade. The major characters of the play attempt to shape their destiny so as to achieve some satisfaction, yet happenstance invariably ensures they are diverted in their aim. Nonetheless, in keeping with the conventions of the genre, by the end of the play all demands have been inadvertently satisfied one way or another. Jack Worthing, upon admitting to Algernon Moncrieff that his financial liability of a brother is a fiction, is shocked to discover that Algernon, altogether more adept in flouting Victorian convention, has likewise invented an invalid friend, Bunbury, whom he visits in the countryside. Algernon coins the term "Bunburying" to describe the connivance. With his new-found knowledge, Algernon poses as Jack's imaginary brother Ernest, so that he might visit Jack's country house and meet his cousin Cecily Cardew and propose to her. Jack has similar plans for Algernon's cousin Gwendolen Fairfax. What unfolds is a series of comical events culminating in the exposure of their game, as well as Jack's discovery of his true identity, which just so happens to be Algernon's elder brother. He exclaims, "I always said I had a brother!" (Wilde, 1895, p. 356). The play therefore, has the structure of a joke in that this revelation retroactively alters the meaning of everything which precedes it. "Moncrieff" is the quilting point which fixes the meaning at the end of the play. Lady Bracknell, newly revealed as Jack's aunt, informs him that he was named after his father. Jack immediately consults the "Army Lists" of the period to find out his father's name and discovers that it is in fact "Ernest," the name he had been pretending to have for the benefit of his fiance, Gwendolen. He says, "Gwendolen, it is a terrible thing for a man to find out suddenly that all his life he has been speaking nothing but the truth. Can you forgive me?" (Wilde, 1895, p. 357).

Another technique utilised in comedy is the reduction of man to his "nature" for comic effect. At this point Zupančič's distinction between "true" and "false", or conservative, comedy is instructive. She draws from Hegel's discussion of comedy in *The Phenomenology of Spirit,* where he distinguishes comedy from the (Greek) epic and tragic forms which represent, via narrative and the mask respectively, the dualism between the concrete and the universal such that (in Hegelian parlance) the universal remains abstracted from the concrete and actual self. Rather than limiting the field of comedy to the leftover or "physical residue" (Zupančič, 2008, p. 26) which could not be sublimated via the narrative or the mask, the comic character or sequence becomes essence in a way which does away with representation (ibid., p. 27). It is not that the universal is undermined by the particular, by human finitude or folly. Zupančič uses the typical example of an aristocrat slipping on a banana peel. What might be considered comical is the coincidence of the comic character's dignified office with what is deemed to be his unavoidable and inevitable human weakness or base nature. This kind of comedy, according to

Zupančič, perpetuates the abstract dualism of the concrete and the universal and is her definition of false or conservative comedy. This configuration appears in part seven of Freud's *Witz* on "Jokes and The Comic". There we find a libidinal economy of the comic which produces its effects via identification or a mirror-stage-like empathy with the comic character. What Freud includes under the heading "unmasking" offers a precise definition of conservative comedy as Zupančič sees it. Unmasking, Freud writes, is,

> the method of degrading the dignity of individuals by directing attention to the frailties which they share with all humanity, but in particular the dependence of their mental functions on bodily needs. The unmasking is equivalent here to an admonition: such and such a person, who is admired as a demigod, is after all only human like you and me.
>
> *(Freud, 1905b, p. 202)*

True comedy produces a different formula. Lacan writes, "if a man who thinks he is a king is mad, a king who thinks he is a king is no less so" (Lacan, 1946, p. 139). True comedy formulates the example of the proverbial banana peel so as to render comical the aristocrat who thinks he is an aristocrat. In other words, the ego-ideal does not escape unscathed to the other side of a dualism of dignity versus human nature, but is itself subjected to comic treatment. Zupančič writes:

> The ego-ideal directly is a human weakness – which is to say that, in this kind of comedy, the process of identification with the partial feature is, by virtue of its comic character, always also the process of disidentification. The point is not that an aristocrat is also an ordinary man. He is an ordinary man precisely as an aristocrat.
>
> *(Zupančič, 2008, p. 32)*

This formula appears in *le Balcon* when Madame Irma mocks the aspirations of the Chief of Police who wants to become a legislator and a leader.

IRMA: *(Worried)* You're crazy. Unless you really do think you're an empire-builder – in which case, you're crazy.*(Genet, 1991, p. 43)*

The comic character, for Zupančič, is the enjoying incarnation of a unary trait presented to us in the form of a passionate and unstoppable attachment to a particular object or activity. We are reminded of Algernon and his "Bunburying". We see Jack, driven to the city in order to escape the tedium of his life in the countryside, reappearing there in full mourning dress to announce the death of his make-believe brother, ready to give up his surplus enjoyment, only to be met with the enjoying incarnation of Algernon, posing as Ernest. A surplus of enjoyment adheres to Jack in the form of an undead brother who is the cause of a series of events which will lead to his final vindication. Comedy proper, as Zupančič delimits it, is closely related to the logic of the drive, demonstrating that subsequent to castration in language, the subject is not simply destined to bemoan the loss of a mythical, pre-symbolic "full" enjoyment, but rather, is driven by a surplus generated by the interface of language and the body which can be reduced to neither one of them.

Turning then to *le Balcon,* the opposition to the play's production in France was hardly surprising according to Lacan, given the state of theatre at the time which he saw as merely representing agreeable characters, pleasing to those there to identify with them. Similarly, Genet considered Brecht to be a didactic voice of the status quo (Lavery, 2010, p. 81). Lacan maintains that comedy always appears during times of crisis; in this instance a crisis of faith, characteristic of the post-war era, in traditional authority figures and institutions such as those which appear in *le Balcon:* The Bishop, the Judge and the General. However, comedy does not function here as an anodyne, nor serve to bolster the identifications of the audience. In his note on how to perform *Le Balcon* from 1962, Genet wrote that the play must have a narrative tone that is always equivocal and shifting. He writes, "the equivocation must be maintained until the end" (Genet, 1991, p. xii). Zupančič's reading of *Le Balcon* focuses on the modern functioning of power satirised there. However, rather than wallow in nostalgia for a golden age of the Name-of the-Father, as Zupančič sees it, comedy reveals this power as always-already restored, its point of impossibility being at the same time its condition of possibility (Zupančič, 2016, p. 222).

Genet's characters appear in all their regalia within the confines of Madame Irma's house of illusions, a brothel where ordinary men come to act out these roles or symbolic functions which, "are respected *because* they're profaned" (Lacan, 1957–1958, lesson 14, 5 March 1958, p. 15). This disavowed enjoyment allows society to continue to function. Common to all the scenarios which unfold in the brothel, the script of the fantasy is agreed upon beforehand and allows for no deviation. The total compliance of the other is required to pull it off, so to speak. "My existence as judge is an emanation of your existence as a thief … You won't refuse to be a thief? That would be evil. That would be criminal" (Genet, 1991, p. 13). The enactments are intermittently interrupted by the sound of machine gun fire coming from the rebellion which is taking place out on the streets. Roger, who leads the rebellion has kidnapped one of the prostitutes, Chantal, to represent the workers. He longs for a rebellion devoid of passion and cannot fathom the fact that the rebels are in fact *enjoying* the uprising; the singing, the gun fire and the bazookas. Roger asks, "What the hell do you want? I didn't pull Chantal out of one brothel to put her into another" (Genet, 1991, p. 55). For Lacan, Roger represents,

> the real man, whose desire no-one doubts as capable of complete arrival, of asserting itself as such, in a harmonious way. Proletarian consciousness has always believed in moral success – it doesn't matter whether it's right or wrong to do so.
>
> *(Lacan, 1957–1958, p. 14)*

Genet's play offers a critique of this "real man" and the notion of an enjoyment-free revolution.

Lacan turns his attention to the Chief of Police who for much of the play has been concerned with the fact that nobody has sought to profane his function. Nobody in the brothel wants to dress up as a Chief of Police. Madame Irma tells him, "Your image hasn't yet acceded to the brothel liturgy" (Genet, 1991, p. 41). The rebellion is quashed by means of presenting the public with the appearance of its failure; the Judge, the General and the Bishop of the brothel are made to stand in for the real Judge, General and Bishop, along with Madame Irma who poses as Queen, all of whom have in fact, been overthrown by the rebellion. At this point, Roger comes to the brothel and asks to play the role of the Chief of Police. In his search for a simulacra that might admit him to the nomenclature of the brothel, the Chief of Police decides that a giant phallus, "a man-sized prick" (Genet, 1991, p. 85) is the most appropriate costume for any role play enacted in his guise. Roger adopts the costume and enacts a scene which culminates in his castrating himself. The Chief of Police declares, "I've arrived! My Image! I belong to the nomenclature. I've got my simulacrum!" (Genet, 1991, p. 94). Zupančič writes:

> Genet's play illustrates how castration (its display) paradoxically functions as the phallic emblem of our times, of modern power … In a strange reversal of the classical logic of castration (as the means of acquiring access to symbolic power), it involves a castration of the symbolic (public) image as a means of exercising and perpetuating one's unlimited power.
>
> *(Zupančič, 2016, p. 231)*

This approximates what we have seen with the feminine masquerade. A lure is offered to both captivate and obfuscate. "Look, I don't have it." However, this display ultimately rests on the presupposition that it, the phallus, is there to be had. It is on the side of phallic jouissance and fear of castration, and does not recognise the phallus for what it is, a semblance. Power's point of crisis is inherent to its functioning and the lure masks this by imitating this impotence (Zupančič, 2016, p. 231).

The distinction between the masquerade and the postiche, which Maria Cristina Aguirre draws out in her reading of Riviere's article, sheds more light on the potential reach of comedy, especially as Zupančič theorises it. The postiche as evocation of the lack is posited as a counterpoint to the postiche which disguises lack, demanding respect and distance (Miller, 2000, p. 22).

ROGER: Is everything exactly right? My costume? My toupee?
CHIEF OF POLICE: He knows I wear a toupee?
BISHOP: (*With a mocking laugh, to the* JUDGE *and the* GENERAL) Everyone knows.*(Genet, 1991, p. 89)*

Aguirre writes, "[T]he phallus worth anything is the one that declares I am semblant" (Aguirre, 2010, p. 87). Once again though, this is not a question of semblance as opposed to the real thing, for the semblance is the mask of nothingness (Miller, 2000, p. 14). However, for a semblance to declare itself a semblance is not necessarily going far enough. As Zupančič and others emphasise, this veiling which highlights does not stop the phallus from continuing to function. Comedy points to this very fact, it holds a mirror up to the perverse structure of society. Everyone knows, as the Bishop says, and yet …

Biographers have attempted to debunk some of the myths Genet created about his childhood. There is no evidence to suggest his mother was a prostitute, and he did not remain in state care until the age of seven. Born in Paris in 1910, his mother abandoned him to the *Bureau d'Abandon de l'Hospice des Enfants-Assistés* six months later. He was almost immediately placed in the care of a foster family with whom he lived until the age of fourteen. Much critique has been made of Sartre's (1952) hagiography *Saint Genet: Actor and Martyr* for colluding with Genet's myth-making. These critiques, in their quest for a purely factual account of Genet's life, never question what function this mythologising may have had for Genet. Much like Lacan's reflections on Gide, Sartre isolates a constitutive moment in this mythology, a fatal instant, the effect of which is the "reciprocal and contradictory envelopment of the before by the after" (Sartre, 1952, p. 2). It is the moment Genet is caught stealing and hears the words, "You are a thief" (ibid., p. 17). It is a falling foul of the Other which will retroactively alter all that came before it, and which will thereafter constitute an essential repetition for Genet. Sartre offers his own version of Freud's "*Wo Es war, soll Ich werden*" (Freud, 1933a, p. 79), by insisting that in this moment, Genet will become that which he is accused of being; a thief. Where one might be left with a question – Am I a thief? Am I a man or a woman? – Sartre believes Genet to have heard an answer:

> Even before he emerged from his Mother's womb, they had already reserved beds for him in all the prisons of Europe and places for him in all the shipments of criminals. He had only to go to the trouble of being born.
>
> *(Sartre, 1952, p. 31)*

This is not so much Sartre's collusion with the fantasy as it is a demonstration of its vociferousness and reach. To ask, "How could it have been any other way?" so emphatically is to suggest precisely that it might have been. If Genet was subject to the infinite destructuration which, according to Lacan, results from being a child who was not desired, the fantasy gives Genet a place. For Sartre, Genet's stealing maintains a veil over his original crime; that of being born. In a formulation which prefigures Lacan's definition of comedy he writes, "[H]e will live this impossibility as if he had created it expressly for himself" (Sartre, 1952, p. 50). Similarly, it is in considering the connection between Gide and comedy that Lacan raises the question, "[W]hat does it mean to enjoy one's position?"

Pierre-Gilles Gueguen critiques Sartre's reading on account of the fact that Genet had begun stealing prior to this designation from the Other, and for the fact that it doesn't take into account what this stealing might have meant as a symptom;

for Gueguen a question of being and having addressed to the Other regarding the phallus. He writes, "[T]he Sartrean reading does not include this element and presents as a free choice something that turns on an effect of the unconscious" (Gueguen, 2009, p. 99). However, whether Sartre, or indeed Genet, attribute this to a conscious, free choice does not rule out the possibility that something of a forced choice, which operated at the level of the subject, took place. Gueguen reads the case of Genet in terms of a foreclosure of the phallus and therefore, as an ordinary or untriggered psychosis.

However, Gueguen overlooks the phenomenon of splitting which Sartre picks up on; an "air-tight partition" (Sartre, 1952, p. 15) that exists for Genet between two disparate and irreconcilable systems of thought. Sartre's reading points to the logic of disavowal, of "I know very well, but all the same ... " Genet later said of the book that it left him feeling stripped naked and unable to continue to write (Gobeil, 1964). André Michels, in his commentary on Wilde and *The Picture of Dorian Gray,* similarly draws attention to the phenomenon of splitting (Michels, 1996a p. 23). He further recognises a provocation of the law in Wilde's decision to take libel action against the Marquess of Queensberry, the consequences of which Wilde maintains rendered him a pariah. He reads the stark dichotomy of truth and appearance which permeated Wilde's life as indicative of perverse structure and consequently, Wilde's work as a curative attempt to inscribe the Name-of-the-Father at the symbolic level (Michels, 1996b). *The Importance of Being Earnest* lends itself quite well to this reading, given the play ends with Jack's verifying the name of his father. Michels would have it that the same dichotomy of truth and appearance is reproduced in Wilde's work.

However, in considering the work of both Genet and Wilde alongside Lacan's discussion of the mask and the masquerade, we have, arguably, seen the opposite. Both *Le Balcon* and *The Importance of Being Earnest* are plays which trouble this strict dichotomy of appearance versus truth. This brings us back to Zupančič's theory of comedy as potentially involving, or at least approximating, a process of disidentification. Wilde's ironically titled satire and Genet's bordello are testament to this. Nonetheless, if the artistic production, much as the symptom, can be considered in terms of an attempt at cure, then how we envisage this cure runs the risk of becoming prescriptive the more readily one accepts some of the ideas put forward in Seminar V. For Zupančič, comedy goes further than bringing about a liberation from the image and in fact produces a disidentification with the ego-ideal, such that the contingency of the subject's identification is brought to light. What comedy can contribute, according to Zupančič, is a conceptual desublimation or demystification of the phallus. Miller's formula of the "true woman" (Miller, 2000, p. 17) as an incarnation of lack which reveals the absurdity of having – as opposed to the woman with the postiche who must hide her lack, both of which can co-exist in the same person – is just one of the ways this absurdity can be revealed. Lacan says that with comedy, the fruit of the subject's encounter with the signifier must come onto the stage (Lacan, 1957–1958, p. 11). It does this in a way which reveals as contingent, that which has historically been taken as necessary.

References

Aguirre, C. (2010). A Lacanian Reading of Womanliness as Masquerade. *The International Lacanian Journal of Psychoanalysis: Hurly Burly*, 3: 85–88.
Chiesa, L. (2007). *Subjectivity and Otherness: A Philosophical Reading of Lacan*. Cambridge & London: MIT Press.
Freud, S. (1905b). Jokes and their Relation to the Unconscious. *S.E.*, 13: 3–249. London: Hogarth.
Freud, S. (1927d). Humour. *S.E.*, 21: 159–166. London: Hogarth.
Freud, S. (1933a). New Introductory Lectures on Psychoanalysis (1933 [1932]). *S.E.*, 22: 1–182.
Genet, J. (1991). *The Balcony*. T. Hands, B. Wright & B. Frechtman (Trans.). Faber & Faber.
Gobeil, M. (1964). Interview with Madeleine Gobeil. *Playboy Magazine*, 44–55.
Gueguen, P. -G. (2009). The Extraordinary Case of Jean Genet. *Lacanian Ink*, 34: 95–105.
Lacan, J. (1946). Presentation on Psychical Causality. In: *Écrits: The First Complete Edition in English* (pp. 123–158). B. Fink (Trans.). London & New York: W. W. Norton & Co., 2006.
Lacan, J. (1957–1958). *The Seminar of Jacques Lacan: Book V, Formations of the Unconscious*. C. Gallagher (Trans.). London: Karnac, 2002.
Lacan, J. (1958). The Youth of Gide, or the Letter and Desire. In: *Écrits: The First Complete Edition in English* (pp. 623–644). B. Fink (Trans.). London & New York: W. W. Norton & Co., 2006.
Lavery, C. (2010). *The Politics of Jean Genet's Late Theatre: Spaces of Revolution*. Manchester: Manchester University Press.
Marivaux, P. (1988). The Game of Love and Chance. In: *Marivaux: Plays*. J. Walters (Trans.). London & New York: Metheun.
Michels, A. (1996a). Oscar Wilde: Aesthete and Homosexual. *The Letter*, 8: 1–16.
Michels, A. (1996b). The Hatred of the Father in Perversion. *The Letter*, 8: 17–32.
Miller, J. -A. (2000). On Semblances in the Relation between the Sexes. In R. Salecl (Ed.), *Sexuation* (pp. 13–27). Durham, NC: Duke University Press.
Riviere, J. (1929). Womanliness as Masquerade. *The International Lacanian Journal of Psychoanalysis: Hurly Burly*, 3: 75–84, 2010.
Sartre, J. -P. (1952). *Saint Genet: Actor and Martyr*. B. Frechtman (Trans.). Minneapolis: University of Minnesota Press.
Wilde, O. (1895). *The Importance of Being Earnest and Other Plays*. London: Penguin Books, 2000.
Zupančič, A. (2008). *The Odd One In: On Comedy*. Cambridge & London: MIT Press.
Zupančič, A. (2012). Sexual Difference and Ontology. *E-Flux*, 32. Retrived from: http://worker01.e-flux.com/pdf/article_8948423.pdf.
Zupančič, A. (2016). Power in the Closet (and its Coming Out). In: P. Gherovici & M. Steinkoler (Eds.), *Lacan, Psychoanalysis, and Comedy* (pp. 219–234). New York: Cambridge University Press.

PART 4

Witz

11

LACAN READING FREUD

On the relationship of Seminar V to "Jokes and Their Relationship to the Unconscious"

P. G. Young

What is at stake in Freud's book on jokes, insofar as it is addressed to the analytic experience of its readers? Lacan reorients psychoanalysis on the basis of this question, in the fifth year of his seminar, entitled Formations of the Unconscious, offered in the winter of 1957 and spring of 1958. Seminar V inaugurates the formulation of the phallus as signifier – signifier of desire, in its unconscious function as desire of the Other. After a brief discussion of this conception as a turning point within the more general syntax of Lacan's series of seminars, I will briefly frame the overall architecture of Seminar V according to its emergence. These indications will ground my approach to the question of how Lacan *arrives* at this fundamental reorientation by means of a primary reference to Freud's analysis of the joke. I offer an introductory examination of the trajectory of this reference in Seminar V. What Lacan explicitly says about Freud's text on jokes is contained in the seminar's first eight lessons. Another aspect of this reference could be characterised as the way Lacan negates it – the aspects of rupture and discontinuity in its deployment, both within and beyond these first lessons, alongside loud omission of prominent elements in Freud's analysis which nevertheless ground Lacan's schema. I will also explore some of these elements insofar as they anchor Lacan's graphic construction in Seminar V.

We can begin with a passage from the seventeenth lesson of Seminar V:

> Just as we've defined the paternal signifier as the signifier which poses and authorizes the play of signifiers in the locus of the Other – well, there's another privileged signifier, having as effect this institution, in the Other, of what changes its nature … this is why the Other isn't simply and only the locus of speech, but, like the *subject*, implicated in the dialectic situated on the phenomenal plane, of the reflection regarding the little other.
>
> *(Lacan, 1957–1958, lesson of 26 March 1958, p. 272)*

In Seminar III, Lacan (1955–1956) had already elaborated the father as a symbolic function, as a signifier that authorises the play of signifiers in the locus of the Other. In Seminar IV (Lacan 1956–1957) he had already approached the psychical incidence of the phallus as lacking, metonymic object. In order to distinguish the phallus as "another privileged signifier" (ibid.) from the paternal signifier, Seminar V introduces a divergence within the phallic function itself, between *object* and *signifier*.

From a summary perspective, what is at stake here is a diagnostic differential. The manner in which Lacan proceeds is telling; Seminar III orients the distinction of psychosis from neurosis around an interrogation of the incidence of the paternal signifier, whereas it is only after the function of the phallus has been amplified as signifier that the concluding lessons of Seminar V reformulate the difference between hysterical and obsessional structure. Once Lacan has established the phallus as signifier, he is able to reorient the differential clinic of the neuroses around the question of the function of the phallus within the transference. He explicitly resumes this question in Seminar VIII, recalling that the purpose of elaborating a difference between the imaginary and symbolic phallus, which Seminar V inaugurates, is to assist our "articulation of the function of the phallus in the neurotic transference" (Lacan, 1960–1961, lesson eighteen, 26 April 1961, p. 4). Lacan never stopped pursuing the consequences of writing the phallus as a signifier. In lesson twenty of Seminar XVI (Lacan, 1968–1969, lesson of 14 May 1969, p. 320) he proposes that the phallus as signifier "is not in the system of the subject, since it does not represent the subject. What it represents, you might say, is sexual enjoyment as outside the system – namely, as absolute." In Seminar XX, he once again renews the phallus as signifier in order to construct the formulas of sexuation (Lacan, 1972–1973, lesson seven, 13 March 1973, p. 78).

Phallus as object and signifier in Seminar V

In order to track the way the phallus shows up in Seminar V, I propose three signposts which divide the seminar into four movements. The first turning point in this series occurs in lesson eight, where Lacan begins to speak about the phallus as object. The second junction arrives in lesson thirteen, where he begins to speak about the phallus as signifier. Our third landmark appears in lesson twenty, where he begins to speak about the phallus as signifier of the desire of the Other. Lacan exploits the subjective genitive with this expression, accenting the symbolic phallus as signifier of lack and desire in the Other, not a signifier of desire for the Other.

The first part of the seminar, made up of seven lessons, is where Lacan offers his manifest commentary on Freud's "Joke Book". Lacan does not mention the phallus in these lessons. What he does mention there is what he calls the "metonymic object" (Lacan, 1957-1958, lesson one, 6 November 1957, p. 9), which he gradually embeds within the structure of demand, as derived from Freud's analysis of jokes. Lacan rereads Freud's examination of joke structure as indicating an absolutely metonymic or displaced object in the denominator of all signification.

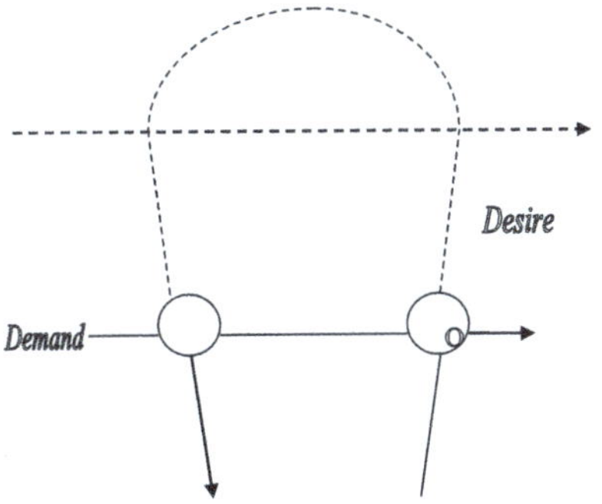

FIGURE 11.1 Adapted from Seminar V, lesson eighteen, 16 April 1958, p. 313.

At the conclusion of lesson eight, Lacan makes his first mention of the phallus by suddenly identifying it with this metonymic object. After the phallus is introduced here as object, the manifest reference to the Joke Book virtually drops out. The meticulous, line-by-line reading conducted throughout the previous lessons comes to an abrupt halt in lesson eight, and nothing is left to remind us of the joke but the schema Lacan has derived from it, which he will use to rewrite the three moments of the Oedipus complex over the course of Part II. Nevertheless, this reminder is itself an intervention, with its own retroactive effect on how we read the Joke Book. Although Freud never directly mentions the Oedipus complex in the latter, Lacan's manner of proceeding positions "Jokes and Their Relationship to the Unconscious" as a book about Oedipal structure.

We can mark the transition from lesson seven to lesson eight by taking a closer look at where Lacan has arrived in his analysis of the joke at the conclusion of Part I, before he mentions the phallus for the first time. Lesson seven concludes with two correlated gestures. The first involves a schematic transformation. Over the course of Part I, we see Lacan deriving the structure of demand from the Joke Book. The schema he constructs to support his propositions is now known as the "graph of desire". The schema in its completed form is composed of an upper and lower horizon, with a third line looping retroactively through both of them. Lesson seven is where Lacan writes an upper horizon on this graph for the first time. According to Lacan, Freud's analysis of the joke obliges us to approach the horizon of demand, the horizon of speech itself, as fundamentally diploid. Lacan says that we must write another, upper horizon, because the structure and procedure of the joke opens up an alterity in the Other, in the big Other: "The first schema … thus transforms, through this development we're giving to the formula of the Other as subject" (Lacan, 1957-1958, lesson seven, 18 December 1957, p. 123). In psychoanalysis, formation of the unconscious opens up a gap in the demand addressed to the Other. It opens up a gap between the horizon of an unbarred Other, as the locus of a virtually consistent code of signification, and the horizon of the Other as subject. In lesson eight Lacan will go on to say that he began his seminar with the Joke Book precisely in order to ground the difference between these two discursive horizons of the Other. In lesson seven he is already writing the unbarred Other on the lower horizon, and writing desire in the gap between the two horizons – the barred Other is not written as such on the upper line until lesson nineteen.

In lesson seven, after developing this first schematic gesture by appealing to a difference between the Other as code and the Other as subject, Lacan suddenly starts talking about comedy. He recommends that we read some Aristophanes and then he launches into a review of a play by Moliere, in order to demonstrate how desire can emerge in the Other, beyond its codification. This is how Part one ends, and it is usually a bit baffling for first-time readers.

What these coupled gestures demonstrate, and what Lacan does not explicitly indicate, is that he is hitching Freud's analysis of the joke to Hegel's analysis of comedy. In Hegel's *Phenomenology of Spirit*, comedy is where Spirit "advances from the form of substance to assume that of subject" (Hegel, 1807, p. 453). Lacan's promotion of the joke as subjectivation of the Other is a way of reminding us that Freud's examination of the joke, which itself turns upon the distinction between subject of the unconscious and preconscious ego, is not without precedent in Hegel's formulation of comedy as subjectivation of Spirit.

Here I am emphasising the proximity of this tacit hitch to what I have called our first signpost, the first appearance of the phallus in the seminar as *object*. As we move through Part II, the manifest reference to the joke falls out, and Lacan uses its residual schema to rewrite the Oedipus complex in terms of three phases or moments. For the purposes of this introductory essay, I would underscore that Part II gradually articulates these three moments to different modes of the phallus as *object*. As Part II progresses, Lacan repeatedly ends individual lessons by postponing discussion of the relationship between the function of the phallus and comedy, which he abruptly introduced in lesson eight. When he finally speaks of comedy again in lesson fourteen, the significance of the phallus is given another twist, and he begins to speak about it as *signifier*. We can therefore say that the respective references to comedy in lessons seven and fourteen literally bracket the Oedipus complex with a differential in the function of the phallus: the phases of the Oedipus complex are gradually knotted to a permutation in the phallic function.

Lacan begins lesson fourteen by introducing the question of jouissance in relation to desire for the first time, and resumes the topic of comedy in the specific context of this distinction. Echoing his strategy in lesson seven, he references a theatrical production, in order to explore this distinction. In this instance, the play is by Jean Genet. In the trajectory of Seminar V, the differential of desire and jouissance is contemporary with the emergence of the phallus as signifier. Over the course of Part III of the seminar – lessons fourteen through nineteen – Lacan increasingly conjugates the phallus as signifier to *desire*, while the question of the relationship of the phallic signifier to jouissance receives comparatively little airtime. This culminates with our third junction in lesson twenty, where Lacan begins to speak about the phallus as the signifier of the Other's desire. In lesson twenty-one he states:

> It's not enough to say that it's a signifier. Which one is it? It's the signifier of desire ... The phallus is the signifier insofar as who doesn't have it? – insofar as the Other doesn't have it ... The phallus situates on the plane of the Other. It's the signifier of desire, insofar as desire articulates itself as desire of the Other.
>
> *(Lacan, 1957–1958, lesson twenty-one, 17 May 1958, p. 318)*

Part IV re-orients a clinic of the neuroses according to this conjugation, and Lacan completes the construction of his graph by nominating its upper line as the horizon of transference, writing the phallus as signifier upon it.

"Jokes and Their Relationship to the Unconscious"

Freud's book about jokes is itself structured like a joke; "it may be read as a sort of joke which perpetually deconstructs itself" (Flieger, 1991, p. 84). In my reading, the book's concluding chapter functions as a thoroughgoing punchline, retroactively reorienting the stakes and thematic trajectory of the preceding text. When we note that this final chapter concerns the *comic*, we can then immediately mark how Freud's formal strategy of composition, his order of exposition, perhaps not unwittingly, reverses what is asserted in the content of the text itself: that the comic only ever functions as preparatory in relation to the *Witz* – the punchline of the joke concludes a previous comic "set-up" in the preconscious. There are many ways in which Freud's Joke Book can be read backwards as well as forwards, insofar as it sustains a short-circuit between form and content, exhibiting the "Janus-like two-faced character" (Freud, 1905, p. 155) Freud attributes to jokes themselves.

It is not until the second section of the final seventh chapter, which localises the comic in and as a preconscious system, that Freud (1905) makes the following explicit statement: "I set great store in clarifying this most delicate point in my arguments – the relation of jokes to the comic" (p. 206). Freud's 1905 exploration of the enigmatic differentiation of *Witz* from the comic not only develops the distinction of ego from subject, his analysis of the comic ego also emerges as a thorough precedent to what he will eventually designate as a differentiating grade in the ego itself (Freud, 1921, p. 129).

Freud (1905) waits until the sixth section of this chapter to formulate the "essence of the comic in a preconscious link with the infantile" (p. 225). The seventh chapter eventually situates this link in the automatism of a differential within ego-representation. Freud resolves the comic into "species" according to the primary psychical route of this automatic process. In contrast to the joke, which engages subjective determinants through an economy of inhibition (*Hemmung*), comic pleasure is the result of either an economy of representation – hinging upon what Freud calls *Vorstellungsmimik*, literally translated as "mimetic representation," and translated by Strachey as "ideational mimetics" (Freud, 1905, p. 192) – or it is the result of an economy of affect via humour. Over twenty years later, Freud (1927) identifies the latter as an instance of the super-ego, itself addressing another instance of the ego as object (p. 165). Freud concludes the book with a brief recapitulation of these three economic registers – joke, the comic of *Vorstellungsmimik*, and the comic of humor – as derived from respective registers of loss.

Freud's 1905 formulation of the comic imaginary – as an ideal image of the body which does not function independently of its anticipatory, or *specular*, relay through the detour of its reflected *semblable* - is a precursor of what numerous post-Freudian clinicians approach as an intrapsychic formation distinct from the super-ego and the ego-ideal: the ideal-ego. Lacan repeatedly referred the formation of the ideal-ego to the "mirror stage" or "mirror phase" (*stade du miroir*). In Seminar V, he writes the *Vorstellungsmimik* of the comic ideal-ego as i(o) (Lacan, 1957–1958, lesson seventeen, 26 March 1958, p. 271). While i(o) renders the ego as specular image of the other, it also harbours ambivalent identification with the absent/present object of the mother's desire.

Freud's analysis implicates these three knotted dimensions – the joke (*Witz*), humour, and the comic – as three core registers of clinical experience. Past and contemporary Anglo-American interpretations of Freud's book on jokes tend to foreground one register of his analysis (primarily that of humour) while eliding the singularity and dynamic interrelation of other registers. This leads to a longstanding climate of research in which Freud's careful distinctions are simultaneously illuminated and telescoped. Freud's composite strategy in "Humour" and "Jokes and their Relationship to the Unconscious" establishes differentiation of *Witz* from the comic, and another "intra"-comic distinction between the comic of *Vorstellungsmimik* (ideal ego) and the comic of humor (super-ego). Noting Freud's eventual articulation of humour as hypercathexis of super-egoic word-representation – "it is really the superego which, in humour, speaks such kindly words to the intimidated ego" (Freud, 1927, p. 166) – we can retroactively read chapter VII of the Joke Book as bracketed by this latter distinction between comic image (ideal-ego) and comic voice (super-ego).

Freud's analysis of the comic in chapter VII of the Joke Book accomplishes a subtle shift: beginning with a dual, mimetic pair of comic persons, the analysis gradually delineates an incongruous pair constituted by a "big" instance of the ego and another "small" ego, both localising as centripetal poles of the preconscious economy of the ego: a "big" Otherness and "small" otherness. The comic procedure emerges as an automatism of the emergent gap or discrepancy between these two forms of o/Otherness. The ego experiencing comic pleasure is enjoying this difference as such. Freud consistently critiques the assumption that this discrepancy is pleasurable insofar as it grants a feeling of superiority with respect to the comic other; his analysis shifts the accent onto the automatism of the discrepancy itself. Freud subordinates manifest aggression to the automaticity of a differentiating grade within the comic ego. This distinction between a "little" other and a "big" Other – a difference which functions both intra-psychically and interpersonally in Freud's analysis – is frequently treated as a specifically Lacanian concept. Lacan's explicit derivation of the other/Other distinction from the Joke Book frames automatism of this differential as constitutive of the preconscious dimension of the clinical relationship, where the unconscious formation opens and closes.

"A joke is made, the comic is found." (Freud, 1905, p. 181). For Freud, what is found in the preconscious is the automatism of big and small instances of the ego, the specular ego and a big "unbarred" or super-egoic Other. The joke's preparation mobilises this comic (dual) dimension, to which the punchline then contributes unconscious "subjective determinants" (Freud, 1905, p. 112). The comic preconscious can function independently from implementation as preparatory phase or façade, girding passage of the joke; the comic already involves a specific psychical order of incongruence, discrepancy, or lack of fit. Freud distinguishes absence and presence of comic incongruity from tension and resolution specific to the joke; in this reading, the discrepancy between the punchline and its comic preparation is the discrepancy between two orders of discrepancy.

Freud reserves the subject for the ternary joke, whereas both the joke and the comic involve the ego itself as an object. In chapter VII the comic is without a subject, emerging as a fundamentally anonymous universe of privatised enjoyment; the comic is nevertheless not without an object. Freud's analysis pluralises the preconscious ego into psychical instances serving the primary task of "accommodating the Other to an object … of obtaining the Other's fixation, discursively fixed, on some metonymic object" (Lacan, 1957–1958, lesson seven, 18 December 1957, p. 105). In contrast, chapter II of the Joke Book, devoted to the techniques specific to jokes, is saturated with names and nomination, indicating a subject of symbolic construction beyond what is found in the comic libidinal economy. As humorous as it may be, the comic dimension of demand nominates neither the ego of the analysand nor the ego of the analyst as subject.

Freud's analysis of the *Vorstellungsmimik* in chapter VII retroactively positions the joke as an apparatus which implements a second degree of the mirror beyond its comic coordinates. The punchline metaphorises the comic lack of the object. It transposes the impasse of ambivalence inherent to the specular image, deprivatises superegoic enjoyment, and propels momentary creation of a new discursive link; according to Freud, a joke involves a "peremptory urge to communicate" (Freud, 1905, p. 143), in contrast to the automatism of comic pleasure, which can be experienced without verbalisation to another. Here we can pose the preliminary question of how the Real of bodily laughter, while variously knotted to each of these three registers, is unique to none of them; from this perspective, the manifest absence/presence of spontaneous or elicited laughter would not necessarily indicate functional action or passion of these registers within the clinical relationship.

Jokes and their relationship to psychoanalysis

Lacan anchors construction of his graph of desire to Freud's attribution of comic architecture to the preconscious system. The relationship of the ego to the image of the other – i(o) – functions as a kind of discursive buttress to the preconscious horizon of the speaking subject, supporting localisation of a big Other. The lower half of Lacan's graph is an attempt to portray Freud's subordination of the preconscious imaginary to the task of accommodating the Other to an object. Comic automatism knots an omnipotent/super-egoic Other to a specular image of the body, itself libidinalised as virtually harbouring absence/presence of an object causing desire in the Other. Furthermore, the graph inscribes this anticipatory envelope – which totalises/idealises the body as imaginary unit – on the psychical axis of the message: the image of the body is a message insofar as it conveys a demand. The 1905 and 1927 analyses of comic structure eventually present the question of a structural relationship between the super-ego and the mimetic specular image (ideal-ego) as a fundamental polarity within the preconscious narcissism of the speaking subject. Formations of the unconscious subvert this comic universality, where the ego of the analysand and the ego of the analyst transact.

Lacan uses the structures implicated in Freud's analysis of jokes in order to reorient phallic determination of the object – beyond the ambivalence of its comic absence/presence – as decisive in neurosis under transference. The object assumes phallic significance beyond the preconscious economy of an essentially anonymous traffic of mimetic word-representation. In the comic phases of psychoanalysis, an initially "non-denominational" phallus begins to circulate as a radically metonymic object in the denominator of signification. The ego of the analysand and the ego of the analyst reciprocally preserve and identify with this phallus, which eventually yields a comic discrepancy, impasse, or lack of fit in the preconscious dimension of the clinical relationship. When the unconscious opens and closes within this relationship, the phallus is functioning as a signifier of lack/lacking signifier, without signification. The formation of the unconscious induces passage between the comic horizon of a consistent Other –reciprocally re-enforced by the ego as its object – and another horizon of the Other as subject of a desire without signified. In 1957, Lacan proposes the phallus in its symbolic function as a signifier of this discrepancy of the horizon of demand from itself, mobilised in jokes and analytic discourse.

While developing these perspectives on the joke – as dynamic knotting of identificatory registers, as permutation in the phallic function – Lacan radically expands the implication of Freud's 1905 analysis by questioning the equivalence of joke structure with speech as such. In this sense, all punctuation is punchline – no sentence, text, narrative, or analytic lesson ends without retroactive effects upon what precedes it. The length of the analytic lesson will vary according to the emergence of these effects. Directly influenced by Freud's analysis, contemporary continental linguistic research continues to treat the procedure of the joke as paradigmatic of discursive and textual structures. Benveniste (1966) and Todorov (1977, 1978) emphasise how the mechanisms Freud rediscovers in the *Witz* (condensation, displacement, retroactivity) are not specific to manifestly humorous discourse. Building upon the work of Jolles (1929) and Morin (1966), more recent linguistic theories of humour – such as Attardo's Isotopy Disjunction Model (Attardo, 1988, 1994) and the General Theory of Verbal Humor (Attardo & Raskin, 1991) – approach jokes as the "embodiment of the most elementary type of narrative structure" (Attardo, 1994, p. 91). These linguistic theories formulate the relationship between preparation and punchline in the joke as arising from concurrent activation of two incompatible scripts, and thus diverge from the incongruity-resolution theories represented by Shultz (1976) and Suls (1972), which approach the punchline as a resolution or elimination of a previously established cognitive incongruity.

Freud (1905) distinguishes the psychical pleasure of the punchline from that involved in the resolution of riddles (p. 150), which move from the unknown to the known. The moment of unconscious knowing is not the arrival of an imaginary knowledge re-enforcing the ego of the analysand or the ego of the analyst as naïve or humorous. From the perspective which questions psychological affinity of the joke with the analytic act of interpretation as such (Reik, 1948; Lacan, 1957–1958; Israel 1977, 1988), we could then distinguish a comic horizon of interpretation, which gratifies insofar as it moves from the unknown to the known, from another moment of interpretation which proceeds from the unknown to the unknown.

As a final remark on the stakes of the divergence and convergence of the joke and the comic, I will cite one brief passage from the second section of the Joke Book's final chapter. Freud (1905) states that "in the case of giving free play to unconscious modes of thought, the convergence of jokes and the comic is a necessary one" (p. 206). We can link this with his observation in the sixth chapter of "Inhibitions, Symptoms, and Anxiety": "it is especially difficult for the obsessional neurotic to carry out the fundamental rule of psychoanalysis" (Freud, 1926d, p. 121). Obsessional neurosis under transference busies itself with the paradoxes, costs, and benefits attendant to undoing the discursive convergence of joking subject and comic ego. By the end of Seminar V we can further translate this as an undoing of the phallus in its function as signifier of an Other desire. What is itself humorously undone here, but whose place remains, is the comedy of passage from one signifier to another.

References

Attardo, S. (1988). Trends in European Humor Research: Towards a Text Model. *HUMOR*, 1 (4): 349–369.

Attardo, S. (1994). *Linguistic Theories of Humor*. New York: Mouton de Gruyter.

Attardo, S. & Raskin, V. (1991). Script Theory Revis(it)ed: Joke Similarity and Joke Representation Model. *Humor: International Journal of Humor Research*, 4(3–4): 293–347.

Benveniste, E. (1966). *Problemes de Linguistique Generale*. Paris: Gallimard.

Flieger, J. A. (1991). *The Purloined Punchline: Freud's Comic Theory and the Postmodern Text*. Baltimore: The Johns Hopkins University Press.

Freud, S. (1905). Jokes and Their Relation to the Unconscious. *S.E.*, 8. London: Hogarth Press.

Freud, S. (1921). Group Psychology and the Analysis of the Ego. *S.E.*, 18: 65–143. London: Hogarth Press.

Freud, S. (1926). Inhibitions, Symptoms, and Anxiety. *S.E.*, 20: 87–165. London: Hogarth Press.

Freud, S. (1927). Humour. *S.E.*, 21: 159–166. London: Hogarth Press.

Hegel, G.W.F. (1807). *Phenomenology of Spirit*. New York: Oxford University Press, 1977.

Israel, L. (1977). *Pulsions de Mort: Seminaire 1977–1978*. Strasbourg: Arcanes, 1998.

Israel, L. (1988). *La parole et l'alienation*. Strasbourg: Arcanes, 2007.
Jolles, A. (1929). *Einfache Formen*. Tubingen: Niemeyer, 1965.
Lacan, J. (1955–1956). *The Psychoses: the Seminar of Jacques Lacan, Book III*. New York: W.W. Norton & Company, 1993.
Lacan, J. (1956–1957). *Le Seminaire livre IV, La relation d'objet*. Paris: Seuil, 1994.
Lacan, J. (1957–1958). *Seminar V. Formations of the Unconscious*. P.G. Young (Trans.). Unpublished.
Lacan, J. (1960–1961). *Seminar VIII, Transference*. Paris: Unpublished.
Lacan, J. (1968–1969). *Le Seminaire livre XVI, D'un Autre a l'autre*. Paris: Seuil, 2006.
Lacan, J. (1972–1973). *On Feminine Sexuality, the Limits of Love and Knowledge: Encore, the Seminar of Jacques Lacan, Book XX*. New York: W.W. Norton & Company, 1998.
Morin, V. (1966). L'histoire drole. *Communications*, 8 *(L'Analyse structurale du recit)* (pp. 102–119). Paris: Seuil, 1981.
Reik, T. (1948). *Listening with the Third Ear*. New York: Farrar, Strauss & Giroux.
Shultz, T. R. (1976). A Cognitive Developmental Analysis of Humour. In A.J. Chapman & H.C. Foot (Eds.), *Humor and Laughter: Theory, Research, and Applications* (pp. 11–36). London: Transaction Publishers, 2004.
Suls, J. M. (1972). A Two-Stage Model for the Appreciation of Jokes and Cartoons: An Information- Processing Analysis. In J.H. Goldstein & P.E. McGhee (Eds.), *The Psychology of Humor: Theoretical Perspectives and Empirical Issues* (pp. 81–100). New York: Academia Press.
Todorov, T. (1977). *Theories du symbole*. Paris: Seuil.
Todorov, T. (1978). *Les genres du discours*. Paris: Seuil.

12

"DID YOU HEAR THAT TOM'S DICK WAS HAIRY?"

Witz, cure, and the transmission of psychoanalysis

Jamieson Webster and Marcus Coelen

Lacan revisits the question of *Witz*, or jokes, in the first few sessions of Seminar V, The Formations of the Unconscious. Most will remember his long analysis of Heinrich Heine's joke about the *famillionaire*—neologising familial, familiar, and millionaire—that Freud had used as the paradigmatic *Witz*. Moving further and further away from the traditional register of jokes as metaphor and meaning towards their more disruptive function, Lacan looks not only at how the *Witz* condenses and economises language in uncanny, upsetting ways, but also how jokes reveal the object as not only diverse and arbitrary, but also potentially dissolvable in language. What we can see in *Witz*, he says, is everything that is left behind in the metonymical chain as waste, and also what cannot be fully realised on the level of metaphor. The *Witz*, thus, while depending entirely on the linguistic mechanisms of metaphor and metonymy, will also show what's left out by them: this might be where its specificity lies among the various formations of the unconscious.

This investigation into the mechanisms of metaphor and metonymy, furthermore, leads us in two directions important for psychoanalysis: towards a concept of transmission and a concept of cure. The first takes us on a search for Lacan's place in his unfolding discourse, increasingly centred on his analysis of the word "*famille*" in relation to Heine's neologism *famillionaire*. Lacan sets up a chain of figures from Freud to Heine to Mallarmé and the French lexicographer Littré. The second direction, that of the concept of cure, takes us to a case vignette where we hope to show you the importance of metaphor and metonymy in a dream and series of *Witz* in sessions. Finally, we will make some comments about this clinical relevance of *Witz* in relation to the stakes of psychoanalysis itself. Seminar V, stretched between the object relation and the question of desire and its interpretation, read closely, provides a surprising look at some of the most supposedly *famillionaire* concepts in Lacan.

That obscure and volatile object

It was Freud's contention that in the end no joke, no *Witz,* no manifestation of witticism is non-tendentious. Freud (1905c) defines jokes as "a psychical factor possessed of power" determined by the tendentiousness "to promote the thought by augmenting it" (p. 132). This fundamental tendentiousness of jokes is not bound to their content. Freud writes that even "if the thought contained in them is non-tendentious and thus only serves theoretical intellectual interests" (ibid.), jokes would still reveal what they are, i.e., a certain psychic *will to power.* Jokes want to be jokes—and by "setting themselves up against an inhibiting" (ibid.) counter force, they are involved in a game of power. Therefore, jokes can never be non-tendentious.

On the level of thought and "intellectual interests" the dialectics of the joke are always at play. Ironically, the last form of jokes that Freud explicitly categorises as "tendentious", before saying that in fact all jokes are tendentious, is the "skeptical" joke (ibid.). Here, witticism shows itself to be "attacking ... the certainty of our knowledge itself, one of our speculative possessions" (ibid.). The sceptical joke takes on the question of what can be determined as true. True, all jokes are tendentious because they promote thought; true, tendentious jokes attack thought itself. So why are you telling me that no joke is non-tendentious while in fact no joke is?

Is witticism then spirit turning against itself? Lacan can be said to have elevated the "attack on thinking" that is the joke, to the level of psychoanalytic speech and the very matter of its enunciation. Teaching the formations of the unconscious does not simply require, so he says, "to speak about speech but to speak wholly in keeping with speech" (Lacan, 1957–1958, p. 23). What teaching witticism requires is a *style*, perhaps "even a few barbs" to touch on the "truth" (ibid.). To touch the self-attacking nature of thought in witticism is not some turning in a vacuum, a procedure in the abstract, since in fact, witticism is, as Freud had said, "the most social of all the mental functions" (Freud 1905c, p. 178). The joke is also the most transient (see Freud 1905c, p. 217) form of thought. Taking these together, it is this trait of excess in disappearance, this attack to the point of vanishing, that Lacan, following Freud, tries to inscribe into the transmission of psychoanalytic experience.

We might let this excess in witticism's disappearance verge on turning psychoanalytic thought itself into a *Witz*. Many have looked at Freud's oeuvre and have wondered how a scientist attempted to found the unconscious on the basis of something as ephemeral as dreams, jokes, and mistakes. Can we save the object from completely collapsing? Lacan seems to think we cannot go far enough in the Real of the *Witz*; that when "we address the other," and express "ourselves by means of witticism," we would, says Lacan, "be all the happier in a way" (Lacan, 1957–1958, p. 23). And he continues to promise that this "is what I try to do in the brief time I have for the discourse I address to you" (ibid.). Psychoanalytic teaching, the transmission of psychoanalytic experience, if structurally affected by *Witz*, is also affected by a certain economy of disappearance.

What is at stake with the *Witz* is its disappearing and the sort of object that can occur with it. Psychoanalytic thought, if it is the thought of witticism, and if it is concerned with its *true* object, must leave itself as the trace of its own dissolution. Lacan posits the *Witz* as the very paradigm of psychoanalytic thinking:

> We centre *esprit* on the *trait d'esprit,* that is, on what in it seems the most contingent, the most outdated and the most open to criticism. It is indeed part of the genius of psychoanalysis to do things like that.
>
> *(Lacan, 1957–1958, p. 13)*

So the *Witz* is difficult, or even impossible, to contain, and it is not easily identified either. If construed as this conundrum, witticism is *the* obscure and volatile object of psychoanalysis itself. It might thus be instructive to see how the witticism is put by Lacan in relation to other formations of the unconscious—especially the parapraxis of forgetting—in order to perceive what effect this approximation of the one and the other has for their exposition. It might allow us to get a sense of how *Witz*—as thought and remainder of its disappearance—allows us to name, grasp, and set free the object of psychoanalysis in its two main social manifestations or institutions, i.e., transmission and the cure.

The *Witz,* the forgotten name, and the devaluation of language

In order to carve out the logic of the witticism, Lacan contrasts it with the forgetting of a proper name. He hones in on the two opening vignettes in Freud's book on *Witz* and his book on parapraxis: *famillionaire* and *Signorelli* (Freud, 1905c; Freud, 1901b). With the latter, "[i]nstead of seeing a word like '*famillionaire*' emerge, we have the contrary— something goes missing" (Lacan, 1957–1958, p. 29). Whereas the witticism produces something new, the forgetting of a proper name opens a hole. Nonetheless, they share a topography: "'Famillionaire' is a positive production, but the point it's produced at is the same hole as the one that the phenomenon of a slip displays ... and what puts us on the track of the lost signifier are the metonymic ruins of the object" (Lacan, 1957–1958, p. 34). It is not the functioning of a *Witz* that needs analytic work really—it's simply funny or it's not. What requires a process of analysis and reconstruction is the repressed content, as we can, according to Lacan, still trace what is repressed in the condensation of "familiar" and "millionaire".

This can be done by examining the metonymic ruins in the same manner as Freud, who, in order to get to the missing name *Signorelli*, had to move through a series of other names that began from the syllable "Bo": the names *Boticelli* and *Boltraffio*, bringing him to *Trafoi* and then to *Bosnia* and *Herzegovina*, in which he found "Herr", to finally reaching "Signor" and thus *Signorelli*. Through this metonymic chain of what Lacan calls "sparks" and "spatters" (ibid.), Freud discovers the motivation for forgetting—namely a series of references to sex and death centred around the "master" or "mister" (*Herr, Signor*) —that touched him recently and which he had cause to forget (see Freud 1901b, pp. 3–4).

As for the "metonymic ruins" of the joke that Heine places in the mouth of his character Hirsch-Hyacinth, Lacan refers to the biographical material alluded to by Freud while expanding it. Freud wrote that there "is not a little evidence to show how much Heine suffered both in his youth and later from this rejection by his rich relations. It was from the soil of this subjective emotion that the *'famillionaire'* joke sprang" (Freud, 1905c, pp. 140–141). And Lacan adds: "In this I am saying no more than Freud" (Lacan, 1957–1958, p. 34). Yet he is saying more than Freud, producing out of the subjective soil from which the word *famillionaire* as a joke sprang, a series of wordplays from *fat-millionaire*, to *infamillionaire*, to *madmillionaire* and *faminellionaire*, that all seem to work (ibid., pp. 35-36).

But if they work as metonymical ruins of an object and word-being, what could it be that is "lost" in it? According to Lacan's hypothesis, it must be another signifier. And he is willing to provide it when saying that we should note that the word "*familial*" was a neologism in the late nineteenth century, denoting a moment when the family, in a kind of decline, can be treated as an object because it required all kinds of new political realities such as the birth of family welfare services (see Lacan, 1957–1958, p. 47). The witticism hovers, gathering into it a series of puns on the relationship between money and family, social class and value, just as the structuring function of the family is in part being laid to waste.

The argument might seem strange at first sight and its value remains hidden. For, one might ask, what does this particular history of the *French* word "*familial*" have to do with the coining of the term "*familionär*" out of "*familiär*" and "*Millionär*" in a joke that is situated at the border of what is considered to be the *German* tongue, using elements of German to create a *Witz* based on a word composition that doesn't properly *belong* to any specific language. The coinage *famillionär* is neither German nor French nor Latin, but rather makes use of these languages to become its own verbal entity. Its metonymical devaluation opens language by playing on the breakage between the linguistic and its beyond. Without these metonymical ruins that fill the pages of the book on *Witz* and the book on parapraxis, we wouldn't have metaphorical creation. Furthermore, with metaphor alone we wouldn't have the object that, paradoxically, we "have" as that which we have lost. Lacan (1957–1958) calls it "verbal being" (p. 35). But he underlines that "a verbal being is still a being, and it increasingly tends to become embodied" (ibid.). And without being able to evoke this "verbal being" we would not be able to produce *analytically*—i.e., to trace or construct—the repressed signifier.

In the sections on the *Witz*, Lacan describes metonymy again and again, more than the esteemed metaphor, pointing to the slippage of language at the edge of the hole, breaking it into pieces, playing with contexts and usage, finding equivalences, to the point where this misuse of language is a devaluation and reduction of it, allowing us to see some truth or touch something real of the object. Metonymy lies at the other end of the dimension of meaning, what he calls, following Saussure, the dimension of value, where "it refers to the diversity of objects already constituted in language, into which the magnetic field of each person's needs, with their contradictions is introduced" (Lacan, 1957–1958, p. 72). Only on this ground can we be led to the flash of meaning in its disappearance best embodied by witticism and those making jokes.

If one were to generalise this juxtaposition of witticism and the forgetting of a proper name, one could say that the latter touches on the very "existence" of the subject and on what he or she can't say, or can only say at the limit about it—death and "the last things" (ibid.). The former, on the other hand, leads into the linguistic fabric, into its ties with the socio-economic and its texture, including the history of how the subject is inscribed into them, coerced to listen to or say elements belonging to that very fabric. In both cases, what *is* being said in the witticism—"*familionaire*"—or half-said in the forgetting of the proper name—the chain of "Bo-", "-elli-", "-i-", and "-or-", names that occur *instead* of the forgotten *Signorelli*—produces a metonymical devaluation of the language that at the same time produces either the pun or the hole as metaphor.

Here, let us wander back to Lacan's surprising introduction of "*familial*" into the equation of the signifiers "*familiär*" and "*Millionär*". Passing through dictionaries, encyclopaedias, city streets, and the remnants of historical imagination, Lacan himself produces the signifier that was "repressed" by the witty creation of poet Heine when coining "*familionär*" (Lacan, 1957–1958, p. 45). Lacan inscribes what Heine repressed. This signifying act is accompanied by a speculation on the possibility that Heine invented his pun "during one of those solitary walks in night-time Paris he would have taken, after the meetings he had … with Baron James Rothschild who treated him like an equal and in a manner that was 'completely famillionairely'" (ibid.). It is this concretism—and thus the *image* of the poet walking the streets of Paris by night—that he is adding to Freud's interpretation of the more general "family background" to the witticism.

Lacan, speaking in Paris, wandering, night and day, the same streets as the poet did, mobilises the history and institutions of the French language to construct his own type of familiarity with the "found footage" of signifiers. He flips the pages authored by Émile Littré, compiler of the eponymous dictionary, famously a source for the poet Mallarmé of whose poetry Lacan gives *en passant* a very clear definition: it is poetry "as a function of its relationship to signifiers" (Lacan, 1957–1958, p. 47). With this definition, he contends that we can find a more rigorous formula of Mallarmé's work than those reverting to idealism or musicality. The formula applied, "it is much less surprising that he took a keen interest in signifiers" (ibid.). This interest is one of the verbal being in its embodiment. The poet is implicated in the poetry signed by his name, "Mallarmé", because it is poetry as relationship (of the subject) to the signifier, albeit in a form that is most remote from personalism and psychologism—its most inhuman form—Mallarmé appearing to be the most abstract and disincarnate of all poets.

If the subject "Mallarmé" found in the dictionary called "Littré" the material for this poetry as relationship to the signifier, the same holds true for Lacan who found out, by means of the same dictionary, that "*familial, -ale, -aux*" was still considered to be a "*neologism*" by the compiler and author of it (Littré, 1873–1874). Lacan, after having provided the scene of Paris by night as the locus of invention for a neologism, further localises the "moment" of the occurrence of the signifier by indicating two dates, 1881 and 1865: "the word '*familial*' was a neologism in 1881. Close consultation of some good authors who have addressed the issue has made it possible for me to date the word's appearance at 1865" (Lacan, 1957–1958, p. 47). The latter year, 1865, is probably meant to refer to the date of publication of the book that is cited in the Littré dictionary as the only source for the lemma, i.e., Marcel Roulleaux's (1867) *Fragments économiques*. The book was in fact only published posthumously in 1867, and received, still in the same year, a review article by the later prime minister and promoter of colonialism Jules Ferry (1867) in *La philosophie positiviste,* a journal edited by Littré himself who, in 1862, had already published a necrology on Roulleaux (Littré, 1862).

The term "*familial*" made it into the dictionary from *post mortem* writing. Current French lexicography, however, dates the occurrence of the term "*familial*", as an adjective derived from the noun *famille,* to around 1830, without further indication of its sources for this (see Rey 2012, vol. I, p. 1315). The date is uncanny, because the 1830s are the years indexed by Lacan in order to add a historiographic hook to the image of the nightly Parisian ambulation by the witty poet: "during one of those night walks in Paris that he had to complete on his own … around the 1830s …." Is it possible that we can confirm Lacan's thesis that Heine's pun "*familionaire*" is equivalent to the newly invented "*familial*", or even that he invented both *at the same time*, immediately overwriting the one with the other?

Also, the other date Lacan indicates, 1881, is curious because one would expect the year of the publication of the last volume of the dictionary as the *terminus ante quem* for the occurrence of the "neologism". The dictionary was in fact published between 1863 and 1874 (though Littré had worked on it for at least for thirty years). So why would the word have been "a neologism in 1881" as Lacan writes? The answer that comes to mind is one that seems to respond to a different question, for it turns out that it was in the year 1881 that Emile Littré died. Are both dates indicating that "[d]eath is the absolute *Herr*" as Lacan would have it, in an expression loaded with pathos and gravity while analysing the forgetting of the name *Signorelli* (Lacan, 1957–1958, p. 32)?

Lacan substitutes 1881, the year of the death of the author, for 1874, the year of completion of the very work in which his name survives. Are we moving into an obscure and abstract space, as if, by speaking and not speaking about "death", a very general idea about the "origin of language" is being illustrated: "when one speaks of *Herr* one does not speak of death because one cannot speak of death, because death is precisely both the limit and probably also the origin of all speech" (Lacan, 1957–1958, p. 5)? But we are not in heaven with pure signifiers, we are in a dimension where the "relationships *to* the signifier" (Lacan, 1957–1958, p. 47) are at stake. In fact, it is Lacan's effort to wrench the signifier "signifier" from linguistics and claim it for psychoanalysis that is at stake.

It is therefore not surprising that one finds that in his most descriptive elaborations, as well as in his most intricate and rarefied formulae, Lacan, like Mallarmé in his sonnets, should be implicated. As he is, for instance, implicated in the "history" of the term *familial* having devoted in 1938 an article for *l'Encyclopédie française* to the "*complexes familiaux*", the "family complexes" (Lacan, 2001). Already then he certainly used some of those "good authors" who according to him whispered "1865" as the year for the birth of the neologism (Lacan, 1957–1958, p. 47). In 1938, Lacan not only used the by then fairly common term "*familial*" in the title of his article, but also presented a conception of "familial things" as woven into the fabric of the social, the economic, the political—and as understandable only as such. These things are not precisely "familionaire" but this pun could be a metonymy for expressing that they are irreducibly familio-socio-economic.

The omission of this text in Lacan's teaching of the seminar might not be significant of anything to anyone, while the omission of a theory of the unconscious and of psychoanalytic practice in the 1938 text itself might have been, however, significant enough for Lacan to omit it from the *Écrits* in 1966. After appearing in the *Encyclopédie française*, a reference book like the *Littré,* it was published only in 1984, to then be republished—posthumously and by members of his family—in Lacan's (2001) *Autres écrits*. The omission of the lengthy 1938 article on "family structures" from the 1966 publication of the *Écrits*, as well as from the Seminar in the 1950s, is obviously overdetermined. Our interpretation is that it has to do with the vicissitudes of the word "familial"—which doesn't contradict, for instance, the Durkheimian approach to the social, the article of 1938 which was eventually replaced by the structuralist anthropology and sociology of Lévi-Strauss.

Yet another omission, or elision, has to be noted then in the vicinities of Lacan's attempt to date and localise the occurrence of the signifier *familial* as what is repressed by the metaphorical creation by Heine. This omission also concerns, how could it not, the question of family. More precisely, however, it concerns the metonymic relation between two families, i.e., the Heine and the Freud families, these agnostic Jews born into the German language, and perhaps Lacan himself, and his first attempts to write himself into the psychoanalytic familial institution with a paper that was poorly recognised.

Freud, in "The Joke and its Relation to the Unconscious", had offered a biographical speculation about Heine being the inventor of the pun, replacing the relation to his own rich family to the one between the character of Hirsch Hyacinth and Salomon Rothschild (see Freud, 1905c, p. 140) using the given name of Heine's uncle "Salomon" as linking material. It is to this relation that Lacan, focusing on the family name "Rothschild" instead, adds Heine's commerce with Baron James in Paris, who indeed treated the poet quite *familionairely*, like he did Chopin, Balzac, and others. Freud only mentions the exclusion of poor Heine from his richer family as a biographical motive woven into the joke. Yet Freud had also offered an autobiographical element:

> I recall a story told by an old aunt of my own, who had married into the Heine family, how one day, when she was an attractive young woman, she found sitting next to her at the family dinner-table a person who struck her as uninviting and whom the rest of the company treated contemptuously. She

> herself felt no reason to be any more affable towards him. It was only many years later that she realized that this negligent and neglected cousin had been the poet Heinrich Heine.
>
> *(Freud, 1905c, p. 140)*

In the familial fabric of the text, Freud is situated very close to Heine. Like Lacan's, Freud's interpretation is not without concretism—on the contrary, not only does he write his own family history and himself into the history of the joke, he also allows us to picture Heine as the "negligent" and "neglected" element of the family, the "uninviting" one: he is"*unappetitlich*" in German, meaning almost "disgusting". He is some kind of familial waste at the table. But why is it not mentioned by Lacan? Or better, is this not Lacan's fate as well when it comes to the Freudian family?

Clinical waste

It is our contention that this focus on metonymy, this waste product in the production of the *Witz*, is of vast clinical value and forces Lacan to come to some surprising conclusions, different perhaps than those of Freud. Freud, Lacan says, seemed to think that the satisfaction provided by *Witz* was simply a cover for aggression, that the *Witz* tricks the other into letting down their censor; and we are at our most rude and aggressive when joking. Lacan, however, is quick to dismiss this theory. Freud wouldn't have gone through the trouble of carefully analysing hundreds of *Witz* if this was the final lesson; examples which, in the end, show us the range of linguistic mechanisms involved in unconscious formations:

> I am alluding here very precisely to this element of transmission which makes it the case that there is something there that, in a way, is supra-individual, and that is tied by an absolutely undeniable community to everything that has been in preparation since the origins of culture. What one is addressing when one attacks a subject at the level of the equivocations of signifiers has, as it were, a singularly immortal characteristic.
>
> *(Lacan, 1957–1958, p. 106)*

This immortal characteristic points to something beyond the flesh and blood person who is drawn into the joke and toyed with. It constructs someone quasi-anonymous who is reached out to in the game of witticism that attempts to attain a form of mutual pleasure that Lacan calls a "very special communion" (ibid.). This communion mirrors the community drawn on by the joke that extends back to the very "origins of culture" (ibid.).

Lacan seemingly moves from the deconstruction of the family, its waste products, to a possible relationship or social bond found in the sedimentation of linguistic material contained by the exchange of *Witz*. This communion, he says, "is no doubt more specifically humanising than any other, but it is humanising precisely because we begin at a level which, on both sides, is very inhuman" (ibid., p. 107). Here, we can see the value of the *Witz* in a flash: contra some interpersonal aggression, he tells us what the joke or witticism is, namely *pleasurogenic*. The *Witz* uses inhibition, prohibition, and repression, in order to pinpoint and make heard what never gets said or heard, to echo back the habitually unsaid and have it reverberate in the unconscious. The *Witz*, he says, opens up an almost infinite distance from need because of the satisfaction that can be found in toying with language alone. A strange communion indeed.

In fact, it seems as if we couldn't be closer to the function of the analyst, even as the notion of a "very special communion" might make the aficionados of analytic abstinence and asymmetry shiver. Shiver away. The humanising function of *Witz* is not only this echo, but also, he says, a work of unmasking, a liberation from the image that wanders off in its way, in order to resolve itself into the pure pleasure of some archaic mythic child and their first play with words, extracted from their relationship to things or even identity. It is also everything that can take place, usually of tragi-comic variety, around the axis called "love". A tall order, for something so small.

> In the case of the joke, through a sort of forcing, a happy shadow or reflection of a former satisfaction is conveyed. An astonishing success, one purely achieved by signifiers. Let's say that something happens the effect of which is, very precisely, to reproduce the initial pleasure of the satisfied demand even as it accedes to an original novelty. That is what the joke, essentially, accomplishes.
>
> *(Lacan, 1957–1958, p. 86–87)*

Relishing in Freud's acerbic tone when he says that "the only joke is one that I myself recognise as a joke" (ibid., p. 89), Lacan will also name this accomplishment *sovereignty*. Like pornography, I know it when I see it. This figure of the sovereign pleasure delivered by the *Witz* that only wants to be what it is, to augment its very nature against thought, is perhaps the same sovereignty that can be offered by psychoanalysis. The *Witz* as that to which we must add the thought: "And yet, I need the other" (ibid., p. 90). Funny.

Witticism and forgetting in the cure: A vignette

Let us dissect the accomplishment of the special communion in the play by play of a clinical moment that begins with a patient's forgetting and ends with an interpretation by way of a joke from the analyst, moving finally to another round of parapraxes. During the late phase of an analysis a patient was working on the question of her attachment to sickness as some earlier symptoms had reappeared—a moment which felt like a first approach to the question of the termination of her analysis. In a particularly poignant dream, her boyfriend was removing something horrific from her leg and said, "It's sickle cell anaemia". She couldn't remember what a sickle was. In the analysis, there is an ongoing concern over her and her partner's mutual attachment to being sick or being stuck, and indeed both look to the other in order to continue hesitating like the prisoners in the prisoner's dilemma; gazing at the other to try and define what you are, unable to move towards the exit. Caught in what Lacan called "the time for understanding", this hesitation can go on seemingly forever (cf. Lacan, 1945).

The analyst now said to her: "You want to see the sick!" This suddenly prompted a spontaneous image in the session. She said,

> I see myself with an L shaped tool in my hand (her father's first name begins with the letter L), you know like the ones that come with whatever you've bought at Ikea. I'm trying to find the place to insert it and it's terrifying me that I can't find an opening. Jamming it against a solid surface. What is that thing called, Jerry, Jerry, it's a man's name, I don't know, I can't remember.

"Allen wrench," the analyst offered. "You were thinking of Jerry Rig?" "Funny," she said,

> that's a word my boyfriend uses—Jerry Rig—when we are in situations where someone's sick and everything is falling apart … I guess the sick is comforting because I know where to go in and start fixing, it's a compulsion, but if I'm just waiting for an opening, there is something completely terrifying. I also hate the mystery of the other— the constant anxiety, "will they do it?"

In the next session she speaks passionately about Chris Kraus's novel *I love Dick* that was turned into a TV series. The story opens with Chris seeing Dick and falling immediately in love, passionately starting Chris's writing process by writing to Dick. Much as the love letters to him reignite desire in the novel's auto-fictional character, including in her marriage, it was likewise reigniting a certain sexual ardour between the patient and her partner. But, she was disappointed in her need for what she called a tool, her vibrator, though she took in the message of the show—that Dick didn't really matter. So anything or anyone could be used to prop up and sustain desire. The analyst said to her suddenly: "Any Allen, Dick or Jerry", and both broke into laughter.

In the next session, she dreamt that she claimed a child from a family whose parents had fallen asleep and failed to care for her. She said, "It's going to be ok. You are mine. She's mine". This came from another TV show, also based on a book, Margaret Atwood's *The Handmaid's Tale*, and the most recent episode featured a handmaiden stealing her baby back and threatening to kill herself and the baby. She ends up being convinced by the main character, *Offred*, not to harm the child. Then she kills herself. She noted that since the handmaidens are named based on the paternal figure to whom they are assigned, *Of-fred*, was the only one that sounded almost like an actual name because of the phonetic fusion in the double "f": Offred. In the other handmaiden's names you could more clearly hear that they were *of* whatever man—*Ofwarren, Ofjames*, etc. *Offred* seems oddly self-possessed, as if she has her own name even when she doesn't. Offred's name is a metaphorical condensation and provides a "family structure" while it also makes her part of a metonymic chain, like all linguistic material. Offred alone seems able to act and in this episode, she rescues this child, telling the handmaiden that she needed to give her daughter a chance to grow up. Children didn't belong to us, but to themselves, Offred tells the other handmaiden. Having seen the show, the analyst mentioned what Offred had said and that the patient hadn't mentioned it. She said she had forgotten that, and then recalled a recent inhibition meeting a colleague because she thought she would take something from her—maybe her ideas, or something of herself, she didn't know.

This led her back to her many symptoms of illness when she first came to analysis and her family's dream that a medical doctor will give you back to yourself by curing the sickness to which all the women are so morbidly attached. "This Drama of doctors!" she squealed. And then added: "and dentists even!" She suddenly remembered something that was so funny to her she could barely contain her laughter and speak clearly. A comedy sketch of a song about how weird teeth are, how they are bones on the outside that you wash; that you can lose them; and that your parents have some arrangement with a fairy to take them away while you are sleeping. She suddenly tried to remember the name of the comedy show, "Unshakeable? No, Unstoppable? No, Jesus, what is it?" The analyst asked her what was somehow like *unshakeable* and *unstoppable*, without being entirely expressed by these terms. "Unspeakable? No, that's not right either". The analyst laughed and told her to say it when she found out what the word was and ended the session. She texted the analyst that night, "It's unbreakable". A few weeks later, she started writing a collection of short stories that she had been hesitating on for years.

Writing witticism

A session or a sequence of sessions like this one is, in its structure, neither of the order of a joke nor of the one of the forgetting of a proper name; it may contain, and almost inevitably does contain, instances of both. It also contains instances and traits of the third formation of the unconscious, the dream, while the fourth formation, the symptom, can be said to provide the framework and playground for the unfolding, self-resisting, exploding, or imploding analytic cure. Also in the cure, the dream remains the *via regia* to the unconscious in as much as the interpretation of dreams provides most clearly the schematism of condensation, displacement, representability.

The material of our vignette would lend itself to a schema where the names that are half-forgotten and make it into a joke appear at the point of the Name-of-the-Father, much like Freud's *Signor(elli)* or *Herr(zegovina)*: Allen, Jerry, Dick, Offred, L. But the *Witz* is also one that makes the name seen for what it is, nothing really, an X, a point of appeal, indeed a tool—Dick, Sickle, Wrench, Rig, Bones. This brings the message of castration to the table. So that while it may be nothing, it can also be seen for what it is, the tool that is language, books, and writing: *I love Dick, The Handmaid's Tale, Unbreakable.* All these "metonymic ruins" play with the configuration of the symptom that pivots in the cure between sick and dick, name and nothing—consistently pointing to pathos—sickness, neurosis, suicide, neglect—in the *Herr*-dimension of death and the familial that governs the production of any witticisms or forgetting. As "unshakeable, unstoppable, unspeakable" they index, however, the drive—this ultimate hypothesis of analysis. And what the forgotten "unbreakable" adds to the chain is the question of the end of analysis, as well as the way that this end is shaped by the infinite, metonymic, material nature of verbal beings in search of objects. Is she sick? Or is she dick sick? Is the patient going to break off, return into sickness, go on, or do something with her tools? Whatever the answer, it is an unknown signifier, different from a lacking signifier. It gives us a point X as place to move towards in the future.

Lacan always indexes this unknown signifier as an "X". This X is essential to the logic of witticism,

> insofar as this X is present, a metaphorical formation tends to be produced ... It isn't because the name isn't grasped that there is a lack. No, the lack is the lack of this name. Searching for the name, we encounter a lack in the place where it should be serving its function and can no longer serve it, for a new meaning is required, one that demands a new metaphorical creation.
>
> *(Lacan, 1957–1958, p. 51–52)*

The cure is a formation in the throw of metonymy that makes a joke out of it, forgets it, dreams it up, throws it away, and then links it, finally, to something that can be transmitted—providing it with a new familial arrangement, a new name, in the pleasurable communion of psychoanalytic work. What it produces is perhaps more ephemeral, the waste of time itself, having touched something on the level of the drive; but it is also, by virtue of that, more pleasurable—unspeakably funny even.

But why "X"? One can say that Lacan's invention and use of pseudo-mathematical writing—his equations, schematisms, and graphs—serves the function of condensing or metaphorising the formations of the unconscious. These mathemes should be taken as a specific form of witticism, already used by Freud when he produced the graphic representation of *Signorelli* and *familionaire* (see Freud 1901b, p. 5 and 1905c, p. 19 rep.).

> This isn't about the loss of the name. It's about the loss of an X that I am introducing here because we are going to learn how to recognise it and make use of it. This X marks the appeal to signifying creation.
>
> *(Lacan, 1957–1958, p. 51)*

In the Seminar, the "X" marks the signifying creation itself, the "sovereign" inscription of this elementary matheme as the witticism of transmission.

Transmission is structured like a *Witz*. It inscribes the material encounter of those who meet in their desire as the "X" which marks the crossing point of their coordinates, coordinates that they have to keep drawing. But doing so, this is the place where communion happens, even when there is no longer a name and no sexual relation to be reported! This may be what makes it so pleasureogenic. X, this less-than-signifier, by being drawn in virtually infinite lines, is also the sovereign mark of psychoanalysis itself— it is dick, nothing, one of these jokes, in the subtle volley between analyst and patient, between analyst and other analysts. Or as Freud put it: "These jokes are not entirely without a purpose; they are a 'take-in'" (Freud 1905c, p. 138, Fn. 1). And we are taken in by it.

References

Ferry, J. (1867). Marcel Roulleaux: Fragments économiques publiés par ses amis. *Revue de la philosophie positiviste*, 1: 289–312.

Freud, S. (1901b). The Psychopathology of Everyday Life. *S.E.*, 6. London: Hogarth.

Freud, S. (1905c). Jokes and their Relation to the Unconscious. *S.E.*, 8. London: Hogarth.

Lacan, J. (1945). Logical Time and the Assertion of Anticipated Certainty: A New Sophism. In: *Écrits: The First Complete Edition in English* (pp. 445–488). B. Fink (Trans.). London & New York: W.W. Norton & Company, 2006.

Lacan, J. (1957–1958). *The Seminar of Jacques Lacan. Book V: The Formations of the Unconscious 1957–1958*. J.-A. Miller & R. Grigg (Trans.) Cambridge: Polity, 2017.

Lacan, J. (2001). *Les complexes familiaux dans la formation de l'individu*. In: *Autres écrits* (pp. 23–85). Paris: Le Seuil.

Littré, É. (1862,April 6). Marcel-Hippolyte Roulleaux, notice nécrologique. *Journal des débats*.

Littré, É. (1873–1874). *Dictionnaire de la langue française*. Paris: L. Hachette. Available at: http://www.littre.org.

Rey, A. (Ed.) (2012). *Dictionnaire historique de la langue française*. Paris: Le Robert.

Roulleaux, M. (1867). *Fragments économiques, publiés par ses amis*. Paris: Guillaumin.

PART 5

Graph of desire

13

ON THE DEVELOPMENT OF LACAN'S GRAPH OF DESIRE

Dan Collins

Readers of Lacan either love or hate his graphs and diagrams. For some, they are illuminating pedagogical tools that condense a great deal of Lacan's thinking into concise schematic representations. For others, the graphs represent only wilful obfuscation, and they are best ignored. The latter camp seems to feel that the danger of the graphs is that they obscure with arcane symbols what Lacan so carefully spells out in the seminar.

Lacan seemed to be aware of his audience's potential ambivalence towards his graphs, and at one point, while elaborating on the difficult Schreber schema in "A Question Prior to Any Possible Treatment of Psychosis", he cautions that "it would be better to consign this schema to the garbage heap, if, like so many others, it prompted anyone to forget, because of an intuitive image, the analysis on which this image is based" (Lacan, 1958a, p. 478). Thus Lacan thinks that the graphs present a danger exactly opposite to that feared by the graph-haters—not obscurity, but a too-facile clarity. He seems to think that an intuitive grasp of the graph might cause one to skip over the steps of his argument: to paraphrase Yeats, "Letters and pointed lines took all my love / And not those things that they were emblems of".

Thinking of the graphs only as a schematic condensation of completed arguments is in fact limiting. It's true that the various graphs are usually presented in a definitive version in one or another of Lacan's published works. But prior to that, they usually go through developmental stages in Lacan's seminar, and during the incremental steps of their development, they're often presented in versions very different from their canonical form. The slow construction of the graphs, then, sheds light on their final form.

This observation may not be of much comfort to graph-haters. I'm arguing that instead of simply forcing oneself to comprehend the definitive version of a graph, one should take the added effort to understand the several forms—many later abandoned—that a graph took along the way. Why? Because the graphs are more

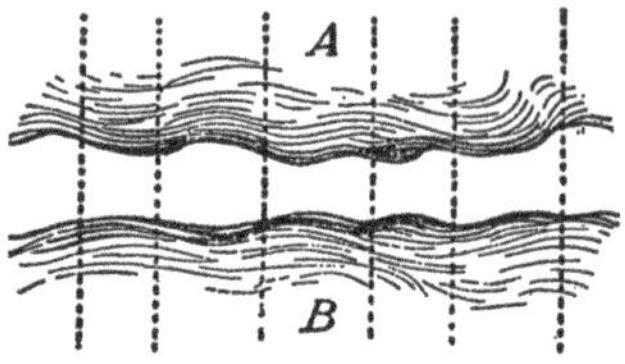

FIGURE 13.1 Schema of the two waves
(From Course in General Linguistics by Fedinand de Saussure, 1959)

than just pedagogical tools. They are the way Lacan thinks. Lacan doesn't just work out arguments in prose and then condense them into graphs. He often works out arguments graphically and then struggles to describe them discursively. The graphs, in other words, are Lacan's laboratory. His graphs are where he carries out his thought experiments, and they provide an opportunity to observe Lacan's thought in motion.

The best test case for this argument is Lacan's graph of desire, or the "big graph", as he develops it in Seminar V. The graph takes on its final form in "The Subversion of the Subject and the Dialectic of Desire in the Freudian Unconscious", a talk that was delivered in 1960 and was largely rewritten for the publication of the *Écrits* in 1966. The graph, as presented in this essay, is the definitive version of the graph that is familiar to readers of Lacan.

In Seminar V, though, the big graph begins its life as a modification of de Saussure's diagram of the waves (see Figure 13.1).

Here, the two levels represent "the indefinite plane of jumbled ideas (A) and the equally vague plane of sounds (B)" (de Saussure, 1959, p. 112), in other words, the level of the signified and the level of the signifier. Language itself is represented by the dotted lines that subdivide sections of the two waves, but more importantly, link them together: "Language might be called the domain of articulations .... Each linguistic term is a member, an *articulus* in which an idea is fixed in a sound and a sound becomes the sign of an idea" (de Saussure, 1959, pp. 112–113).

Lacan mentions his borrowing specifically at the beginning of *Seminar V*: "The signifier's relation to the signified ... led me to refer to Ferdinand de Saussure's famous schema in which you see the double parallel flow of signifiers and signifieds, distinct and destined to perpetually slide over one another"

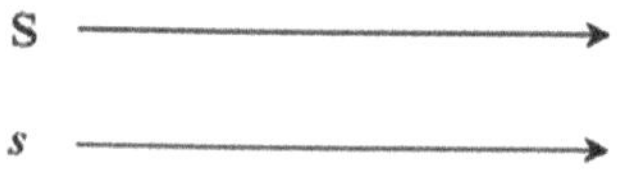

FIGURE 13.2 The schema of the two waves simplified

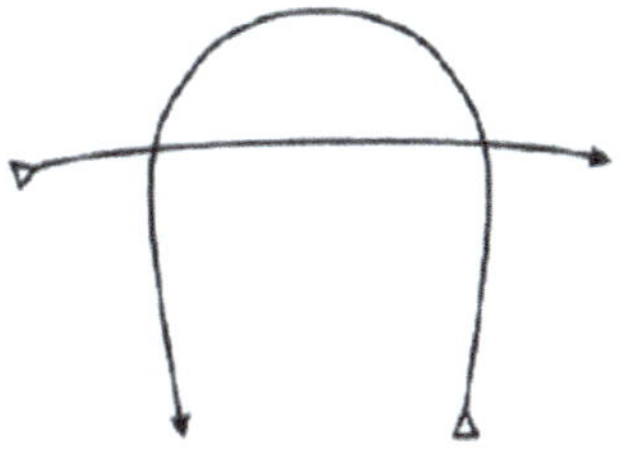

FIGURE 13.3 The first cell of the graph of desire
(Adapted from Lacan, 1957–1958, p. 8)

(Lacan, 1957–1958, p. 7). And so, we could say this is the very first version of the big graph (see Figure 13.2).

Lacan reverses Saussure's "indefinite plane of jumbled ideas [signified] and the equally vague plane of sounds [signifier]" (de Saussure, 1959, p. 112) as he habitually does, and he places the signifier (S) on top.

Next, Lacan bends one of these lines so that it intersects the other twice (see Figure 13.3), but he immediately clarifies that they no longer represent the signifier and the signified:

> Note that you cannot confuse what these two lines previously represented [in de Saussure's diagram]—namely the signifier and the signified—with what they represent here, which is slightly different, for now we are going to place ourselves entirely at the level of the signifier.
>
> *(Lacan, 1957–1958, p. 9)*

The first line now represents the signifying chain "insofar as it remains completely permeable to the properly signifying effects of metaphor and metonymy, which implies the possible actualization of signifying effects at all levels, down to the phonemic level in particular" (Lacan, 1957–1958, p. 9). The other line, which

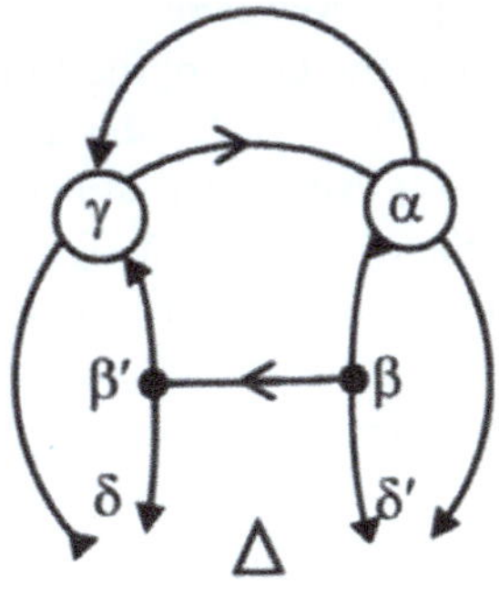

FIGURE 13.4 The first draft of the graph of desire
(Adapted from Lacan, 1957–1958, p. 10)

loops backwards and intersects the first line twice, is that of "the discourse of reality we all share … Most of the time, this discourse only consists of a subtle mixture of received ideas" (Lacan, 1957–1958, p. 10).

These definitions are already somewhat different from what we would expect from the definitive version of the graph. The first line, that of the signifying chain, seems to be describing the specifically combinatory—we could even say the automatic—effects of language. In the hand-drawn figure that accompanies the transcript of the seminar, this line is specifically labelled as a chain of phonemes. The intersecting line seems to have much in common with Heidegger's notion of "idle talk" (*Gerede*) (Heidegger 1962, pp. 211–214, ¶ 35). In the transcript, this line is labelled as a chain of semantemes. Lacan also describes it as "empty discourse" (Lacan, 1957–1958, p. 10).

The first line, then, involves the strictly unconscious signifying chain, and we could even say that Lacan's brief description of it suggests a similarity to his later notion of *lalangue*. The line that intersects it twice is specifically associated with "the individual subject's concrete discourse" (ibid.). We could even describe it as the conscious discourse of the subject.

The more complex version of the graph that Lacan gives in the first session of the seminar is a first rough draft of the canonical version—at least of the lower level of the canonical version. This "draft version" (see Figure 13.4) labels the intersections at α and γ and for the first time includes what will come to be known as the imaginary short circuit from β to β'.

It must be noted that there is very little need here for the Greek letters as the points on the graph will be redefined and relabelled throughout the seminar, but this is perhaps the point. Lacan can refer to the intersection at α, for example, in a number of ways before he labels it definitively.

Lacan first designates the intersection at α as a "bundle of usages" (Lacan, 1957–1958, p. 10), which implies that the combinatory effects of language are at least in part habitual, conditioned by the everyday discourse of the intersecting chain. Lacan calls this intersection the place of the "code" (ibid.), borrowing the term from linguistic theory, but throughout the seminar he'll undermine the notion of a code and will specifically reject it in the "Subversion" essay: "the one-to-one correspondence between sign and thing is not preserved here" (Lacan, 1960, p. 682). What's more important for Lacan is that this is the place of the Other "insofar as it's the companion of language" (Lacan, 1957–1958, p. 11). This may strike us as odd wording, but what seems important to Lacan is that the big Other is not simply the symbolic, or the language system, or even the treasury of the signifier. It is all that, but it must be *an* Other, an incarnated Other. It must be someone who is appealed to. Language is invoked whenever we address this Other, and Lacan says that it's sufficient if there is only one living Other because there is "not only one Other but even two" (ibid.), that is, the Other of language and the incarnated Other. In the sixth session of the seminar, Lacan will say that the Other must be "made of flesh", but must also be "quasi anonymous" (ibid., p. 106).

At the intersection γ, we have the message. Again, *code* and *message*, are terms borrowed from linguistic theory, but Lacan complicates the idea of the message, suggesting that it's the "conjunction of discourse with the signifier as the medium that creates meaning" (Lacan, 1957–1958, p. 11). So the speaker isn't just relying on his or her linguistic competence, or knowledge of a code, to produce meaningful utterances. If meaning is born here, it's because everyday discourse has become entangled in the unconscious signifying chain. Lacan even says that truth is announced here, which is a value that usually plays no part in any communications theory of code and message. Indeed, Lacan will account for what allows the place of the message to take on the value of truth (ibid.).

Most of the time, though, our speech doesn't rise to this level. This is an important point. Most of the time, our concrete discourse *doesn't* intersect with the signifying chain: it's "the pure and simple purring of repetition" (ibid.). Most of the time our discourse takes the short circuit represented by the line between β and β'. The point β is identified as the *I* of the discourse, and Lacan specifically calls it the "place … of the one who is speaking" (ibid.). At point β' is the metonymic object (ibid.). I think we could read this short circuit grammatically and say that what links the *I* as subject and object is a verb. So the line β-β' represents our relation—whether it's a relation of love, or hate, or ignorance, or use, or neglect—to our objects. Lacan is quite clear that "[t]his is everyday discourse, words put together for the purpose of saying nothing, owing to which you reassure yourself that you are not simply dealing, opposite you, with what man is in his natural state, namely a ferocious beast" (ibid.). This point shows again how far Lacan is from linguistic theory, which is only concerned with language competence and language performance and doesn't ask whether speech is full or empty. Later in the seminar, Lacan will ask us to imagine what it would mean if language were only a code and the signifier were "simply a kind of conditioning" (Lacan, 1957–1958, p. 435). In principle, he says, we'd have the "ideally functioning society" that "has always been dreamt of by utopians", one that attains "the satisfaction of each according to his needs" (ibid., pp. 435–436).What, then, interferes with this perfect society? What normally prevents speech from attaining truth? And when it does, what marks the meaning delivered in the place of the message as true?

Lacan gives a clue in his critique of the utopian society. In this society, everyone is satisfied according to their needs, but, he says, "One adds, to be honest, that everyone participates according to their merits, and that's where the problems start" (ibid., p. 436). What's suggested here is that language can't be universal, can't be simply a communication system to which we're conditioned, because we're all invested in it differently. We all have different libidinal investments in our metonymic object.

This Lacanian insight is illustrated by the great example of the seminar, Freud's example of Hirsch Hyacinth's joke of the millionaire. Heinrich Heine's humorous character wants to claim with pride that when he met Salomon Rothschild, the millionaire treated him quite *familiarly*. But, Lacan points out, Rothschild is, for Hyacinth, already a libidinal object; he is "my millionaire" (Lacan, 1957–1958, p. 17). Thus *millionaire* and *familiar* "meet and come together in the message at γ, to form 'famillionaire'" (ibid.). This implies that between the position of α, which is

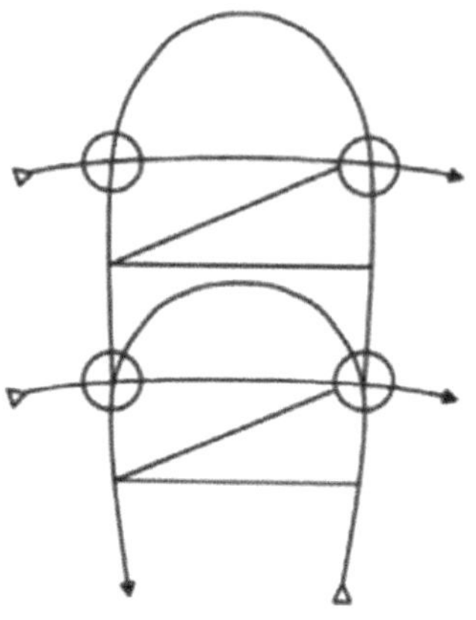

FIGURE 13.5 Homology of the two triangles
(Adapted from Lacan, 1957–1958, p. 193)

the code, and β', which is the metonymic object, there's a connection, and a diagonal line could be drawn connecting the two. In fact, in the seminar as it has been printed in both the French edition and English translation, this line appears in only one rendering of the graph and in quite a different context (see Figure 13.5).

But this connection between object and Other is implied throughout the seminar. This is how our involvement in language goes beyond mere conditioning by a code. Lacan is clear here: the message that gets deposited at γ is "not in the code .... [I]t's manifestly in violation of the code" (Lacan, 1957–1958, p. 18). *Famillionaire* isn't a lexical item in English, or French, or German. And yet, we all understand what has been said. The human use of language, then, can invent new usages beyond the code.

We should note that this is not how a joke or a slip of the tongue is usually represented for pedagogical purposes. Normally we talk about the interference of the unconscious chain of signifiers in conscious discourse (see Figure 13.6)

Lacan's graph is already a much subtler mechanism in that it tells us *how* this interference occurs. It's because we're libidinally invested in the object of our discourse that the code can be interfered with, violated. Lacan says that the "specific signifying function of [famillionaire] is to designate not only this or that but also some sort of beyond" (Lacan, 1957–1958, p. 59). I would say that the word *beyond* is in fact the most important word in the seminar.

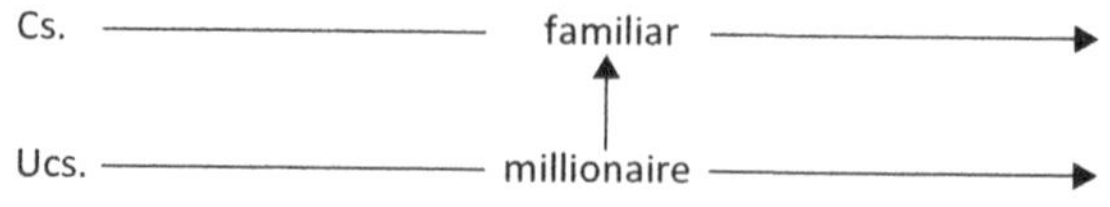

FIGURE 13.6 Diagram of a slip of the tongue

In fact, I even think we find in the suggestion that libido interferes in the code a hint of something that is very current in Lacanian theory today, the suggestion of a symbolic unconscious and a real unconscious. In the fourteenth session of the seminar, Lacan says:

> The unconscious discourse is not the last word of the unconscious, it's supported by what truly is the ultimate mainspring of the unconscious and which cannot be expressed in any other way than as the subject's desire to be recognized.
>
> *(Ibid, p. 240)*

And so, in the seminar we have a beyond of the code, a beyond of the unconscious, a beyond of language, and we'll have a beyond of demand, a beyond of the mother, a beyond of suggestion, and a beyond of the Other. I think that part of the value of following the development of the graph is that we see plainly how Lacan reaches, or is compelled to advance to, each of these *beyonds* in succession. As the seminar proceeds, Lacan will leave behind the joke, which only takes up the opening sessions, and consider the Oedipus complex, the Name-of-the-Father, the symptom, and the diagnostic structures of hysteria and obsession. Meanwhile, during the course of the seminar, he writes both "On a Question Prior to Any Possible Treatment of Psychosis" and "The Signification of the Phallus." In spite of accomplishing all this in the course of 1957–1958, Lacan also has, in retrospect, some remarkable lapses. As of Seminar V, he doesn't yet have a clear notion of desire. He's developing one, but desire in this seminar is largely a matter of a natural tendency towards objects. He also doesn't yet have a notion of the drive as distinct from desire. And yet he incorporates the inscriptions for both desire and drive into the upper level of his graph. Lacan's graphic representations here are outrunning his theory. It's literally as if he develops the graph first—especially at the upper level—and then figures out what inscriptions should go in what places. This may seem like a rather ad hoc procedure, but the graph, in effect, teaches Lacan what desire is and what fantasy and the drive are.

Lacan introduces the upper level of the graph in the seventh session of the seminar, and with the purpose of representing "the Other subject" (Lacan, 1957–1958, p. 111). The idea seems to be that the subject has its own level of the graph, so the Other should have one, too. The most important feature of the upper level of the graph is introduced immediately. Since the upper level represents another subject, the two levels of the graph are superimposable: "I am thereby indicating the superimposition of the system of the Other subject onto the system of the first" (ibid.). The positions at the two levels of the graph, then, are the same. But since the Other already has a place on the original graph, Lacan starts from that position of the Other and stacks the second level on the first. He even identifies the positions with the same Greek letters. And what he emphasises first is that the Other has its own chain of discourse along the line β to β'. At the upper level, this becomes beta double-prime (β'') and beta triple-prime (β'''). Lacan draws the lesson from this immediately, that as subject, the Other has its own libidinal objects and its own discourse in relation to them. As he puts it, "everyone has, as they say, his own little idea" (ibid., p. 121). This is a crucial point for the development of the Oedipal conflict because although the child takes the mother as object, the mother has her own preoccupations. This is why the entire upper level of the graph becomes the schematisation of an Other desire.

It's not until session seventeen of the seminar, some months later, that Lacan develops the "formulas of desire" (cf. Lacan, 1957–1958, ch. XVII) that provide the inscriptions that will populate the completed graph. Here, for the first time, we see the formulas for the drive, for fantasy, and for the signifier of the lack in the Other, although they're not identified as such immediately. And it's something of a mystery why and how Lacan develops these formulas. They're presented in linear form and they are in fact *not* immediately inserted into the graph. Nor does Lacan seem to understand them very well at first. His first gloss of the formula for fantasy is that

> human desire is not directly implicated in a pure and simple relationship with the object that satisfies it, but that it's just as much linked to the position that the subject adopts in the presence of this object as it is to the position he adopts outside his relations with the object, in such a way that nothing in his relations with an object is ever completely exhausted.
>
> *(Lacan, 1957–1958, p. 301)*

This description is not yet Lacan's later notion of fantasy, but it does summarise one of the major developing themes of the seminar: that demand always asks for more than simple satisfaction. It asks for recognition from the Other, and the gap between simple need and the demand that represents it is where desire emerges. In the contemporaneous "Signification of the Phallus" essay, Lacan will put this succinctly: "desire is neither the appetite for satisfaction nor the demand for love, but the difference that results from the subtraction of the first from the second" (Lacan, 1958b, p. 580). The date of this essay is given very precisely as 9 May 1958. In the session of 7 May, Lacan says that desire is "the margin or result of the subtraction, as it were, of the requirements of need from the demand for love" (Lacan, 1957–1958, p. 362).

Thus the well-known formula for fantasy, $\$ \lozenge a$, and the formula for drive, $\$ \lozenge D$, are, in their first elaboration, conceptually closer than they will appear to be later. The formula for fantasy seems to emphasise the subject's relation to the object, while the formula for drive seems to emphasise the subject's relation to the signifier, in the form of the demand. In session twenty-two of the seminar, Lacan tries to tease out the difference between the two levels by focusing on the demand as constitutive of the subject. At the lower level of the graph, the subject is constituted by A, the big Other as law. At the upper level though, the subject's relation to demand takes this position, and determines subject beyond the determination of the Other, suggesting that the subject is not completely constituted by A, and is "never a pure and simple subject of knowledge" (Lacan, 1957–1958, p. 373). Thus the message at the upper level is that the Other is incomplete, S(Ⱥ). It's in the next session that Lacan draws a distinction, suggesting that the formula $\$ \lozenge a$ might represent the function of fantasy, which he doesn't seem to have yet differentiated from concrete fantasies: "I believe that at this place [$\$ \lozenge a$], the schema presented to us here opens up the possibility of locating and articulating the function of fantasies" (Lacan, 1957–1958, p. 386). He's only slowly making the distinction between fantasies and the unconscious fantasy in these very sessions:

> This notion of fantasy as something that undoubtedly partakes of the imaginary order, but which, at whatever point of its articulation, only ever functions in the economy through its signifying function, seems essential to me .... I would go further—I do not believe there is any other way of conceptualizing what are called unconscious fantasies.
>
> *(Lacan, 1957–1958, p. 388)*

Lacan's formulation of drive in the seminar also seems unfamiliar to readers familiar with the later Lacan. The closest we get to his later formulations arises only when he considers the demand for analysis. The subject has a relation to his own articulated demands, of course, but what about the demand for analysis? Lacan says, it's a renewal of the subject's demands (Lacan, 1957–1958, pp. 416–417). Simply by entering analysis and free associating, the subject revives old demands: "It's insofar as this demand is formulated in archaic signifiers that we speak, for example, of oral or anal regression" (Lacan, 1957–1958, p. 417). This is how the place of the drive at the upper level of the graph is also a treasury of signifiers. It's the collection of those drive signifiers that represent the subject's stereotypical, and archaic, ways of enjoying. Still, Lacan hasn't completely sorted his concepts, because a few moments later, he'll claim that drive is just "a technical term" for desire (Lacan, 1957–1958, p. 418).

With that much of a reading of the big graph accomplished, however incompletely, we can return to our original question. Do the developmental stages of the graph help us in understanding the final presentation of the graph? Does an understanding of the steps Lacan takes help us to understand where he arrives? Ultimately, every one of us has a style of reading Lacan, and it helps us to understand Lacan if we compare our understandings. Even if we know Lacan very well, we can always be surprised by someone else's insight into some detail of Lacanian theory. We can always say, "I never thought of it that way". At the very least, the developmental stages of Lacan's graph provide us with one more insight, one more reading, one more understanding—Lacan's own.

References

de Saussure, F. (1959). *Course in General Linguistics*. W. Baskin (Trans.). New York: Columbia University Press.

Heidegger, M. (1962). *Being and Time*. J. Macquarrie & E. Robinson (Trans.). New York: Harper and Row.

Lacan, J. (1958a). On a Question Prior to Any Possible Treatment of Psychosis. In:*Écrits: The First Complete Edition in English* (pp. 455–488). B. Fink (Trans.). New York and London: W. W. Norton & Company, 2006.

Lacan, J. (1958b). The Signification of the Phallus. In:*Écrits: The First Complete Edition in English* (pp. 575–584). B. Fink (Trans.). New York and London: W. W. Norton & Company, 2006.

Lacan, J. (1960). The Subversion of the Subject and the Dialectic of Desire in the Freudian Unconscious. In: *Écrits: The First Complete Edition in English* (pp. 671–702). B. Fink (Trans.). New York and London: W. W. Norton & Company, 2006.

Lacan, J. (1957–1958). *The Formations of the Unconscious Book V.* J.-A. Miller (Ed.). R. Grigg (Trans.). Cambridge: Polity Press, 2017.

PART 6

Paternal Metaphor

14

FATHER LOVE

From Oedipus complex to Paternal Metaphor

Megan Williams

Like Freud, Lacan did not cease to work the question of the father, despite his critique of Freud, the father of psychoanalysis, having made too much of father-love, both clinically and theoretically. Lacan moved from the father as symbolic, through his imaginary effects, to the real effects of the paternal function. Freud wrote of *Vatersehnsucht*, father-longing or -passion, as universal: the longing one has for a father as master of, and protector from, the forces of reality and of the psyche (Freud, 1923b, p. 37; 1927c, p. 18; 1930a, p. 72; 1939a, pp. 109, 148). Lacan spoke scathingly of this image, representing a father instead as a humiliated, tireless, and possibly ineffective worker for the family; asking what there is to love in that (Lacan, 1969–1970, p. 100). He extracted from the poor person of the father the normativising function essential in engendering subjectivity. Yet, with a sleight of theory, he returned to love as the catalyst necessary to the realisation of the function. So he, too, makes love for the father approach a universal. This left him in the horns of the dilemma he had implicitly critiqued in Freud: how can psychoanalysis retain the bones—the essential function, catalysed by love—whilst dissolving the neurotic complex? He first dealt with it by attributing the neurotic effects of the Oedipus complex to a conflation of symbolic function with personal love and/or hate for that imaginary father who can appear as "old fogey" or tyrannical god (Lacan, 1959–1960, pp. 307–309). The Oedipus complex itself he came to regard as no more than family drama or myth, unusable by psychoanalysts in this form (Lacan, 1969–1970, pp. 98–130). Only its functional elements were of use: castration and the paternal function. By the time of his twenty-second seminar, *RSI*, however, it could be argued that he viewed the function itself as neuroticising (Lacan, 1974–1975, Seminar XXII, lessons of 21 January & 11 February, 1975), and his question became how an analysis could tie the knot of subjectivity differently, doing without the father even if the skeleton was made of him. This trajectory took him from the Oedipus as myth to the father as symptom; from the father as symbolic Name to he who, by assigning names, makes the Symbolic emerge from the Real (ibid., lessons of 21 January and 13 May, 1975). Throughout it, the aspect most difficult to shake free of theoretically and clinically was the one he found most derisory in Freud: love for the father. Whether from love or some other grip, the father did not let either Freud or Lacan alone, and each of them tried to theorise this hold. This chapter takes as its primary focus the early days of the trajectory: Lacan's work on the father in his Seminar V, The Formations of the Unconscious, which he gave from 1957–1958. Here he proposes the "Paternal Metaphor" as the foundational and structuring formation of the unconscious (Lacan, 1957–1958, Seminar V, lessons of 15 & 22 January, 1958), echoing Freud's nomination of the Oedipus as the nuclear complex of the neuroses, but emphasising the father as a symbolic element or signifier functioning to structure subjectivity. Where not otherwise indicated, references made in this chapter will be to these two seminar lessons.

Lacan arrives at his formulation both from Freud and from a survey of the psychoanalytic literature after Freud, from which he isolates two key elements. One of these is Klein's work on the presence in the psyche of the Oedipus complex—particularly the phallus of the father—at very early ages. Lacan takes this as confirming its retroactive function, which in turn confirms its foundational structure in relation to the unconscious. The Oedipus complex weaves through and structures all experience, including that which may be thought to pre-date it. As Freud emphasised, this function pivots around the phallus as signifier of sex. Lacan, as we will see, will formulate this as the castration complex giving all of psychical life the form of O/δ the signification of the phallus (Lacan, 1958, pp. 464–65).

The second key element that Lacan extracts from the literature is that the Oedipus complex is held to result in three outcomes, comprising relations to reality, and both the moral character and sexual identity of the subject; aspects in which are to be recognised three functions of the psychical apparatus identified by Freud: ego, superego and ego ideal. Lacan will relate each of these to the prohibiting or prescriptive aspects of the paternal function.

For Lacan, the paternal function is a key component of the ego, in furnishing the kernel of its ideals and designating it a named "one" with a singular identity. Beyond that, he is concerned with the subject of desire and the constitution of an unconscious, to whose emergence the father is essential. Singularity implies separation, which the father effects by prohibition and recognition (and psychoanalytic clinical work testifies to the demand for recognition so frequently addressed to a father). The father's link to nomination is thus apparent, and the Lacan of the 1970s will make it the essential paternal function—having an ego requires a name that differentiates one from all others. In 1957–1958, this comes into effect via the primary Name, the Name-of-the-Father. As for the superego, Lacan finds there an imaginary confusion of function and person resulting in hatred for the father for, in his later words and echoing Freud, the impossibility of making jouissance enter the Other (Lacan, 1959–1960, p. 308; 1962–1963, lesson of 13

March 1963). The ego ideal, on the other hand, is born from love for the father, and gives the subject a sexual identity at the culmination of the castration complex.

How, then, does the father function in the complex? Lacan says that he first enters as an intruder into the bliss of the imaginary triad in which child and mother are intricated.

The imaginary triangle

In this first imaginary triangle, the mother is the only Other of the child and thus not separable from the big Other of the symbolic order. Lacan has elaborated elsewhere that a baby is helpless in the symbolic order: the mother takes its first cries as enunciations and determines their meaning—that it is hungry, wet, and so forth (Lacan, 1960, pp. 680–693). The child is thus inserted into language, but the significations are the mother's: it receives its own message in inverted form from this Other and is captive within her universe of significations.

Nevertheless, Lacan still calls this a triad rather than a dyad, because the mother in the normal case evinces, by her speech and her absences, "a desire for something other" than the child (Lacan, 1957–1958, Seminar V, lesson of 15 January 1958, p. 16). In representing her alternating presence-absence, the child is first subjected to something beyond the mother: its own signifying chain (*fort—da*!; gone—there!), albeit one still grounded in the mother. The child doesn't know the meaning of the mother's desire but the unknown is signified—"what is she wanting beyond me?" This "what?", signifier of the desire *of* the mother, makes the third position of the triangle as a result of the child's desire *for* the mother. It is occupied by an image—the phallus—which is sketched out for the child as a result of the mother's unconscious position as castrated, or subject to phallic signification. For the child, however, the mother is still omnipotent, uncastrated, in that this phallus is not something she is deprived of but something she has.

As for the child, in attaching itself to this phallus, it already desires "something other". It's demand for need satisfaction has become a demand for love, which makes the child dependent on the mother's desire. To be loved by her is to captivate her desire, and Lacan depicts their first bliss together as involving the child playing at being her "something other", her phallus. This triangle is called by Lacan "imaginary" (Lacan, 1957–1958, Seminar V, lesson of 22 January 1958, p. 2) to differentiate it from the symbolic relation in which he locates any adult speaker: a ternary composed of speaker, interlocutor and the universe of language on which speech relies, the big Other. For the child, the mother *is* the big Other, which is thereby limited to her significations. The child is *assujetti*: a neologism which combines the notions of being subject to, in this case, the significations or fantasm of the mother, and of being an "a-subject", that is, not a subject in his own right (Lacan, 1957–1958, Seminar V, lesson of 22 January 1958, p. 13). There is also an implicit reference to the object *a*. An object *a* is not a phallus. The latter is a signifier that can be identified with, convoking prestige and desirability, whereas the former is unrepresentable, disposable, potentially horrifying. One cannot assimilate being an object *a* to one's ego. Beyond the bliss of this mutual seduction, then, the child is subject to the maternal desire as if to a law which is singular, capricious, and doesn't guarantee him a place in his own name. The question is thus how to separate mother from law: to bring into being an Other beyond the mother to which she would also be subjected, in order that the subject have a separate existence and its own (unconscious) universe of signifiers.

As Lacan developed in the previous year, the separation is thrust upon the child by the Real which emerges from inside its body and psyche and finds no representation in the mother's significations: jouissance which is not oral or anal (which are signified) but sexual (Lacan, 1957–1958, Seminar IV, lesson of 13 March 1957). Lacan depicts a gulf developing between what the child apprehends that the mother desires and this Real that it has but cannot offer to the recognition of the Other, and of which it might ask, "what does it want, here inside?" (Lacan, 1960–1961, Seminar VIII, lesson of 19 April 1961, p. 8). At this point the mother's turning to the child becomes anguishing rather than blissful; doubly so in that, once alerted to the Real at stake in sexuality, there is also the unknown of, "what does she want of me?" These unknowns open the chasm of anxiety, splitting the subject between what it has and what it must offer the mother in order to be her phallus; between being nothing in itself (*asujetti*) or nothing of value for her. It is the chasm which, in the absence of the father's Name, a phobic signifier may metaphorise: the tiger under the bed or the biting horse convoking both the anguishing unknown that threatens identity from inside, and the maw of the mother's desire insofar as the child is unable to satisfy it. Thus Lacan observed that a chasm opens for little Hans when he grasps that his mother desires something Real—in that she has a baby—and that the only Real he has to offer her is inadequate—in that she rejects his display of his penis to her (Lacan, 1956–1957, lessons of 13 & 20 March, 1957). There is an urgent need for a signifier to represent two unknown desires, on the side of the body and of the mother. This the phallus will do insofar as it is brought by the father as a signifier and no longer an image in the field of the mother.

In what follows I will address the Paternal Metaphor as an operation in which the father's prohibition of these unknowns constitutes them as desires, for whose representation he then furnishes an ideal. In doing so I will examine three elements: the prohibition of real satisfaction, the prohibition of the mother, and the privation of the mother.

Prohibition of the real satisfaction

It would seem that, in order to come to the normative position of desiring "something other", the child must be prohibited from achieving satisfaction with that which is in its own disposal, by masturbation. This is the first sense of the passage concerning what Lacan calls "prohibition of the real satisfaction" (Lacan, 1957–1958, Seminar V, lessons of 15 January 1958, p. 11 & 22 January, p. 13).; "real" here indicating immediate and bodily. It would also include the oral and anal jouissance of the real objects at play with the mother. What is at stake is an interdiction, imposed not necessarily by the father, but by a real agent—mother, father, teacher. The prohibition concerns what Lacan has elsewhere characterised as too close to home to participate in the field of social relations. It is a way of referring to a jouissance which occurs in the body and thus apparently in the child's "home", yet which the prohibition will make foreign by its effect of constituting "home" as the shared symbolic-imaginary field of discourse. Echoing the Freudian threat, Lacan calls this operation "castration", meaning a symbolic act (prohibition) causing an imaginary wound—in that what is castrated is not the imagined organ but an unrepresentable jouissance (Lacan, 1957–1958, Seminar V, lesson of 15 January 1958, p. 10-12). The prohibition effects a turning outwards: jouissance must be sought via desire, in the field of social relations recognised by the Other. Or, as Lacan asserted two years later: "[C]astration means that jouissance has to be refused in order to be attained on the inverse scale of the Law of desire" (Lacan, 1960, p. 700).

However, there is also the sense in which the prohibition functions as a naming of the anguishing unknown which comes from "inside". It will only be a few years until Lacan emphasises that what is involved in the first manifestations of sexual arousal is less satisfaction for the child than anguish, insofar as the Other doesn't sanction this jouissance with recognition. The previous year's commentary on the case of little Hans, as well as the later "Geneva Lecture on the Symptom", propose that jouissance of the child's "own" sexual organs is traumatic if not given phallic signification—as lacking and desired (Lacan, 1989, pp. 15–16). In other words, the prohibition is necessary, not to forbid satisfaction, but rather to close the chasm which has opened; to knot with meaning something that demands from inside, yet is already lost to a subject of language. It gives phallic signification to the void that jouissance makes in the symbolic Other by being unrepresentable. The term "Real" here is therefore a precursor to Lacan's later conception of the Real as impossible, and also references Freud's observation that the real object of the drive is always already lost to representation.

The phallus coming to bear as signifier depends on the next two logical components of the Metaphor as well, but rests on this first prohibition, since phallic signification concerns that which is represented as lost or wanting; the object *a* signified as what one *n'a plus* (no longer has), as too close to home to be apprehended in the symbolic field of the big Other and therefore *unheim* (literally, un-home), uncanny (Lacan, 1962–1963, Seminar X, lesson of 19 December 1962). The function of the father will be to symbolise that this loss of jouissance is the Law, whose other side is desire. The jouissance named phallic by the prohibition is then held in reserve to make the real of phallic sexuality, which would otherwise be a matter solely of signifiers and images. It is a reformulation of Freud's theory of the various aspects of infantile sexuality being drawn together under the rubric of the phallus to make the infantile entrepreneur ready to invest its sexual capital (Freud, 1905d, p. 207; 1900a, p. 561).

Although Lacan schematically separates the prohibitions of masturbation and of incest into two logically distinct moments, they overlap: "[Castration] ... is ... profoundly linked to the symbolic articulation of the prohibition of incest" (Lacan,

1957–1958, Seminar V, lesson of 15 January 1958, p. 10). Freud indicated that a child's masturbatory jouissance is clothed in fantasies of incestuous relations of love and desire—this is the sense of his psychical reality (Freud, 1950a, pp. 260, 267, 276). If the first prohibition signifies the phallus as something which the child doesn't *have* at its own disposal, it is not separable from the prohibition of those relations in the second logical moment, where it will also become something which the child cannot *be* for the Other.

Prohibition between mother and child

The father's intrusion into the imaginary triangle has the key, symbolic function of prohibiting incest, understood as that relation in which the child desires to fulfil the image of the mothers' desire (to be her phallus) and the mother is satisfied by the child as object *a* or phallic image. The key point is that, whether in the so-called primal scene, or by a telephone call, his intrusion claims the mother as belonging to him *by right*; that is, by his name as father. By this symbolisation the child is frustrated in its possession of the mother and the real objects found in her. The mother is also frustrated in her enjoyment of the child insofar as she is not only mother but a woman who desires the child's father and accepts his claim on her.

The prohibition of incest depends on the mother recognising the father's right—or the right of some instance beyond her. If she accepts his speech claiming her and drawing her away from the child, the effect is to signify to the child that there is something to which she, too, is subjected; that there exists a symbolic universe beyond her. Evidently this depends on the paternal function and the prohibition of incest being already inscribed in the unconscious of the mother. Ultimately, this apprehension that the mother is dependent on something beyond her symbolises to the child that there is a Law which subjects her; one which is universal, neutral and, unlike the mother's whims, uninfluenced by anything that the child *is*. It thus relieves the child of anxiety along with its imagined possession of the mother.

Privation of the mother

This aspect goes beyond the castration of the subject to the castration of the Other and is the key to the constitution of the child as subject of desire with an unconscious—and thus a name, we could say—of its own. It is the moment in which the "something else" of the mother's desire is removed from her disposal and placed under the rubric of the father. It occurs, says Lacan, insofar as the father shows himself, and is recognised by the mother, as potent; that the child encounters the mother's desire for the father as a man. It is her desire which, in the symbolisations of the child, endows the father with the phallus.

If that occurs, the mother appears as being deprived of what she desires and dependent on an object which the Other has or doesn't have. Lacan observes that the father, endowed with the phallus by the mother's desire for it turned towards him, is thus imagined by the child as having deprived the mother of it, even though in fact what he deprives her of exists only as a symbol. In the child's eyes, the mother joins the universe of beings who must seek to satisfy the desire for what they do not have via the Other. She appears in a state of privation. For Lacan, this is the nodal point of the castration complex, understood as the co-operation of castration, frustration and privation to make the Paternal Metaphor. It culminates in the child subjected in its own name to the desire for something other—other than the mother and other as such.

The Paternal Metaphor

The child's question about what the mother desires, urgent because of its dependence, requires a signification. However, linguistic structure is such that a signification cannot be pinned to a signifier because a signifier can only ever produce more signifiers, a chain, none of which say the thing itself. It is impossible to say what the mother desires, an impossibility attested to by the incessant questioning of small children, whose inexhaustibility points to the lack of satisfaction that each answer brings. There is a lack or void in the Other of the signifier, which is to say that there is no Other of the Other: no arbiter to whom the child might refer for the final meaning of the speech it receives.

For Lacan, the intervention of the paternal function doesn't provide a final answer but nevertheless makes a halt to the inexhaustibility of the question. This occurs in the linguistic operation of metaphor, where the child's signifier, Desire of the Mother, is pinned not to a signification, but to another signifier that intrudes from outside, the Name-of-the-Father. The result is the emergence of a new signified, the phallus—in its turn, also a signifier, since a signification cannot be pinned to a signifier. The Paternal Metaphor signifies to the child in the first instance that the mother desires *what she doesn't have* and that she *turns to the father for it*, not to the child. The term that Lacan has been using of the mother, "a desire for something other", is key. "Something other" *is* the phallus, a signifier designating that which is other *as such,* which one desires and *doesn't have.* It stands thus in the void of the inexhaustible question of what the Other desires, no longer as image or object but as a signifier which links to others to make new chains, always leading elsewhere like a ferret darting through speech. It also stands for what one *n'a plus* as prohibited, making that fallen jouissance the reserve of the phallus. The Metaphor makes the structure of desire the universal law of speech: that any other, including the mother, seeks jouissance by desiring the phallus, which can be had only in signified ways.

The castration complex, via the father, thus co-constitutes the lack in the mother and in the Other and knots it to desire directed away from the child, towards the phallus and the father as its bearer. In receiving this signification, the child's Other is castrated, and the child is castrated of the jouissance which attached it there. The Paternal Metaphor thus depends on the child's acceptance or refusal of the privation of the mother, which is dependent in turn on the mother's desire for the father and her regard for his speech, signifying him as potent or having.

In sum, the Paternal Metaphor is the operation of a signifier which is Other to the mother's signifying chain. Lacan goes so far as to use the term "Other of the Other" (Lacan, 1958–1959, Seminar VI, lesson of 8 April 1959, p. 7), even though he will come to say, no doubt deriving the conclusion in part from this present work, that there is no Other of the Other. This is the function of the father as exception. From the child's point of view, he has possession of *the mother* and thus the father from whom issues the Law that prohibits incest is excepted from it. He is exception also in that he intrudes from a place "above the signifying chain" (Lacan, 1957–1958, Seminar V, lesson of 22 January, 1958, p. 16) that the child has made from the mother's speech. In constituting a Law beyond the mother, his Name brings into being, for the child, an Other separate from the mother-Other. Where she had been signified to the child as omnipotent, she becomes not-all, an other subject and not the Other.

It is pertinent to note that Lacan's distinction between function and person allows him to define the Name-of-the-Father as anything which can fulfil the functions outlined of being above the signifying chain in a metaphorical position and the one who mediates the Law recognised by the mother. Any instance satisfying these conditions will have this function, whether or not there is an actual father in the family.

Sexual identity

There is then a turning point between being the phallus—in imaginary games—and having it. The effective privation of the mother renders it futile to try *to be* the phallus for her so the path opens to *having* it, the mode of which determines the sexual identity of the subject. This occurs, Lacan emphasises, because the child's love, under the influence of the mother's privation, turns from her to the father. Having the phallus becomes the aim *par excellence* and so the father who bears it is idealised and introjected as an ego ideal. For the Lacan of 1958, the final step of the Metaphor resolves the complex in the Freudian way. The boy trades the desire of the mother for the "deeds" (Lacan, 1957–1958, Seminar V, lesson of 15 January 1958, pp. 10-11; lesson of 22 January, p. 15) which say that one day, like his father, he will bear the phallus and be able to give another woman (note that the mother thus joins the series of women) what she desires. The girl turns from the mother who has been unable to give her what she lacks to obtain the phallus from the later substitutes of the father in the form of love, desire, and children. Both cases, Lacan emphasises, depend on love for the father as potent, as protecting them from the anguishing desire for, and of, the mother by putting them aside (into latency) and giving an identity that doesn't depend on satisfying the mother. The child's anguish is (in the ideal case) further resolved by the function of a universal Other signifying to the child that the sexed places are determined not by choice, character, or fault, but by a universal distribution in which each one has a place.

It is implied here, though not made explicit until subsequent years of Lacan's seminar, that the phallus as signifier of desire knots something of the Real of jouissance such that it can be recognised by the Other—that is, signifies it as lacking, desired, and sought in the sexual partner. The lost object *a* becomes the reserve of infantile sexuality which erects the phallus—the singularity of a jouissance whose adhesion to the body of the mother has been cut and knotted to the universal of a position taken in relation to the phallus.

Thus love for the father determines the eventual sexual identity of the child and his Name plays a role in all of the turns which establish subjectivity: the mother being symbolised to the child as castrated, the child grasping what it has (its sexual identity) and its sexuality being put out of play of the field of the mother. Lacan's notion of the Oedipus complex is therefore not so much a Freudian story of incestuous desire prohibited, as an operation that rescues the child from its captivation by the mother's unconscious signifiers in order that it become subject to a desirous signifying chain of its own: a move from being *asujetti* to being subject. By the Paternal Metaphor the child becomes a named one amongst others.

It ought to be noted in passing that Lacan will later theorise femininity as having a relation to the lack in the Other beyond that of phallic signification (Lacan, 1972–1973, pp. 64–89). He will also develop a theory of psychosis as a failure of the paternal function and therefore of phallic signification (Lacan, 1958, pp. 445–488). In Seminar V he is outlining what he regards as the normative position. Subsequent developments in his work on the neuroticising effects of the paternal function and love for the father will also expose to what extent the present depiction is an ideal one.

Father love

It is at this third moment of the Paternal Metaphor that love for the father is crucial, and Lacan will later call the salvation found there *père-version*: turning towards (*vers*) the father's *version* of sexuality (Lacan, 1982, p. 167). The ideal father of the Metaphor represents sexuality as a matter of *having* rather than *being something for* an Other; of desiring rather than seeking to be loved. *Père-version* will make the father not an ideal for the ego, but a model for the unconscious of how to do with jouissance—by making a father-symptom. We have seen that sexuality concerns more than signified identity as a man or woman—it also involves the "real satisfaction". The father's prohibition makes fall those maternal objects *a*—gaze and voice—which endowed the child as beloved object. Other objects of real satisfaction had already been prohibited. What Lacan adds to his later version is that the potent father knows how to find sexual satisfaction by electing a woman into the place of these objects in order to fix his jouissance there by the repeating letter of the symptom. This is his *perversion*.

If the Paternal Metaphor symbolises the father as bearing the phallus which makes him desired by the mother, it is implicit that the father is loved by the child insofar as he is a man who takes the mother as a woman. What the child has of signified relations is with a father and a mother, so the Metaphor necessitates the paternal, but then makes the bridge between father and man, mother and woman: from the familial into the social. Thus it needs the paternal yet requires its annihilation and replacement by the masculine; requires the establishment of the place of an exception, but also its effacement by the series. It is in this respect that it is not only normativising but potentially neuroticising, leading to the anguishing and depressing effects of the castration complex which Freud and Lacan both outlined in their work. Love or hate for the father as exception to castration testifies to the hope of attaining that place. It entrains masculine anxiety and inhibition of believing in the phallus of the Father, feminine disappointment in seeking the Father rather than *a* man, or the feminine madness of believing in Man as exception (Lacan, 1990, p. 40).

How then can a subject exit *Vatersehnsucht*? How, having identified with an exception, can a subject become one of the series of men and women? This is one of the orienting questions of Lacan's later work.

References

Freud, S. (1900a). *The Interpretation of Dreams. S.E.*, 4–5. London: Hogarth.

Freud, S. (1905d). Three Essays on the Theory of Sexuality. *SE.*, 7: 125–245. London: Hogarth.

Freud, S. (1923b). The Ego and the Id. *S.E.*, 19: 3–69. London: Hogarth Press.

Freud, S. (1927c). Future of an Illusion. *S.E.*, 21: 3–58. London: Hogarth Press.

Freud, S. (1930a). Civilisation and its Discontents. *S.E.*, 21: 59–198. London: Hogarth Press.

Freud, S. (1939a [1937–1939]). Moses and Monotheism: Three Essays. *S.E.*, 23. London: Hogarth Press.

Freud, S. (1950a [1887–1902]). Extracts from the Fleiss Papers. *S.E.*, 1: 175–282. London: Hogarth Press.

Lacan, J. (1956-1957). *The Seminar of Jacques Lacan, Book IV: The Object Relation 1956-1957.* L.V.A. Roche (Trans.). Unpublished manuscript.

Lacan, J. (1957–1958). *The Seminar of Jacques Lacan, Book V: The Formations of the Unconscious 1957–1958.* C. Gallagher (Trans.). Karnac Books.

Lacan, J. (1958). On a Question Prior to Any Possible Treatment of Psychosis. In:*Écrits: The First Complete Edition in English* (pp. 455–488). B. Fink (Trans.). New York and London: W. W. Norton & Company, 2006.

Lacan, J. (1958–1959). *The Seminar of Jacques Lacan, Book VI: Desire and its Interpretation 1958–1959.* C. Gallagher (Trans.). Karnac Books.

Lacan, J. (1959–1960). *The Ethics of Psychoanalysis 1959–1960: The Seminar of Jacques Lacan Book VII.* J.-A. Miller (Ed.), D. Porter (Trans.). London: Routledge, 1992.

Lacan, J. (1960). The Subversion of the Subject and the Dialectic of Desire in the Freudian Unconscious. In: *Écrits: The First Complete Edition in English* (pp. 671–702). B. Fink (Trans.). New York and London: W. W. Norton & Company, 2006.

Lacan, J. (1960–1961). *The Seminar of Jacques Lacan, Book VIII: Transference 1960–1961.* C. Gallagher (Trans.). Karnac Books.

Lacan, J. (1962–1963). *The Seminar of Jaques Lacan, Book X: Anxiety 1962–1963.* C. Gallagher (Trans.). Karnac Books.

Lacan, J. (1969–1970). *The Other Side of Psychoanalysis: The Seminar of Jacques Lacan Book XVII.* R. Grigg (Trans.). New York & London: W. W. Norton & Company., 2007.

Lacan, J. (1972–1973). *On Feminine Sexuality, the Limits of Love and Knowledge 1972–1973. Encore: The Seminar of Jacques Lacan Book XX.* J.-A. Miller (Ed.) & B. Fink (Trans.). New York & London: W. W. Norton & Company, 1998.
Lacan, J. (1974–1975). *The Seminar of Jacques Lacan, Book XXII: R.S.I., 1974-1975.* C. Gallagher (Trans.). Karnac Books.
Lacan, J. (1982). Seminar of 21 January 1975. In: J. Mitchell & J. Rose (Eds.), *Feminine Sexuality: Jacques Lacan & the École Freudienne* (pp. 162–171). London: MacMillan Press.
Lacan, J. (1989). Geneva lecture on the symptom. *Analysis*, 1: 7–26.
Lacan, J. (1990). *Television: A Challenge to the Psychoanalytic Establishment.* J. Copjec (Ed.) & J. Mehlman (Trans.). New York & London: W. W. Norton & Company.

PART 7

Obsessional

15

"WHY CAN'T A WOMAN BE MORE LIKE A MAN?"

The obsessional and the signifier

Nadezhda Almqvist

In Seminar V Lacan asks, "if the phallus is encountered in the barred form where it has the place of indicating the Other's desire, what about the subject?" (Lacan, 1957–1958, p. 329). In a highly condensed form Lacan here touches on several important ideas concerning neurotic subjectivity including the phallus as a signifier, repression, castration, and the desire of the Other. This essay is a commentary on Lacan's thought in Seminar V concerning the obsessional subject's relation to the signifier and simultaneously to desire. As a means of illustrating Lacan's thought, I will use the example of the obsessional linguist, Professor Henry Higgins from George Bernard Shaw's play *Pygmalion* (1912) and its Hollywood remake *My Fair Lady* (1964). While this short commentary will not, and cannot, give a complete overview of obsessional neurosis, it will attempt to draw on what I believe is essential to Lacan's thought on the subject at this moment in his teaching. Indeed, if the obsessional is, as Lacan says, "a man who lives amongst signifiers" (Lacan, 1957–1958, p. 446), or someone who "clings to everything that belongs to the verbal order" (ibid., p. 396), an exploration of the linguist Professor Higgins may offer a useful point of reference for reading Lacan's ideas.

Speaking Barbarian

When George Bernard Shaw's play *Pygmalion* (1912) was first performed, the science of speech and the comparative study of languages and dialects were already well developed. Shaw, himself a keen linguist, drew on these sources and his Professor Higgins was inspired by linguists and inventors with complex family histories, such as Alexander Melville Bell, Alexander Ellis and Henry Sweet (Shaw, 1916, p. 109). Linguists, of course, were not the only ones concerned with speech, and during this time Freud's theory and treatment of neurosis was already well known. For Freud, as Lacan notes, "man is constituted as a subject of speech" (Lacan, 1957–1958, p. 383) and adds that "desire is obliged to be mediated by the signifier" (ibid., p. 335). In the introduction to the Rat Man case, Freud makes some preparatory remarks which are important for understanding and contextualising Lacan's elaboration on how desire is structured in the locus of the Other (ibid., p. 418). Freud noted that "the language of an obsessional neurosis - the means by which it expresses its secret thoughts - is, as it were, only a dialect of the language of hysteria" (Freud, 1909, pp. 156–157). For Lacan too "in man's relationship to signifiers, the hysteric is a primordial structure" (Lacan, 1957–1958, p. 344).

Professor Higgins, to paraphrase Lacan on the obsessional, is "a man who lives amongst signifiers" (ibid., p. 446). Phonetics is more than a job for Higgins, it is also his hobby and since he is a confirmed old bachelor, there isn't that much going on outside of it (Shaw, 1912, p. 30). His house, equipped with everything that a highly cultured man like him could desire, could be described as a kind of temple to the Word. It is to this temple that Eliza Doolittle, a native English speaker, comes for English lessons and becomes his protégée. Higgins dismisses her at first, but something in Eliza fascinates him and out of curiosity he makes a bet with his colleague, Colonel Pickering, stating that in six months he can "make a duchess of this draggletailed guttersnipe" and teach her to speak properly (Shaw, 1912, p. 24). Eliza is more than a bet for Higgins but indeed a chance to demonstrate his notion that inequality is a result of speech, and that his knowledge of phonetics can help resolve class differences and open middle class opportunities for the poor. The Professor, however, is no simple altruist and his attitude quickly moves between compassion and hatred. In *Pygmalion* when Higgins first sees Eliza, he says: "A woman who utters such depressing and disgusting sounds has no right to be anywhere - no right to live" (ibid., p. 16).

Higgins's obsession with speech and social difference is not uncommon, and for many societies and theorists language remains a distinct mark of class difference. Among the ancient Greeks for example, speech was a key trait of civilisation and those who couldn't speak Greek, or spoke Greek badly, were called *barbaroi*. A barbarian, derived from the sound *bar bar,* is someone who speaks incomprehensibly with grammatical errors, confusion, non-sense and slips (Levine Gera, 2003, p. 192). If the word "barbarian" is defined in opposition to comprehensible speech, could we not say then that in this word we discover division; on the one hand the conscious, articulate speaker, and on the other, the subject *(bar)*barred by the signifier? Indeed it may be no coincidence that in his bet with his friend Pickering, Higgins refers to Eliza in the film as a "barbarous wretch" (Warner & Cuker, 1964). In other words, Higgins discovers a speaking barbarian, marked by the phallic signifier, and via this identification he will discover himself as (*bar*)barred subject: "insofar as the Other's desire is barred [that] the subject will recognize his own barred desire, his own unsatisfied desire"(Lacan, 1957–1958, p. 345). Yet for Lacan, the speech articulated by the split subject is barred not so much for the others but barred to himself.

Civilising myths

If speech constitutes the barbaric, does it also constitute what we think of as "civilised"? Indeed, where do these observances lead us if not to the heart of Freud's theory concerning the origins of civilisation? For Freud, civilisation begins with a barbaric murderous thought, the killing of the father by the primal horde, represented in the Oedipus complex with the result of repression (Freud, 1913, p. 146). The death of the father in the Oedipus complex emphasises his function as a signifier substituting for the maternal signifier, which, as Lacan further develops it, has a normalising effect for the subject (Lacan, 1957–1958, p. 152). Lacan's reading of *Totem and Taboo* (Freud, 1913) emphasises the death of the father who becomes a signifier, which organises the rest of the signifiers, hence "the close link that exists between death and the emergence of signifiers" (Lacan, 1957–1958, p. 292). Dismissed by many as poor speculation on Freud's part, Lacan sees the event as hugely important as in this work he links desire and the signifier. However, sometimes the father, who is the agent, supported by civilisation, for one reason or another doesn't exercise his function of prohibition in the complex. As a result the Oedipal scenario doesn't take place and the father is not hated and killed. The prohibition of the father, or whatever the subject can make use of in the absence of a father in the complex, introduces the child into a discourse beyond the desire for the mother. In Seminar V Lacan refers to three moments that take place in the Oedipus complex which when successful allow the child to move away from the position of an object for the mother in the primordial phallic stage (ibid., p. 186). In an attempt to symbolise the mother's lack, her presence and absence, the subject enters language. Without the desire of the mother, the subject never becomes alienated by the signifier. The consequence of this failure affects the subject in a profound way. The body, which is a gift of the word, remains unsymbolised and the drives unmediated by language abandon the human body to a primal and traumatic satisfaction. Without the desire of the mother, the development of the ego and the narcissistic identifications also become problematic. From the beginning, the life of the subject, beyond its physical existence, is dependent on the space of lack brought by the speech of the mother. Lacan notes that the child's desire aims not at the mother, but towards the mother's desire. Beyond satisfaction the child discovers that there is something left for the mother to desire. It is this desire of the mother, the mother as lacking, that becomes the prioritised object. If the child succeeds in becoming the imaginary phallus, the place of lack will be closed off and the subject will lose any sense of being since the sense of being is supported by lack. The lack in the Other becomes the necessary condition for the formation of the subject. If there is space preserved for lack in the discourse of the mother, the child, via this lack, is in a position of the object of desire. Without it, the child's destiny is to become an object of jouissance for the mother. Of course, the Oedipal myth is a myth inherited from Ancient Greek civilisation, and other cultures have their own myths (Malinowski, 1927) and sometimes the complex can be resolved under a different signifier (Chekurova,

2013). The subject can make use of any signifier, substituting for the father and resolving to an extent the problem with maternal desire (Lacan, 1957–1958, p. 292). In the classical Oedipus complex, the father intervenes and prevents this from happening by separating the child from becoming the imaginary phallus for the mother. Evidently, as part of this process, the father is feared, hated, and rebelled against, since he prohibits the mother and this gives a rise to the murderous thoughts against the father and the desire for the mother becomes repressed. In turn, the subject identifies with the dead father, the signifier. For this precise reason Freud believed that pushing away these murderous and incestuous desires into the unconscious and strengthening the prohibition to such an extent by internalising it in the voice of the superego was what made a man civilised. From this we can expect to discover the mother as an object that dominates the unconscious of every civilised man (Freud, 1912d, p. 163- 175).

Peony or daisy? The mask beyond the flower

It might help to illustrate the above discussion through some reflections on Higgins's relationship to Eliza. In a discussion with his mother Higgins states:

> I can't be bothered with young women. My idea of a loveable woman is something as like you as possible, I shall never get into the way of seriously liking young women: some habits lie too deep to be changed.
>
> *(Shaw, 1912, pp. 43–44)*

Although Higgins's characterisation is almost identical in Shaw's *Pygmalion* and the film *My Fair Lady* (Warner & Cuker, 1964), the Hollywood remake is more centred on the love story between Higgins and Eliza than on the relationship between Higgins and his mother. The play and the film in this way present us with two kinds of loves and perspectives on Higgins's desire. The director of *My Fair Lady* highlights this question in the opening scene of the film where we see a sequence juxtaposing images of two flowers. The images of the flowers shift from one to the other as if asking a question, posing a dilemma. Peonies are beautiful, rich in colour, decadent, and glamorous, like the dresses of the ladies leaving the theatre. The daisy, on the other hand, is from a species most often referred to as the common daisy, the kind of flower which, like desire, can grow in places where it is not necessarily planned, almost like an unwanted weed. Yet, the daisy is also the flower through whose petals the question of love is raised.

Just a couple of years before the play *Pygmalion* (1912), Freud had already drawn attention to the importance of such an opposition in two essays, "A Special type of Choice Object Made by Men" (Freud, 1910h) and "On The Universal Tendency to Debasement in the Sphere of Love" (Freud, 1912d). Here he explores the question concerning what kind of object governs the love life of neurotic men and discovers a division noting that "[w]here they love they do not desire and where they desire they cannot love." (Freud, 1912d, p. 183). In *Seminar V* Lacan revisits debasement in love life as a discovery "which stems from the depths of the Oedipus complex" (Lacan, 1957–1958, p. 308). This phenomenon occurs for men who have not sufficiently abandoned the mother as a love object, conditioned as preferred by the fact that it has been prohibited. Its occurrence is so common that Freud concludes that "a certain amount of this behaviour does in fact characterize the love of civilized man." (Freud, 1912d, p. 184). In other words, the dissociation between love and desire is marked by splitting. The mother is split in two separate halves - the affectionate feelings are kept for one woman that will be loved and respected but not desired, and another, the opposite of the mother, the prostitute type who will embody the sensual side. If once again we return to the opening scene in the film we see how the peony could stand for the loved woman. The idea that the daisy stands for the debased object for Professor Higgins is suggested also by its name - *Leucanthemum vulgare*. In many respects Eliza stands for the prostitute type since she comes from a lower class than Higgins, uneducated, and with suspect morals. It may be no coincidence that in the scene where we are first introduced to Eliza, due to her misunderstanding of Higgins's interest in her speech, she defends herself against the imagined accusation of being a prostitute and declares herself as a "good girl" (Shaw, 1912, p. 13). This idea that Eliza represents the prostitute type is best captured in Higgins's words: "she is so deliciously low - so horribly dirty" (ibid, p. 23).

In Lacan's reading, the significance of the prostitute as a mother substitute derives from the observation that she appears under a mask. It is exactly through this notion of the mask that unconscious desire appears to the extent that to Lacan they are identical (Lacan, 1957–1958, p. 306). In this line of thought we can say that Higgins is interested in Eliza not simply as the proper lady she becomes, represented by the peony, or as a common girl, represented by the daisy, but by the very situation that he cannot pin her down to one or the other. Eliza captures his desire insofar as she wears the mask, insofar as she doesn't reveal herself and remains ambiguous, an enigma to him. Paradoxically, in a short space of time this common girl not only enters his home, but manages to make the Professor neglect everything else and treat her as the most important thing in his life. Indeed, he falls in love with Eliza.

Women as punishment for some men

In *Seminar V*, discussing castration, Lacan says:

> It's palpable at every moment in this observation that the solution to the analysis of the obsessional is that he comes to discover castration for what it is, that is, the law of the Other. This Other that is castrated. For reasons that have to do with his mistaken implication in this problem, the subject feels that he himself is threatened by this castration at a level that is so acute that he can't come near his own desire without feeling its effects.
>
> *(Lacan, 1957–1958, p. 413)*

Higgins's behaviour after winning the bet and the resultant shift in his relationship to Eliza may be a useful way of unpacking this discussion. Higgins's life becomes disrupted in such a way that he cannot carry on as usual. Eliza, who until this point was happy to play along, now that the bet has been won and she can speak like a lady, doesn't find space for herself as desired by the now satisfied Higgins. Her reaction is not that unusual as psychoanalysis shows the effects satisfaction can have on desire. As if forgotten by all, Eliza appears to be more like a trophy of his victory, fallen from a place of being a cause of his desire to a cause of his satisfaction, which leads her to what Lacan refers as a narcissistic demand for love in hysteria (Lacan, 1957–1958, p. 348; p. 361; p. 376). She confronts him and they have an argument in which the professor loses his temper and Eliza leaves the house. Until this point, he more or less had successfully managed to annul her desire by reducing it to a demand in the way he deals with the other woman in his life, such as his mother or his servant. After the scene with the bet he is not able to do so anymore. What is it that Eliza, a common girl, wants beyond a warm bed, new opportunities, or her beloved chocolates? Whatever it is he falls in love with her. If Lacan says that beyond demand there is something that cannot be articulated and cannot be reduced to a demand, it is here that Higgins discovers it in Eliza's discourse. Once again, he unsuccessfully tries to reduce her desire to a particular demand when she tells him: "I can do without you" (Shaw, 1912, p. 77). This surprises him since his entire life is organised avoiding confronting the desire of the Other (hence - we might interpret - the original title of the Shaw's play *Pygmalion*, derived from another Greek myth where the hero falls in love with a beautiful but lifeless statue). In other words, Higgins tries to undo her desire so that he can be what she desires but he becomes the prey of his own destruction.

In the encounter with desire via Eliza's speech, Higgins experiences subjective division or what Lacan refers to as "the dimension of hysteria latent in every kind of human being" (Lacan, 1957–1958, p. 441). On the one hand Higgins seems to be an (extra)ordinary man since no human struggle touches him: "I can do without anybody. I have my own soul: my own spark of divine fire" (Shaw, 1912, p. 78). His lack of strife leads him to spend his days in solitude and doing exactly what he wants, which happens to be reading books and listening to the way people speak. When Eliza confronts him with desire he lays down on the couch (just like an analysand) and starts grinding his teeth, experiencing feelings that are reserved only for women or brought on by them. In his words: "I find that the moment I let myself make friends with a woman, I become selfish and tyrannical. Women upset everything" (Shaw, 1912, p. 29). The space opened up in Eliza's discourse for desire makes Higgins experience repressed anger, half-jokingly he even tries to strike her. Why is this? One answer is simply to state that Henry Higgins is a misogynist. But answers like this are mere labels which provide answers rendering it unnecessary to listen anymore, and moreover still doesn't explain why he hates women. There is one thing that he hates even more than women and these are the feelings brought to the fore by women. Let's not forget that he is the kind of man who is very conscientious of not letting insulting remarks slip out of his mouth, which clearly suggests the existence of such insulting thoughts. If Higgins is the kind of educated man Freud discusses, and if he experiences Eliza's desire as Oedipal, this desire then reactivates the repressed problems with the father, namely the signifier. From this perspective the hatred and troubles with women are underlined by repressed anger and hatred for the father as a prohibition. Avoiding women is a way therefore to avoid what is repressed, unconscious desire.

Higgins's ambivalence towards Eliza is hardly unique and the idea that women are an endless source of problems is neither new nor uncommon. We only have to remember the stories of Adam and Eve or Prometheus, who stole fire from the gods and brought it to mortal men. The gods were not pleased and woman, a beautiful evil, was created as a punishment (for e.g., Hesiod, 1964, *Theog.*, l. 565–612). What could potentially become problematic for obsessionals such as Higgins is that through sexual difference the subject encounters castration anxiety. The myth of Prometheus then can suggest an Oedipal reading: the creation of women by the gods as a punishment for men has little to do with hatred for women but a lot to do with repressed hatred for the father. What this myth emphasises is the destiny of *desire stuck in prohibition* and all the troubles that this brings to the life of an enlightened man. The gods of Ancient Greece already knew a lot about the conditions of human desire and how to be cruel; they gave men what they wanted. As a result they were confronted with the most intolerable feelings in the life of civilised man.

From destroying to restoring the other and beyond

For Lacan the relation of the obsessional subject to desire is marked by contradiction. Often the subject attempts to resolve the problem with desire by making it forbidden (Lacan, 1957–1958, p. 393). Is it a coincidence that Higgins's entire life is dedicated to what can very well be Lacan's idea of the obsessional restoration of the Other, in Higgins's case - maintaining demand? The problems with the father are brought up by the lack in the Other and are directly implicated in what Lacan calls regression to demand (ibid., p. 392). This regression can be understood as an obsessional's complicated strategy of dealing with desire by simultaneously destroying it and preserving it. The obsessional treats demand as precious and important in so far as what is beyond it is nothing other than the subject's desire. In the obsessional mode of existence the subject has entered language and with this has discovered the desire of the Other. The shift that highlights the predominant relation to the Other via demand, takes place when he encounters the (*bar*)barred Other Eliza, whose words make him experience himself as a (*bar*)barred subject. His strategy in order to avoid dealing with the effects of castration, is to *make peace by making it forbidden*, hence he is a confirmed bachelor. Therefore the paternal deficiency in the complex is resolved to some extent via the fabrication of neurosis as a way of sustaining the necessary space for desire. In order to prevent completing the Other and with this disappearance of desire, the subject's relationship to the other is *articulated at the level of demand*, for the reason that desire can never be fully articulated in demand and therefore is destroyed. As long as the relationship with the other is restored to the level of demand, desire will remain alive. Professor Higgins's life is a good example of someone who is quite happy to work very hard. His dedication to the Other, noted by Lacan in relation to the exploit, is so observable that even his own servants regard him a slave. Working very hard indeed could be one solution to avoid castration anxiety. Lacan comments:

> The obsessional subject is caught in this contradiction. He is constantly occupied in maintaining the Other and making him subsist through imaginary formulations which occupy him more than anyone. They are established to support the Other who is perpetually in danger of falling, of succumbing to the demand for death, for this Other is the essential condition for him to maintain himself as a subject.
>
> *(Lacan, 1957–1958, p. 459)*

Freud (1930a) had already stressed the importance of neurotic guilt in "Civilization and its Discontents" which Lacan also discusses in relation to the obsessional's demand for death. Guilt reveals a subject who is fixated on a *demand stuck in prohibition*, prohibited for the reason that threatens the necessary condition of lack. The restoration of the Other can be understood as emerging from the same place of *fear of death of demand* as Lacan, following Freud, notes that for the obsessional, the most troubling demand is the demand for death, where the subject loses his/her words (Lacan, 1957–1958, p. 468).

The more the Other is destroyed, the more he becomes a subject to guilt, the more he enslaves himself in the service of the Other. In some respects, Higgins's behaviour can be reduced to this idea of preserving the signifier, the divine speech, because it sustains the place for desire. If his religion is the *science of speech*, suggested also by the scene where he first appears, namely under the columns of St. Paul's Church, then is his behaviour a form of blasphemy or what Lacan refers to as verbal "destruction of the Other?" (ibid., p. 445). Perhaps out of this guilt for undoing the desire of the Other in the fantasy, he becomes someone who devotes his life to repair the Other via speech by teaching the poor how to speak properly and overcome the effects of class difference (notwithstanding how overcoming class difference can be another form of disavowal). In this line of thought his behaviour in society demonstrates another path that this destruction can go. Although an educated man, his manners are rude, which is even more significant considering how important they are for the society in which he lives. He often appears with inappropriate clothing for an occasion which has a strict dress code or has a disrespectful attitude that worries his mother. What are these behaviours if not a form of destruction of the Other at the level of the signifier? The bet with Pickering to pass a flower girl for a lady follows a similar logic. Having a common flower girl in the same room together with aristocrats is scandalous for society's unwritten rules of behaviour. Does this not degrade the rank of the aristocrat's title to the rank of the ordinary, the peony to the daisy? Or perhaps his behaviour stands for a refusal to limit his discourse to that of a society which doesn't question its own values and where ultimately one's acceptance is based on shallow and artificial behaviour? A discourse where the subject is not treated like a speaking being but rather as a presentable object in the eyes of society? Perhaps his obsession with language and the mechanical way in which he treats human speech, devoid of any desire, is underlined by this alienation. Or perhaps this is his attempt to separate from the demand of the Other, often heard in relation to the demand that children speak, dress, and behave properly? Isn't it emblematic that he recommends Eliza's father, who appears to be the most immoral character, to become a leading moralist? In this way Higgins's choice to live surrounded with books is a way of expanding beyond the shallow discourse of his immediate society and an attempt to search for different values.

Conclusions

As a way to avoid confrontation with castration due to unresolved Oedipus complex, Shaw's character Higgins preferred to deal with the Other at the level of demand, which brought him to discover the *(bar)*barred subject ($\$$). His decision to keep his distance from women is grounded by the same problem. To him women are irrational and therefore difficult to deal with precisely because they are different. Women confront him with something that he cannot completely make sense of. Unlike the other people in his life that he destroys and serves, there is something about Eliza that he can neither destroy nor serve, something that he cannot fully articulate, explain, or rationalise. Different from the rest who make more or less sense in his life, she becomes an enigma and leaves a man otherwise quite content with his life, wondering. In this line of thought Freud also had recognised this enigma attached to the desire of the obsessional and wrote: "I must confess that I have not yet succeeded in completely penetrating the complicated texture of a *severe* case of obsessional neurosis" (Freud, 1909, p. 156). In other words something in the obsessional mode of subjectivity resisted being understood completely, preserving space beyond the significations for the Other. In Seminar V Lacan proposes that desire is an x beyond meaning that the question makes (Lacan, 1957–1958, p. 307). The question mark points towards something like a riddle that remains not fully resolved and hence cannot be reduced to demand. A question which may sound like Higgins's "*Why can't a woman be more like a man?*" (Warner & Cuker, 1964). Perhaps this is another way of raising Freud's question: "*What does a woman want?*"(Freud quoted in Jones, 1955, p. 468).

References

Chekurova, N. (2013). *A Name Which Is Not Oedipus? The Subject in a Society Without Fathers.* MA thesis, Independent Colleges Dublin.

Freud, S. (1909). Notes Upon a Case of Obsessional Neurosis. *S.E.*, 10: 150–250. London: Hogarth Press.

Freud, S. (1910h). A Special Type of Choice of Object Made by Men (Contributions to the Psychology of Love II). *S.E.*,11: 164–175. London: Hogarth Press.

Freud, S. (1912d). On the Universal Tendency to Debasement in the Sphere of Love (Contributions to the Psychology of Love II). *S.E.*, 11: 177–190. London: Hogarth Press.

Freud, S. (1913 [1912-13]). Totem and Taboo. *S.E.*, 13: 1–162. London: Hogarth Press.

Freud, S. (1930a). Civilization and its Discontents. *S.E.*, 21: 57–146. London: Hogarth Press.

Hesiod. (1964). *Hesiod, The Homeric Hymns and Homerica.* E. White (Trans.). London: Harvard University Press.

Jones, E. (1955). *The Life and Work of Sigmund Freud. Volume II.* New York: Basic Books.

Lacan, J. (1957–1958). *Formations of the Unconscious: The Seminar of Jacques Lacan, Book V.* J.-A. Miller & R. Grigg (Trans.) Cambridge: Polity, 2017.

Levine Gera, D. (2003). *Ancient Greek Ideas on Speech, Language, and Civilization.* New York: Oxford University Press.

Malinowski, B. (1927). *Sex and Repression in Savage Society Volume IV.* London and New York: Routledge, 2002.

Shaw, G. B. (1912). *Pygmalion.* Pennsylvania: Pennsylvania State University, 2004.

Shaw, G. B. (1916). *Androcles and the Lion; Overruled; Pygmalion.* New York City: Brentano's.

Warner, J. L. (Producer), & Cuker, G. (Director). (1964). *My Fair Lady* [Film]. United States: Warner Bros.

16

OBSESSIONAL DESIRE IN SEMINAR V

The exploits of Tantalus

Lorenzo Chiesa

The contradiction of pure desire

In many regards, Seminar V stands as a crucial moment in Lacan's oeuvre. Moving from the general assumption that the unconscious is structured like a language – that it fundamentally consists of repressed signifying chains (Lacan, 1957–1958, p. 410) – it is in Seminar V that he provides his most extensive updating of Freud's Oedipus complex (in terms of both individual ontogenesis and universal structure), as well as of the latter's psychoanalytic approach to the formations of the unconscious (especially jokes and dreams). It is also here that Lacan first develops his well-known "graph of desire", which goes together with a careful dialectical differentiation of the notions of need, demand, love, and desire. As Moustapha Safouan puts it, "The Formations of the Unconscious represents the end of a stage in Lacan's teaching – that of his linguistic 'return to Freud'. Had he left us only these first five seminars, we should already attribute him a considerable oeuvre" (Safouan, 2001, p. 105). We also have to bear in mind that four of Lacan's seminal *écrits* were drafted during Seminar V and rely on it: "On a Question Prior to any Possible Treatment of Psychosis", "The Youth of Gide", "The Signification of the Phallus", and "The Direction of the Treatment and the Principles of its Power".

Commentators have explored, at least in part, all these aspects of Seminar V (Chiesa, 2007; Dor, 1998; Evans, 1996; Fink, 1995). But, surprisingly, what has so far been mostly overlooked is the fact that the final third of this long Seminar is devoted to a punctual clinical application of the densely theoretical lessons that precede it. For Lacan, it is a matter of putting into practice the dialectic of desire and demand in the day-to-day treatment of neuroses (Lacan, 1957–1958, p. 399).

In this chapter, I aim to provide an in-depth reading of two lessons from Seminar V (XXII and XXIII) that explicitly focus on the obsessional neurotic's desire. I will also draw on lessons XXIV to XXVIII, where obsession remains one of the leitmotivs. Lacan defines obsessional desire as marked by a "profound contradiction" and as eventually an "impasse" (Lacan, 1957–1958, pp. 401–402, p. 485, p. 494). On the one hand, the obsessional looks for his desire in a "beyond" that corresponds with "desire as such" (ibid., p. 393, p. 400). On the other hand, this very movement is inextricable from an attempted "destruction of the Other" and, more specifically, of his desire (ibid, pp. 401–403, p. 468, p. 472, p. 484). Commenting on Maurice Bouvet, and criticising him, Lacan argues that the analyst should always bear in mind this general contradiction when, in directing the cure, he observes the phenomenology of obsessional desire, and its revolving around a set of recurrent destructive behaviours – if not symptoms – traditionally explained by psychoanalytic literature in connection with incorporation, aggressiveness, sadistic fantasies, not to mention guilt.

I will not deal with Lacan's critique of Bouvet's case studies. Suffice it to say that the latter would miss not only the contradiction on which the obsessional as a subject is as such structured, but also, in close relation to this, his failure to undergo castration. I also wish to specify that this article focuses on the clinical aspects of Seminar V to the extent that, for Lacan, the treatment of neurosis presupposes the recognition of obsession and hysteria as unconscious "modes of subjectivation" (ibid., p. 395, p. 431) on which the entire phenomenology of neurotic behaviours and symptoms is based. I will not tackle Lacan's – quite sporadic but precious – remarks on the direction of the cure, e.g., the handling of the transference; its distance from suggestion; the positive role of resistance; the actual coordinates of regression; etc. (ibid., pp. 443–45, p. 434, pp. 413–14).

***

Lacan's most basic point in Seminar V is that both obsessional and hysterical neuroses revolve as such around a problematic subjective orientation towards *sexual* desire (ibid., p. 396, p. 406, pp. 383–84). It would not be inaccurate to suggest that he generally understands desire as located *in between* need and demand; quite explicitly, "desire takes its place and organises itself … in between the call for satisfaction and the demand for love" (ibid., p. 406). Against superficial accusations of "idealism", Lacan does not deny the existence of sexual need on a level that, for the sake of simplification, we could call "natural" or "instinctual". In the case of *Homo sapiens*, need is, however, always already filtered, fragmented, and isolated by language. In other words, need cannot be separated from the dimension of *demand* as something that structurally exceeds it. This is already witnessed to by the fact that the incessant demands of a child tend not to stop when he is granted access to the objects he demands, that is, when he is satisfied of his needs (which, for psychoanalysis, invariably involve a sexual element). Demand thus eventually amounts to an unconditional demand *for love*: "Demand is fundamentally a demand for love – a demand for nothing, no particular satisfaction", but for what the Other "brings by means of his pure and simple answer to the demand" (ibid., p. 381).

In this context, on the one hand, desire originates from the unconditional horizon opened by the demand for love; it amounts to a desire for desire. More precisely, desire turns the unconditionality of demand into an "absolute condition" (ibid., p. 382) – absolute in the sense that it has "no measure or proportion with the need for any object whatsoever" (ibid.). On the other hand, desire nevertheless *recuperates* the sexual content of need, which is bypassed by the pure demand for love, within the same linguistic horizon. Throughout Seminar V desire is indeed often qualified as "sexual desire" (in later seminars this will be articulated in terms of the *drive*). Commentators usually underestimate this second characteristic of desire but Lacan could not be more adamant about it: "Desire … is not simply sexual instinct [yet] of course [it] does not eliminate the existence of tendencies" (ibid., p. 374); "Desire … is located beyond demand [in that it] gives back the margin of deviation marked by the incidence of the signifier on need" (ibid., p. 381); even more conclusively: "in relation to the demand for love, *sexual need becomes desire* … How could we produce our desires if we did not borrow their primordial matter from our needs?" (ibid., pp. 382–83, my emphasis).

In the lesson that introduces his discussion of obsession, Lacan reiterates that desire lies in "a field beyond demand" (ibid., p. 393). It is precisely in this beyond – to be understood as a negation, or sublation, of the negation carried out by demand with respect to need – that desire emerges as "sexual desire" (ibid.). To stress a distinction without which the entire treatment of neuroses in Seminar V would remain obscure, desire is not only beyond demand as a specific demand for the satisfaction of a particular need (as seen, demand itself is already beyond this level; hence here it would be impossible to distinguish desire from demand). Desire is first and foremost beyond demand as a demand essentially determined by the *de*sexualised demand for love – again, desire recovers sexual need in the very linguistic field that the demand for love opens beyond sexual need.

***

To put it in a somewhat crude fashion, according to Lacan, neurotics fail to appropriately assume the dialectical beyond of demand as the field of sexual desire. Because of this they experience all sort of concrete difficulties in relating sexually to their counterparts. The least we can say is that such a failure involves a certain confusion of demand with desire to the detriment of the latter, as well as an insufficient appreciation of the fact that the field of desire stands primarily as the field of the Other's desire, whose inscrutability cannot be reduced to the logic of demand and response. The desire of the subject as a subject split by language – and hence unconscious – is famously for Lacan the desire of the other (as desiring the other, being recognised by him, and ideally occupying his place), but in turn it more structurally depends on the Other's desire (initially in the guise of the Mother's desire) as the cipher of the Other's *own Spaltung* (ibid., p. 394). The Other, which ultimately consists of the impersonal locus of speech and the battery of signifiers as the presupposition for intersubjectivity, is itself split in the sense that language cannot fully represent sex: "Insofar as the human being is caught in the signifying dialectic, there is something that does not work [with respect to] finding the other sex" (ibid., p. 381; p. 383). This ontological disharmony is at bottom what the neurotic cannot cope with – *not even unconsciously*, unlike "complete"-as-split human subjects, Lacan banters at one point (ibid., p. 394). In other words, the neurotic does not undergo castration, that is, the symbolic operation through which the Other's *Spaltung*, or inconsistency, is partly signifierised.

In the case of hysteria, the subject can find a foothold, support, or prop [*point de appui*] for her desire only by short-circuiting it with the very inscrutability of the Other's desire (ibid., p. 396). The latter is thus in turn "supported" (ibid., p. 397) as an "enigmatic point" (ibid., p. 407) but also eclipsed in that the hysteric attempts (in vain) to reduce it to *her* desire as related to an imaginary counterpart (or *o*ther). As Lacan will put it in later seminars, the Other's desire therefore turns into a desire for the Other to be One, an alleged Master, with which the hysteric *identifies* in order to be herself One. This also means that the hysteric's emphasis on the Other's desire as an indecipherable x – her being "on the level of the Other" (ibid., p. 400) – does not serve the *opposition* between demand and desire as its beyond, but, on the contrary, endeavours to accommodate desire on the plane of the demand for love (ibid., p. 397).

In the case of obsession, the subject assumes a different relation to the Other's desire, which Lacan deems to be slightly more complicated (ibid., p. 398). While the hysteric "searches for her desire in the Other's desire" (ibid., p. 401) – as the desire she attributes to the Other only to limit it – the obsessional evidently "pushes through *his* desire above all else" (ibid., my emphasis). Like the hysteric and every other subject, the obsessional is constituted as a subject only by orienting himself towards desire; but what he aims at is "desire as such", his own desire "in a pure state" (ibid., pp. 400–401). This causes a "negation" and even an attempted "destruction" of the Other, on the levels of both demand and desire (ibid.). Most importantly, given that the subject's desire necessarily depends on the Other's desire, to which alone pertains the title of desire as such, it follows that the obsessional relation to desire is structured like a "profound contradiction" (ibid., p. 401). The obsessional aims at desire as such *without* the Other's desire, that is, without *desire as such*. To put it plainly, he desires a desire that would really be his desire. We are dealing with "the desire to have one's desire" (ibid., p. 430) and thus to make One as a subject. Or better, following the more comprehensive formula of Seminar XVI, the obsessional *paradoxically* aspires to *be One in the field of the Other* (Lacan, 1968–1969, p. 253, p. 260).

In order to explain obsessional subjectivity, Lacan resumes and develops his definition of desire as "beyond demand" (Lacan, 1957–1958, p. 400). As seen, on the one hand, desire goes beyond demand in that it recuperates the sexual need that the demand for love marginalised, and in this sense negated (from this perspective, Lacan can also speak – somewhat confusingly – of desire as "falling short of" or "on this side of demand" [*en deça de la demande*], since as demand for love demand "goes beyond all the satisfactions it calls for" and aims at "the Other's being" (ibid., p. 406)). Here we may say that desire *drives* sexual need back to the subject as a subject of language, by means of a negation of negation. Yet, on the other hand, desire surpasses demand also insofar as it transforms the *unconditional* character of the demand for love into something *absolute*. This is the side of desire that, when isolated as not dialectically articulated with the recuperation of sexual need, accounts for obsessional subjectivity – which is why Lacan speaks of *pure* desire with respect to the obsessional.

Lacan introduces his argument by focusing on "a child who will become an obsessional" (ibid., p. 400). For the sake of simplification, he considers the future obsessional's peculiar kind of demands at an ontogenetic stage at which desire is still embryonic. While other children demand *x*, and then *y*, and then *z* as contingent variables that only sustain the demand for love, the future obsessional presents a "fixed idea" (ibid.). He demands *x* (or *y*, or *z*) in such an insistent way that his parents find it "unbearable" (ibid., p. 401). This child already goes beyond demand in that he "negates the element of otherness included in the demand for love" (ibid.). To expand on Lacan, what matters to the future obsessional is not the demand for love – "It is not this or that I need; I demand to be loved" – where demand still relates negatively to the satisfaction of a particular need dependent on the Other. Rather, what matters to him is precisely the fixed idea – "I absolutely want *that*! I am not demanding to be loved" – where demand is in turn negated, or better, its unconditional character "persists" only as "transferred to *need" in language* (ibid., p. 400, my emphasis).

This re-emergence of need in desire should not surprise us if, with Lacan, we understand desire as a negation of demand's negation of need. However, the problem for the adult obsessional is that the negation of demand's negation of need exclusively coalesces as what Lacan very pertinently calls at one point the "*absolute form* of need" (ibid., p. 401), and not as a dialectical articulation of sexual need in language. In obsession, "desire is the absolute form of need, of need passed to the state of absolute condition, to the extent that it is beyond the unconditional demand [*exigence*] for love" (ibid., my emphasis). The future obsessional's "I *absolutely* want that!" prefigures the adult obsessional's "desire *as such*", which cannot be appropriated, and as always elusive is thus at odds with sexual desire.

***

Let me restate this crucial point. The obsessional's desire as "pure" desire is not strictly speaking a *sexual* desire. Or, it is a sexual desire that unfailingly privileges *desire* over the sexual object, even when it finds it after long detours. In Seminar V Lacan unpacks this issue by dwelling at length on the obsessional's contradiction with regard to desire. As seen, the obsessional's promotion of his desire, as desire as such, is "internally" (ibid., p. 401) contradicted by the fact that it goes together with an attempted destruction of the Other, on which desire inevitably depends. As evident in the example of the child who will become an obsessional, the Other is already vehemently negated on the level of demand, in the name of a nascent desire as beyond demand. But Lacan does not fail to remind us that "desire as such necessitates the support of the Other" (ibid., p. 402), and, more specifically, of the Other's desire: "The Other's desire is not one of the ways of access to the subject's desire, it is rather tout-court the place of desire" (ibid.). This contradiction generates a veritable "impasse", Lacan says, for the adult obsessional's desire (ibid.).

While the future obsessional – contradictorily enough – directly expresses his desire by means of an unbearable demand, which still requires the Other, albeit as negated, the adult obsessional – whose entire subjectivity amounts to a contradiction – represses his desire's fundamentally destructive nature and substitutes it with a host of apparently non-aggressive demands to his counterparts, or "good intentions", which Lacan also calls "obsessional culture" (ibid., p. 417, p. 402). Yet the obsessional continues to be "inhabited", and even "infested" (ibid., p. 402), by pure desire as a desire for the destruction of the Other. In the course of the treatment, if the transference is handled correctly, obsessional culture "does not last long" (ibid.). Outside of the psychoanalytic cabinet, the impasse of the obsessional's desire resurfaces most clearly when, "from time to time, taking his courage in his hands" (ibid.), the obsessional sets off to look for the sexual *object* of his desire. What regularly happens in these rare circumstances is that, first, the obsessional does not recover it easily, and, second, he "incurs the most extraordinary accidents" (ibid.), which immensely complicate his approach to the object.

For Lacan, it is not sufficient to account for these accidents in terms of the prohibiting agency of the superego, which would put a leash on the aggressive tendencies. In addition to that, we witness here something much more structural that concerns again the contradictory status of obsessional desire and is perceived even consciously in the "psychology" of the obsessional subject (ibid.). Namely, the more an object plays the role of the sexual object of desire, the more the obsessional experiences a "decrease of libidinal tension" in moving towards it (ibid., p. 402, p. 412). This is consonant with the fact that the obsessional aims at "desire as such" (ibid., p. 402), a desire for desire that is devoid of objects because it is itself its own object, or, as Lacan helpfully puts it, a "desire in its constitution as desire" (ibid.), a desire constantly in the making and eventually aimed at making One. As for the destructive aspect of such a pure desire, predictably, whenever the obsessional manages to reach the sexual object – not without debasing it (ibid., p. 468) – the attempt to eradicate the Other's desire immediately turns into a "disappearance" of the subject's own desire: "At the moment he has this object of his desire, [for the obsessional] nothing exists any longer" (ibid., pp. 402–403).

The obsessional can thus only subjectivise himself as "a Tantalus", self-condemned to eternal non-satisfaction all the more satisfaction appears to be within his grasp (ibid., p. 412).

Obsessional behaviours

Starting from the end of the first lesson on obsession and throughout the second, Lacan draws on the structural contradiction and subsequent impasse of the obsessional's desire in order to elucidate what he himself designates as typical obsessional "behaviours" (Lacan, 1957–1958, p. 403, pp. 419–20, pp. 474–75). The discussion centres on four ordinary and readily observable phenomena: the obsessional's overall abiding by the practical imperative "Do not do to others what you would not wish to be done to yourself" in everyday life (ibid., pp. 416–17); the mutual implication of his continuous asking for permission and having it refused (ibid., pp. 412–15); the "performance aspect" of the obsessional's activities, that is, his "exploits" (ibid., p. 403, pp. 417–420); and the ultimate proof he requests to corroborate an otherwise temporary and occasional "passionate love" (ibid., p. 421).

Here one cannot but be struck by how all these "cultured" behaviours – especially the first two – appear to assuage the obsessional's aggressive tendencies aimed at destroying the Other. At the beginning of lesson XXIII, Lacan unequivocally states that the obsessional's "access to [his] desire" is based on a "*dependence* on the Other" (ibid., p. 407, my emphasis), to an extent unmatched even by the hysteric. At first sight, this is quite stunning considering that in the previous lesson he contrasted the obsessional's pushing through his desire against the Other with the hysteric's initial being on the level of the Other. Lacan's basic argument becomes clear if we understand that the adult obsessional manages to sustain his unconscious "desire as such" to the detriment of the Other's desire only by "preserving at all costs" (ibid., p. 419) the Other through demand, in a way that is at least partly conscious. The attempted and never successful eradication of the Other's desire as irreducible to signification (as "real", using Lacan's later terminology) for the sake of the subject's absolute desire structurally necessitates the desperate "maintenance of the Other [as the locus] where things are articulated in terms of signifiers" (ibid.; see also pp. 471–2). (In the terms of Seminar XVI, the obsessional can try to keep at bay the *inconsistency* of the Other as real only by overestimating its *consistency* as symbolic.) Because otherwise the obsessional would have nowhere else to "*show*" his desire (ibid., p. 403, my emphasis), Lacan hints in passing, as confirmed on the few occasions in which he openly embraces it as directed against the o/Other only to see it decrease and disappear.

Obsession as a structural contradiction between "desire as such" and the destruction of the Other's desire (on which desire as such relies) thus also manifests two contradictory sides in its very phenomenology. The behaviours I listed above – all originating from an inaccurate dialecticisation of need, demand, and desire – make such a contradiction increasingly evident and unbearable.

1. *"Do not do to others what you would not wish to be done to yourself"*. Up to a point, the obsessional effectively camouflages his destructive intentions and his desire with them. On this level, orchestrated as a "moralising standpoint" (ibid., p. 416), he by and large relates to the Other as an *other*, or imaginary counterpart, and endeavours to reduce desire to a reciprocal recognition of demands. He accordingly tends to altruistically submit to the other's demands. But precisely because of his avoidance of the unbridgeable gap between demand and desire, he also at the same time contradictorily demands that his *desire* be recognised by the other. That is, the obsessional asks the other to

"*consent*" to his desire (ibid., my emphasis). Given the latter's being beyond demand, consent cannot, however, be obtained, as it would have to be granted "in a fashion completely different from the answer to a demand" (ibid.). Consent is an "illusion", a "fantasy" (ibid.), which is even within the conscious reach of the obsessional, yet he prefers to "elude the problem" (ibid.). He does so by soon turning the good intentions of the "It is enough to reach an agreement … to find happiness in life" into a far less uplifting "Do not do to others what you would not wish to be done to yourself" (ibid., pp. 416–17). This should in turn be read as an already rather disturbing "It is enough not to inflict on others the frustrations of which one has oneself been the object" (ibid, p. 416). All in all, the obsessional concretely lives most of his existence following the ambivalent principle "Spare the other!" (ibid., p. 417). His symptoms – "a whole series of ceremonials, precautions, detours [but also of] tricks, schemes, and intrigues [*manigances*]" (ibid.) – should be led back to it. (Lacan adds two important clinical specifications. First, directing the treatment of the obsessional along the lines of respectful "oblativity" as a correct access to "genital maturity" (ibid., p. 416) only reinforces his already oblative fantasy and, at best, displaces the symptoms. Second, and in relation to this, if it could ever be really implemented, the categorical imperative "Do not do to others what you would not wish to be done to yourself" would assuredly be completely beside the point "when it is a question of a realisation such as a sexual union" (ibid., p. 417). In brief, sex can never be fully consensual. This most topical and ideological matter would require a book of its own – especially when read in conjunction with the nowadays equally pervasive "tolerant" principle "Spare the other!")

2. *Permission/Refusal.* The obsessional is always asking the other for permission. He is vividly aware of that when he describes his symptoms. Evidently, "to ask [continuously] for permission, is precisely to have as a subject a certain [peculiar] relationship with one's demand" (ibid., p. 412), which obscures one's desire. Placing oneself in "the most extreme dependence" (ibid.) on the other insofar as he speaks – and thus on the Other as the locus of the signifying articulation – is here clearly meant to "*reinstate* the Other" (ibid., my emphasis) – or preserve and maintain him – on the level of demand precisely to the extent that the obsessional subject contradictorily puts him "in question" and "in danger" on the level of desire (ibid.). Again, for the obsessional, his desire as "desire as such" goes together with the attempted elimination of the Other's desire, which would, however, also bring about the disappearance of the subject's own desire. Asking for permission should therefore somehow compensate for this predicament. Yet, with a further dialectical twist that surpasses the dimension of the demand for a direct "agreement" – soon to be moderated by the categorical imperative – what is actually pursued in the request for permission is nothing but *refusal*. For the obsessional, "refusal and permission imply each other" (ibid., p. 413). The obsessional concretely puts himself in situations where asking for permission solicits refusal, for instance,

by repeating his request in order to specify it, or to receive a confirmation that the permission has been granted (this point remains implicit in Lacan's reasoning, but I think it directly follows from it). Paradoxically, this is what allows him to overcome the frustration-control level to which the failure of a straightforward "agreement" with the other consigned him; the "pact" that is now being refused is in fact given against the background of what he – wrongly – perceives as a "promise" (that *his* desire may eventually be recognised; that he may be One in the field of the Other) (ibid.). This is sufficient for the obsessional's "desire as such", or desire to have one's desire, to be tentatively *articulated* in the guise of a contradiction; at this stage, all "he *needs* [is] an *unsatisfied* desire" (ibid., p. 415, my emphases) (the use of "need" in this context is, for what we have said, far from coincidental). In other words, here the obsessional partly "solves the problem of his desire's evanescence by turning it into a *forbidden* desire, [as] supported by the Other's *interdiction*", i.e., the refusal (ibid., my emphases). But this status quo unavoidably remains itself "ambiguous" (ibid.); desire is accessed by the obsessional only as an *unsatisfied* desire sustained by the Other's interdiction; he thus desires more and more to make it performatively *present* to the Other and against him.

3. *The exploit.* The obsessional "inflicts on himself all sorts of particularly difficult and testing tasks"; more to the point, he "very brilliantly" succeeds in carrying them out (ibid., p. 418). For the obsessional, "work is powerful"; he would much deserve a "little holiday" (ibid.), during which he could do what he wishes, but work is actually there to liberate him from the time of rest, which he considers as time lost. On a first level, the exploit appears to be quite openly aggressive. It addresses the counterpart or imaginary other seen as an "adversary" – e.g., the slacker colleague – whom the obsessional "seems to defy" (ibid., p. 419). In this sense, the exploit amounts to a "won performance", or a "sprint" (ibid., p. 418). But, on closer inspection, the "prowess" of the exploit evidences nothing more than a "sport game" and always remains "fictitious" (ibid., p. 419). The obsessional merely "plays with the other" (ibid.). In other words, he is not a Hegelian master involved in a struggle to death. The "risks" he takes are always "limited" – in this sense, the obsessional "opposes absolute virility" (ibid., p. 403) – which is why, thanks to a "wise economy" (ibid., p. 418), he thrives in the confrontational exploit as what he, often consciously, desires to do. However, on a second and more fundamental level, the exploit is addressed to the Other as a "spectator", who "keeps the score" (ibid., p. 419). Here lies the "real danger" (ibid.) for the obsessional as the contradiction and impasse of his desire take centre stage again, and more strikingly. On the one hand, the obsessional demands the Other – the locus of signification – to recognise his aggressive desire as conveyed by the exploit; he demands that his remarkable achievements be "witnessed to", "registered", and thus "realised" as "well deserved" (ibid.) – something the negated counterpart could never grant him. Yet, on the other

hand, and more importantly, the obsessional's desire as "desire as such" cannot at all be symbolically contented with a "little reward" (ibid., p. 418) (in Lacan's French, the *petite couronne*, or coronet, of a "Good job!", we may add). Beyond his dialectic of permission and refusal, which privileges refusal in order to articulate desire as unsatisfied desire, the obsessional also more daringly and antinomically tries to obtain *permission* from the Other for his *desire* to be *presented* as such precisely through the lack of satisfaction. To put it bluntly, what he is after is not, or not only, a work promotion (which would simply reignite and escalate the exploit), but a paradoxical promotion and acknowledgement on the part of the Other of the subject's *desire at work*, of a desire both always in the making and destructively oriented towards being One in the field of the Other. The aggressive exploit as a victorious, albeit short-lived, defiance of the other thus soon turns into a deadlocked challenge to the Other's desire. "In the exploit the subject dominates and even domesticates [the] fundamental anxiety" (ibid.) caused by the enigmatic character of the Other's desire; yet, at the same time, in having to register the exploit, and more generally "inscribe his history" (ibid., p. 419) of feats, the obsessional ends up trying to "validate" (ibid.) his pure desire in the very disputed place of the Other, which he no less zealously strives to maintain. Insubordinate bravery gives way to an adhesion to "everything that is of the verbal order, the order of computation, recapitulation, inscription, and even falsification" (ibid.). The impasse of obsessional desire means that ultimately defiance betrays a "defence mechanism" (ibid., p. 420) and the endeavour to performatively display the subject's desire as such calls for nothing other than an – impossible – reinforcement of the "Other's presence" (ibid.).

4. *The proof of love.* As seen, obsessional desire as "desire as such" and "pure" desire lies, by definition, beyond the demand for love. However, the obsessional is in equal measure contradictorily prone to the *proof* of love – the obsessional's desire "is beyond the unconditioned exigency of love, of which on occasion it can come to be the test [*épreuve*]" (ibid., p. 401). The proof of love stands as the point at which the impasse of the obsessional's desire emerges most neatly as the return of the repressed. It occurs on the unusual occasions when the obsessional subject attempts to reach the sexual object, and the more he approaches it the more he experiences a decrease of libidinal tension. In order to avert the imminent disappearance of his desire, which the possession of the sexual object as the supposed destruction of the Other's desire structurally entails, the obsessional stages the proof of love. Here the subject does not only ask the other/Other to give him "what is beyond every possible satisfaction, his very being" (ibid., p. 406) – which amounts to love tout-court, that is, giving what one does not have, as aimed at in the demand for love. Rather, the obsessional passionately requests this "essential presentification" (ibid.) of the Other to prove, or certify in the verbal order, the presence of the subject's own being of desire *at the very moment of its utmost destructive exposure as concomitant evanescence.* We could provisionally phrase this

as "Give me what you do *not* have, your being, so that *I* can finally be the want-to-be (*manque-à-être*) I *am*!". At bottom, the subject is here asking the other/Other for *permission to destroy* him – as a desiring being. Of course, such a request causes for the obsessional all sorts of "extraordinary accidents" (ibid., p. 402) vis-à-vis the sexual object, which nonetheless prevents him from not "exist[ing] any longer" (ibid., p. 403) – as instead happens when he possesses the sexual object.

Later in Seminar V, Lacan summarises the contradiction inherent to the obsessional behaviours we have described so far through the humoristic formula "To be or not…", interrupted and incessantly repeated since the subject has in the meantime forgotten what follows. The obsessional wants *to be* his desire, but, faced with the lack of a foothold on it ("or not"), he always falls back into a unilateral compromise with the Other that represses desire ("…"), only to start again the same movement: "'To be or not…', and the chap scratches his head in order to be able to continue, 'to be or not…, to be or not…, to be or not…', etc." (ibid., p. 474).

What we have designated as the "proof of love" amounts to a final and frantic effort to enunciate this botched formula as the full-fledged Shakespearean question "to be or not to be?", and to solve it positively in terms of being (we should recall that Lacan's lengthy analysis of *Hamlet* in Seminar VI dwells on obsession). "I am not where I am (my always elusive desire) but there where I should be I am no longer (my desire's disappearance). Am I? Tell me that I am!". Interestingly, at one point, Lacan speaks of a specific instance in which *desire* itself, not demand, "calls for an absolute answer" (ibid., p. 406) – the "You are!" never to be given.

Because of the subject's assumption of *the* question "to be or not to be?" in the proof of love, Lacan also tends to closely associate its request for an absolute answer with *acting out* (ibid., p. 421). Although the proof of love functions as a last barrier that protects the obsessional subject from the most extreme consequence of acting out, that is, the disappearance of his desire as soon as he secures the object, it also shares with acting out a concrete reference to a "material" sexual object (ibid.) – which is otherwise avoided by the obsessional. (This is the case in spite of the fact that what is primarily at stake in both acting out and the vicissitudes surrounding the subject's request for the proof of love, is *not* the material sexual object. In this sense, Lacan speaks of this kind of passionate love as not focusing on a partial object but as being itself a "*partial love*" (ibid., p. 421, my emphasis); what we are dealing with is *desire* through love. Along similar lines, elsewhere in Seminar V Lacan also highlights the strong connection between acting out and a "*problematic* falling in love" (ibid., p. 447, my emphasis).)

Yet like the categorical imperative, the search for refusal, and the exploit, the proof of love is a symptomatic compromise eventually aimed at "pleasing" the Other (ibid.), albeit in the radical form of asking for a *permission* to destroy him. The acting out stands instead as an active "attempt at solving the problem of demand and desire" (ibid., p. 420), by exacerbating it and bringing it into the open in the guise of an enigmatic signifier, the phallus.

Against their customary psychoanalytic definition as "bungled actions", for Lacan all the above-mentioned obsessional behaviours are actually "successful acts", in that they "clearly let transpire a tendency" (ibid.) – namely, the obsessional's pure desire as contradictorily articulated in demand with respect to its attempted destruction of the Other's desire. In opposition to these "illusory solutions" – and independently of whether it finally appropriates the object or eventually succumbs to the proof of love – acting out consists of a veritable bungled action that works as a positive "hint" for the analyst (ibid.). It is, strictly speaking, a "paradoxical act [that] reveals that every relationship [the obsessional has] to demand is fundamentally inadequate", since it does not allow him "to access the effective reality of the signifier's effect on him, that is to say, to put himself on the level of the castration complex" (ibid., p. 421).

***

Two broad and crucial issues – also treated in the same lessons of Seminar V – remain to be explored elsewhere. First, we would have to investigate the precise coordinates and reasons of the obsessional's inability to undergo castration due to the particular role the phallus assumes for him in the fantasy. Lacan's very first reference to obsession in Seminar V already clearly delineates the crux of the matter: in obsession, the phallus "as an *imaginary* element" (φ) is "prevalent", whereas castration requires the phallus to be fully unfolded as a *signifier*, that is, turned into a *symbol* (Φ) (ibid., p. 385, my emphasis). Second and in relation to this, we would have to assess the scope and limits of the psychoanalytic solution to this impasse as advanced in Seminar V. On the one hand, the aim of psychoanalysis is to promote the obsessional's "acceptance" of castration as a "signifying function" (ibid., p. 437), yet, on the other, castration "can be articulated in the consciousness of the subject only up to a certain point" (ibid., p. 394) – and this applies to each and every subject, not only obsessionals or neurotics in general.

References

Chiesa, L. (2007). *Subjectivity and Otherness: A Philosophical Reading of Lacan*. Cambridge MA: MIT Press.

Dor, J. (1998). *Introduction to the Reading of Lacan: The Unconscious Structured Like a Language*. New York: Other Press.

Fink, B. (1995). *The Lacanian Subject: Between Language and Jouissance*. Princeton NJ: Princeton University Press.

Evans, D. (1996). *An Introductory Dictionary of Lacanian Psychoanalysis*. London: Routledge.

Lacan, J. (1957–1958). *Le séminaire. Livre V. Les formations de l'inconscient*. Paris: Seuil, 1998.

Lacan, J. (1968–1969). *Le séminaire. Livre XVI. D'un Autre à l'autre*. Paris: Seuil, 2006.

Safouan, M. (2001). *Lacaniana: Les séminaires de Jacques Lacan: 1953–1963*. Paris: Fayard.

APPENDIX: TRANSITORY SEXUAL PERVERSION IN THE COURSE OF A PSYCHOANALYTIC TREATMENT

Ruth Lebovici[1]

Having had the opportunity to treat a patient suffering from a character neurosis with phobic manifestations for more than five years, we have been able to witness the birth and development of a transitory sexual perversion within the framework of the transference and the actions outside the transference. After a brief survey of the case and the general development of the psychoanalytic treatment, it seemed interesting to us to dwell longer on the origin of this perversion. Its manifestations centred around voyeurism, which expressed itself essentially in a pre-genital mode, and its disappearance coincided with the analysis of the genital and pre-genital aggressive drives that had been transferred onto the analyst.[2]

Part 1: Account of the clinical case

1. Diagnosis

The twenty-three-year-old patient (we shall call him Yves) was referred to Dr Lebovici by Dr Mignot with the following note:

> This patient experiences, without genuine anxiety yet with intensity, the feeling of being physically laughable and this results in fact in an extremely troubling inhibition. Strictly speaking, it does not concern an obsessional of the psychasthenic type, still less a melancholic anxiety patient. The neurotic attitude to which the disorder bears witness deserves to be analysed. I believe that this subject should only be given psychoanalytic treatment. A letter he had written to his parents testifies to an attitude of anger with sado-masochistic explosions, in which he finds pleasure.

This young man, who was a trainee helmsman in the merchant navy, had to abandon his profession because of an obsessive idea that haunted him: he thought he was too tall and felt laughable. In fact, he was indeed a very tall young man, of about one metre and ninety centimetres. He eventually locked himself up at home, where he remained inactive. He hassled his mother and did not stop asking her whether he was really too tall. To reassure him about his physique and to distract him, his mother procured him a mistress, whom he went to see every night.

Before the psychoanalytic treatment, the clinical survey was drawn up as follows: the patient sought help for an obsessive idea, "the fear of being too tall and therefore laughable". This obsessive idea can be classified within the framework of the phobias, since the essential mechanism that seemed to govern the formation of this symptom was the displacement of anxiety and the avoidance of the phobogenic situation. Furthermore, other minor phobias existed, which were essentially related to clothing: the fear of shoes being too small, jacket sleeves being too long, trousers not being in conformity with a given model. The development of the drives seemed to have taken this subject up to the Oedipal stage, but this stage seemed largely impregnated by pre-genital pathogenic fixations, in particular sado-masochistic ones. Amongst other things, the letter addressed to his parents mentioned by Dr Mignot bears witness to this – a letter full of scatological terms.

At the end of the treatment, the diagnosis of phobic manifestations developing on the basis of a character neurosis with pre-genital fixations seemed to correspond best to the structure of the case, as we shall see later on.

We shall firstly discuss the biography of this subject as we were able to complete and reconstitute it at the end of the treatment. Then we shall give a brief synopsis of the development of the transference, dwelling in particular upon the transference manifestations.

2. Anamnesis

Yves is an only child. His father is the only son of a country doctor who was often mentioned at the start of the treatment. Indeed, the paternal grandfather, a widower for many years, lived with a cousin who looked after his house. Yves spent his holidays with him. He found a parental couple there that was quite different from that of his parents. His mother was spoken of very badly and his father was reckoned to have made a misalliance by marrying a woman from an inferior social milieu and whose morality was said to be doubtful. The grandfather also disapproved of his son for not having studied, being without ambition and being content with a modest income. Indeed, after the war, our patient's father worked as a wage labourer in a garage. He seems to be a fairly weak character, completely under his wife's control, and from time to time showing explosions of violent anger for mere trifles. If this father appeared through Yves' analysis as very weak, he nonetheless ensured his domination over the entire family through manifestly obsessional character traits: incessant worries about his car, about the location of the furniture, extreme care about his clothes, calligraphic writing, etc. Finding the sharp criticisms of his son difficult to bear, he tried to bring him to his senses. He seems to have had difficulty tolerating the intimacy that existed between his wife and his son.

Indeed, the mother has always had a hold over Yves. It seems that she derived great satisfaction from her domination of her son. Yves always describes her as giving orders to his father as well as to himself. He deplores her habit of concealing his own mistakes from his father, which enabled her to exercise a real emotional blackmail over him. For instance, she did not reveal a theft he had committed from the till of the family cafe. Later, when he fell ill, she never encouraged him to work. Instead she provided him with a mistress from whom she rapidly tried to take her son back. To sum up, it is no surprise that Yves conceived her as a phallic maternal image, insofar as his relations with his mother, relived in the treatment, explain this way of looking.

Yves was born in a small fishing port in Normandy, where he lived for three years. At first he remembered nothing about this period. As the treatment advanced, he did however recall the house, the toilet at the back of the garden where it was dark, and above all a servant to whom he was very attached, despite the fact that she would get rid of him and his toys by sending him to the stairwell. Yves' family moved to a nearby village, where he lived from the age of three to the age of five. His memories of those years are limited: he remembers a transient phobia of red meat and being forced to take a drug called Marinol. He thought he was a spoilt child and he spoke pleasurably about the little car he used to steer around the garden.

Next Yves' parents started running a cafe and tobacco shop in a big city in the West of the country. As soon as Yves arrived at his third residence, which we shall call L, the child was sent to school. He enjoyed himself there and loved boys' games. He was the goalkeeper in a junior football team. But his mother kept watch. She thought that he came home too late at night and that he was too dirty. She prohibited those games and she often sent him on errands to the neighbourhood shops. From this time onwards she often repeated to him that he used to be so sweet when he was little and that he had become more and more unbearable when growing up. Yves' mother ruled over her house, the cafe, the father, the son, and eventually also a widowed uncle who joined the family when it moved to L. This uncle, whom Yves thought was, or had been, his mother's lover, appeared more virile to him than his father, despite the fact that he accepted ungrudgingly the remarks and the authority of his sister-in-law.

Yves' room was next to that of his parents. He remembers that at the age of seven, his mother reprimanded him for urinating on the floor. He told her that she knew very well from her own experience that the penis is stiff in the morning and it is impossible to avoid accidents like that. When he was ill, his mother put him to sleep in the conjugal bed, where he remembers masturbating. He recalls with horror the coverings in which he was afraid of suffocating and the frequent enemas his mother gave him. He loved animals but felt aggressive towards them: he shot arrows at his dog and spat on his parrot. When the parrot died, his mother accused Yves of killing it with spit. Yves believed her because he had faux croup at the time and he imagined that he was contagious and a danger to the bird.

When he went to secondary school, he had some intimate contacts with friends in the dark corridors of the neighbouring houses. This coincided with the discovery of pornographic magazines, which he used constantly in order to nourish his solitary masturbation. He became timid with girls and started avoiding them in the park, whilst being interested in them from a distance.

He spent his holidays with his grandfather, whom he thought very virile, a great hunter and a very commanding figure. His grandfather and he clashed one day apropos of a racing wheel for a bicycle and his grandfather gave in. Yves was very proud of this victory over a man he judged powerful, and from then on the image of the grandfather slightly lost its value. As for his holidays, he remembered spending long periods under the table, where he delighted in looking up the skirts of the cousin and the maid.

In 1940 his father was drafted into the army. A very important memory for him dates back to this period: when paying a visit to his father, together with his mother and a fishmonger whose husband had been detached to the same area, he watched this woman urinate and this really turned him on.

It was not until the very end of the treatment that Yves revealed to us an important detail of his life at the time: during the time of his father's mobilisation, he regularly shared his mother's bed. He was thirteen years old then.

At the time of the German advance, he went to his godmother, ahead of his parents, in a city that was less at risk of attack than L. The cafe was hit by a bomb and the family moved to a farm that belonged to the grandfather. Yves went to the college nearest to the farm and subsequently, when his father had gone to work in Chartres, he became a boarder there and obtained his baccalaureate. This is where his father became involved with a mistress. When Yves and his mother went back to L, after the liberation, his father did not follow them. Yves witnessed, indifferently he believes, scenes in which his mother would scold his father's mistress. During this time he got the date wrong for presenting himself for the entry exam at the school for trainee helmsmen. He was relieved when his father returned home, but he did not want to believe that his father came back for him, as he had confirmed. The following year he left for Caen for his studies. He lived there with a friend he protected and helped, and to whom he was very attached. When he left his school, he started working as a sailor.

From the age of fifteen he felt quite uncomfortable because he was always the tallest of his class. But this feeling was exacerbated during the entire sailing period because his friends did not stop pestering him about it. He became depressed and sought solitude. During a period of sadness he wrote the aforementioned letter to his mother. When his ship moored in his hometown, he decided to call in sick and did not go back on board.

The analysis started a couple of months later: he was twenty-three years old at the time. He lived with his parents who, after the war, and in their confinement to L, had only found a room and a kitchen to live in. Promiscuity was rampant and Yves slept in a metal wall bed that was spread out in the kitchen at night. He was completely inactive and avoided going out during the day owing to his size. He remained stretched out on his parents' bed and masturbated frequently. At the time, the uncle lived in a room in the city, but he came over to share the meals with the family. We have seen that his mother procured a mistress for Yves who was fifteen years his senior, with whom he spent his evenings and with whom he had also adopted the habit of staying for the night.

We shall now very briefly describe the development of Yves' psychoanalytic treatment, which lasted, let us remind the reader, slightly more than five years. We shall follow the treatment from year to year, relating first the subject's life and then the course of the analysis.

3. Development of the psychoanalytic treatment

The patient regularly came to Paris twice a week for two consecutive sessions and a third session separate from the two others. Because of this arrangement, he had to spend one night in Paris. Friends of his parents, who lived in the Paris suburbs, were happy to put him up.

He arrived at his sessions with his body bent forward and this posture worried his parents so much that they wrote to us during the course of the treatment in order to ask us whether it was necessary to consult an orthopaedic surgeon. Before lying down on the couch, he removed his jacket, which he folded carefully. He spoke very little and with effort, repeating before every sentence: "I think that". His position on the analytic couch was always the same: one of his lower limbs was bent vertically, the other bent and resting on the couch.

During the first year Yves remained lazy. He spent his days on his bed reading pornographic magazines, then rapidly he started leafing through the works of Freud. He frequently argued with his parents and his mistress. During this first year, his paternal grandfather died.

Despite his difficulty with speech, the patient presented material during these sessions that was quite rich, especially in terms of dreams. We can only relate briefly their most salient aspects, those we shall utilise in our theoretical discussion. Already, it will be seen, there appeared fantasy material in which the elements of a perversion of the voyeuristic type is clear and which undoubtedly constitutes the basis for the elaboration of perversions during the treatment.

Dream (concerning a dream-pursuit, Yves talks about this repetitive dream): a man in armour attacks him from behind with a kind of gasmask, which brings to mind a fly-tox spray and which would suffocate him.

Dream: "I am at the window with Yves Montand who wants to offer me a cocktail. Then, Yves Montand is standing up naked in front of my mother who is not embarrassed at all. His genitals are much larger than mine. I am naked on the floor under a blanket." (In his associations he will say that his mistress does not think his genitals are long enough and that the night before she gave him an enema when he was stretched out on his back on the floor.)

Later, he will talk about his nocturnal ejaculations after reading pornographic magazines. He has a great deal of masturbatory guilt. Various elements of voyeurism appear: he thinks about the graffiti he is looking for in the urinals and about masturbation among homosexuals. He imagines a prostitute who is masturbating. At the same time he will reveal that in Chartres, during the period when his father had a mistress, he masturbated and dressed himself as a woman. Here he will also recount that until the age of seven he was convinced that women had a penis.

During the second year, when he also remained lazy, an extremely important dream should be mentioned at the onset. In the salon of a cafe Yves notices a big woman whose thighs he spreads out and who has three penises. He sucks and caresses one of the penises and wakes up with an ejaculation. During the same night he has a second dream in which he has sexual intercourse with his mother.

From the start of this year he talks on various occasions about the stories he invents and writes in order to masturbate. The general theme is the following: a young girl with whom he identifies is being initiated sexually by an older woman.

At this moment he sees in numerous dreams how women urinate. At the same time masturbatory fantasies appear that are often supported by drawings: indeed he draws crouched women who are urinating, or he imagines a woman seeing him when he is masturbating in a urinal. She is very aroused and gives herself to him. Later, the end of this fantasy will be recounted in a slightly different way, since he will suck the woman's genitals. At the same time a compulsive idea manifests itself to urinate on the psychoanalytic couch, an idea contemporary with the following fantasy: he urinates on remnants of the analyst's faecal matter.

Some time later we were able to give him an interpretation of the relationship between his Oedipal guilt and his retreat into voyeuristic fantasies. This happened in particular on the occasion of the following dream: he wants to ask the fishmonger, who is a family friend, to have sex with him, but he is stopped by the sight of her maid. In the course of his associations he will tell us that he had seen the fishmonger urinating, as we mentioned above in the discussion of Yves' biography. He tells us that he was in love with the maid in the dream, but that he was afraid of her husband. We were thus able to give him the following interpretation: it was less dangerous for him to watch, as he had done, this woman urinate than to desire having sexual intercourse with a woman whose husband scared him.

The third year saw Yves going off to military service: the analysis was interrupted for three months, at the end of which the subject was declared unfit. On the advice of a friend who was a tax officer, he decided to prepare for the exam that would lead to a job at the Treasury. Yves had reckoned his military service would give him a good opportunity to break up with his mistress and on his return he stopped living with her. He often went out with his friend and the latter's fiancée. During his walks he was tormented by frequent desires to urinate: it was a way of defending himself against the desires he had for his friend's fiancée because, according to him, he led her to suspect that he was suffering from a venereal disease. At the end of this third year he was recruited as an assistant in the same administrative service his friend worked in.

Using his fatigue as a pretext, he asked for the first time to cancel a session. After his desire for passivity had been interpreted, for he knew very well that he would not obtain any satisfaction from us and that he would in this way be forced to come to the session as before, lots of material emerged in which his passivity was expressed as a desire for enemas. Yves associated the enema tube with the maternal penis that featured in the dream of the woman with the three penises. On the one hand, his fear of positive feelings in the transference brought passive desires with it. On the other, it was at the origin of new fantasies with a voyeuristic basis: he found himself in a toilet whose partitioning wall with another toilet had a hole pierced in it. He exhibits his genitals, watches the woman next door urinating and wants to kiss her genitals.

Let us mention another two dreams from the end of this period: in the first, Yves appears in the station of L, wanting to go to Paris for his analytic session. Loaded with two suitcases he risks being crushed by an engine. In his associations, he is surprised that this "steel monster" is driven, he thinks, by a man who looks like him. He is prompted to think of the dream of the woman with the three penises. With hindsight he appreciates the force, the power and the threat she represented for him. In the second dream, he is a little boy who is being tended by his mother on a table. We pointed out to him his regressive position vis-à-vis his mother, as well as towards his mistress and ourselves. What followed was a period during which Yves did not stop repeating that the treatment would not be over until he had had sexual intercourse with the analyst. We told him that he was playing a game of making himself afraid of an event which he knew would never happen.

During the fourth year Yves lived with his family, about which he continued to complain. He felt dominated by his mother, towards whom he would show occasional gestures of independence, which consisted in following young girls in the street, which meant that he came home at irregular hours. Sometimes he accosted them, but he gave up pushing his luck as soon as he learnt about the existence of a fiancé or some friend in the young girl's life. He said that at home one could only make jokes about flatulence and he deplored the fact that his father could only manifest his presence in that way. His mother encouraged him to go hunting and, armed with the gun his grandfather had left him, he found an activity there which manifestly substituted for his sexual relations with his mistress.

At this moment, there developed, with all its intensity, the voyeuristic sexual perversion which will be studied in greater detail. Yves started masturbating in the toilets of a cinema whilst imagining that he was watching women who were urinating. Later, when watching a film, he was afraid of being caught when he fiddled with his fly, and he attributed to this emotion a jaundice that appeared soon afterwards. He eventually discovered a cinema where his perversion could be well nourished. Entering by chance on the side of the women's toilets, he discovered a hole in the partition wall separating two cubicles and from now on he came to occupy his observation post every week after an evening performance, waiting for the arrival of female spectators who came to urinate.

In the spring of that year he came sixth in his exam out of a total of two-hundred candidates.

This is the development of the treatment during this period. We were able to give him a first interpretation of the relations between aggressivity and love. This relation translated into his desire to drink the urine of a woman he was in love with, that is to say, to take something from her in his belly. Indeed, at the same time as having this fantasy, he often produced associations about the danger a man could encounter in his contact with a woman, in particular with reference to the engine (end of the third year): the latter was in fact imagined to be a dangerous woman because she had a penis in her belly.

He is talking so much about his fantasy of masturbating whilst watching a woman urinating that we suggest to him that the fishmonger, from whom his mother wanted to divert his attention while she was urinating, was only a screen memory.

We can also point out to him that he feels the analyst to be more authoritarian than his mother, because the latter supported his regressive activities: jokes concerning anality, encouragement to go hunting.

When the treatment was interrupted due to the analyst being ill, he heard about an obituary of someone with the same name. On his return he recounted how he feared failing his exam because he spent too much time chasing young girls instead of working. An interpretation of Oedipal guilt repeated in the transference was given to him: when his father was drafted, he lived alone with his mother and made a mistake about the date of his exam. Now he imagines that the analyst's husband is dead and he is making sure not to succeed in his exam, so great is his fear of having a manly success when being alone with her. Soon he had an impression of smelling urine and he expressed a desire to drink the analyst's urine. Soon after, he recalled that when he was little he frequently heard his mother urinating during the night in a hygienic bucket and scrumpling up paper. At the same time he expressed an intense fear of dying if he let himself drink women's urine.

We gave him an overall interpretation of his repressions relating to the pregenital drives at the end of this year of treatment. As he observed with relief that his mistress was not losing her appetite despite his having abandoned her, he explained how dangerous he thought women with an empty stomach are. We pointed out to him that he was afraid of being devoured in return, by the women from whom he desired to incorporate something. He then recounted a dream in which his mistress had a penis which he saw himself sucking. He produced associations concerning the insensitive breasts of his mistress and his own, which were by contrast very excitable. Then he talked about the seat worms that made him suffer, as well as about his excessive and unpleasant perspiration. He talked again about the woman with the three penises from his past dream. In this way he expressed his fantasy of exchanging incorporated objects. The woman with the empty stomach ventures to devour him. When he wants to incorporate the maternal penis in the form of urine he wants to drink, he runs the same risk: he sees himself obliged then to restore the bad things he has inside himself. He points out, for that matter, the equivalence between white sperm and urine, presumably corresponding to the fantasmatic equivalence between the breast and the penis. During this session he recalls with emotion that he had never dreamt about genital intercourse with a woman; it always concerns masturbation or oral coitus. He himself underscores the importance of the mouth. The analyst pointed out to him, then, that this is how his fear of talking can be explained, and he admitted, very moved, that healing had always secretly appeared to him as defined by the possibility of "rediscovering the use of speech".

The last year of the treatment was marked by Yves' return to his mistress, whom he took away from a rival. At first he often had nocturnal ejaculations because he avoided having sexual intercourse with her. Then he progressively had a normal sexual activity, in which he took real pleasure. During the strikes of August 1953 he took an active part in the struggle of the trade unions.[3] After a not very brilliant start, he became a fairly capable hunter. He adapted himself very well to his work. When he was given a permanent job, he had no difficulty coming to Paris for three days during a certain period of time. Then we changed to two weekly sessions. The end of the treatment was envisaged at the beginning of the sixth year and the analysis finished a couple of weeks after the resumption at the end of the summer holidays.

During this period he had much less pleasure in frequenting the toilets of his regular cinema. Yet he still often went there spontaneously and we pointed out to him that he found a compensation there for the frustrations we imposed upon him. He replied that when he watched women urinating, or when he imagined intercourse via the mouth, this meant being active and virile for him, because he liked taking more than giving.

On the occasion of a dream, we saw the maid of his childhood re-appear in a blue blouse with a broom and a bucket of water, and he recalled the memory of vague feelings of being attracted to her, linked to the anger and the discontent of being pushed away. At this point in his analysis, he attached great importance to the choice of shoes and clothes. He had talked on various occasions about his purchase of shoes and his fear of having his foot squeezed. But when the shoes were too big, he complained about his lack of balance. When the treatment continued with two sessions a week, he complained a lot about this frustration, which occurred at a moment when he really started desiring the analyst. He often talked about the naughty look he believed he had in the street. Similarly, he said, his mother thought he was sweet only when he was little. We risked bringing this memory into connection with his symptom (the fear of being too tall) and the fear of buying shoes that are too small. He then produced the association of the memory of an effort he had made to penetrate his mistress: he was afraid of wounding her and, as he said, of "wrecking the apartment". We interpreted his fear of having shoes that are too small as the fear of his penis being wrecked. At the same time as desiring to be squeezed by shoes that maintained his balance, he sought and feared a narrow vagina for his penis.

Before the holidays, he declared that, in order to finish, it would be better to have sexual intercourse with his analyst. At this moment he dreamt that from a urinal he heard a friend say to a woman, whose husband was in Indochina, that nothing was happening on the front. Now, this dream was exactly contemporary with the battle of Dien Bien Phu.[4] When we made this remark to Yves, he was surprised by this contradiction and was prompted to reveal the memory of a period during which nothing was happening on the front, during the "phoney war" when his father was drafted: he slept in his mother's bed.

After the summer holidays, he insisted on his desire to end the treatment. He said that he had nothing to learn about himself anymore. We stopped at a mutually agreed date: about six weeks from then. He had been treated for varicose veins and he did not pay for the last session – with the money he went to see a prostitute. The treatment ended then.

At the end of the treatment, from a professional point of view, Yves worked regularly. He got on well with his colleagues and with his boss. He intended to present himself for the higher level exam.

He was still living with his mistress, with whom he had a satisfying sexual relationship. But he was also aware that this liaison had no future. As a matter of fact, he claimed that the treatment prevented him from conquering younger women, whilst at the same time he could not afford the luxury of a room in the city. Indeed, despite our heavily reduced fee, the price of his train pass was high for his salary. Since he got his permanent job, he had actually paid his parents a maintenance allowance, which came as a great relief to him.

He was no longer suffering from his phobias and no longer embarrassed by his size. His speech was easier. His environment and his friends showed him that he had become jolly and that he was making jokes with the young women in the office.

We have had no news from Yves since October 1954, when his treatment ended.

4. Development of the transference

The transference was initially of the maternal type. Despite material that was often Oedipal, Yves had to defend himself against a pre-genital aggressivity he felt towards us: prolonged silences out of fear of being naughty with us, as with his mother and his mistress; fear of using strong words; sharp criticisms of the anal gift through endless discussions of the issue of the fee and delays in payments. Then came the fear of a positive transference: he had to remind himself all the time that we were a therapist and not a woman. He dreamt that we were naked on his knees, but that it was extremely unpleasant. The first flight from this positive transference was into homosexuality: he dreamt that instead of going to Paris, his train headed for Caen where, as we recall, he had a friend he liked a lot. At the time, we were able to show him that his material suggested that seeing our husband would have been more pleasant and less dangerous for him. Since he tried to perceive us as severe, demanding and prohibitive, we suggested to him –

concerning the fear of a man who might strangle him in the dark, and the repeated evocation of the man in armour associated with a feeling of being suffocated during the sessions – that he was scared of us just as he had been scared of the man in armour.

This interpretation of the transference-situation merits discussion: we can indeed ask ourselves whether the material that alluded to a fear of being attacked by a man could be translated as a transference of the paternal type, as the flight into homosexuality mentioned above seemed to suggest, or rather concerned a maternal transference in which the fear of a phallic mother was relived.

This is exactly how the material developed during this period of the treatment. After having manifested his fear of expressing positive feelings toward us, he insisted for a long time on the difficulties he was having in identifying with his father, because the latter could not represent a valid virile image for him. But since his mother was completely unbearable, he explained extensively, as we have seen, how he took refuge in friendship with boys. In all the dreams of this period, he was with one or more "comrades". It was at this moment that he talked about his fear of being mugged in the dark: the treatment gave him the impression that he was left in the dark and his associations prompted him to make explicit his fear of being attacked in the darkness from behind. We were able to remark that it was us that was precisely behind him. A couple of sessions later, he explained that he had the impression of suffocating during the session and he returned to his dream in which he had been sprinkled by the fly-tox spray of the man in armour. He actually associated it with the sensations of suffocation he would have experienced when he came down with faux croup around the age of six. Our second intervention was situated there, according to which his fear of us reminded him of his fear of the man in armour.

The question arises whether this interpretation was appropriate: we had indeed explained to him some time before that he would have preferred being treated by our husband and one could suppose that he was encouraged to defend himself against the fear of a positive maternal transference by the outcome of material indicating a passive homosexual fear transferred onto our husband.

We chose another solution: that of interpreting the transference situation for him as being structured around his fear of phallic women and in particular of his mother. For this orientation we based ourselves especially on the importance of the aggressive pre-genital drives which had coloured his Oedipal feelings since the start of the treatment. The outcome of the singular material that followed this interpretation seemed to have justified it: first of all the dream about Yves Montand mentioned above, then that of the woman with the three penises, finally the memory of seeing his mother at the age of seven. In the course of subsequent sessions, he protested against his passivity toward us: desire to, and fear of, urinating on the analytic couch; the fantasy of urinating on our bowel movements; complaints about our stubbornness in keeping him for three sessions. This stubbornness reminded him of the coercions his mother imposed upon him: ingestion of Marinol; wrappings that would include his arms; tube for enemas. This material was certainly inscribed within the maternal transference, and the object was conceived as phallic. Nonetheless, we can discern a number of new elements there which translate into a more developed Oedipal situation: the importance of the pre-genital drives, which were exteriorised, for example, in the fantasy of urinating on the psychoanalytic couch, should not make us forget that voyeurism was transferred onto the analyst, of whose legs Yves regularly tried to catch a glimpse. More precisely, one will recall that the voyeuristic desires had been interpreted previously as a retreat from Oedipal desires prohibited by the paternal image (dream of the fishmonger). At this moment, Yves, who took off his jacket in a mechanical way before lying down, expressed his fear of being surprised by our husband in such an intimate situation. In this way, it is clear that a triangular situation is being broached in which the paternal image plays above all a prohibitive part.

This Oedipal situation, however discrete, could not fail to determine profound regressions. This is where the fantasy of drinking a woman's urine entered the transference in the form of a perverse fantasy. He developed a fear of this desire, which he considered extremely dangerous – he could die from it. His desire to urinate on the analytic couch was then interpreted to him as the desire to eliminate the bad things he desired to incorporate. The transference was then re-genitalised. He had cramps in the legs, which he interpreted as substitute erections. He dreamt that his analyst kissed him on the mouth. He experienced anxieties of an Oedipal character, after having insinuated that our husband chose female patients in order to cheat on us.

From the fifth year, he criticised his voyeuristic curiosity concerning our legs, treating it as a "ridiculous pleasure". He was still afraid of his oral desires toward us and he defended himself against the desire for vengeance which he attributed to us by relieving himself in order "to eliminate what he had eaten" before coming to the session.

Little by little, he demonstrated, then suppressed, what he called a genuine desire. Yet in his worry of being pushed away he tried to be pitied, then contented himself with words that ensured a continuity in our relation with him and which, whilst still being a regressive activity, appeared as an adaptation.

After this retreat from the Oedipus, he lived the Oedipal relationship by strongly demonstrating his desire for the analyst. This time he was afraid of the spouse and recounted with much affect that he shared his mother's bed during the time of his father's draft.

To sum up, the greatest part of our relations in this treatment took place according to a pre-genital mode. Yves had intense oral and anal desires which made him very passive toward us, but also very aggressive. By analysing these desires in the transference he moved to a genital aggressivity and was able to realise himself in social life. However, from the start of the treatment, the pre-genital drives expressed themselves through the Oedipal desires, and we have seen on numerous occasions the role of the paternal imagos. We can therefore say that the pre-genital desires were above all interpreted in the transference as regressive desires. Nonetheless, the analysis of the pre-genital aggressivity in the transference was broached from the start of the first year of the treatment, at the moment when we chose to interpret his fear of the analyst as a repetition of his fear of a phallic mother.

In this fairly long analysis, the transference neurosis was no doubt running the risk of becoming interminable. In fact the patient, who had hardly any spare cash at the age of twenty-eight, was tempted to content himself with his transferential investments. The analysis of the transference was nonetheless sufficiently effective for Yves to gain sufficient insight, at the end of the treatment, into the ridiculous nature of the desires he felt for his psychoanalyst and it is possible to assert that the dissolution of the transference neurosis required no external measure whatsoever. Above all, it took place under the influence of the genitalisation of the transference, which prompted the subject to renounce his adaptation to the oral regressive situation imposed by the psychoanalysis.

Part 2: Perversion

After this brief account of Yves' biography, his entire psychoanalytic treatment and the development of the transference during its course, it seems possible now to broach the problem that we proposed to discuss, in particular that of the genesis and manifestations of a sexual perversion essentially centred around voyeuristic desires.

We shall first of all study the development of this perversion, on the one hand by surveying the perverse tendencies that could have existed before the treatment, on the other by specifying these manifestations within the framework of the transferential fantasies and extra-transferential acts.

We shall subsequently try to specify how the perversion manifested itself within the transference, because of the very development of the transference neurosis and the counter-transferential elements that we were able to notice.

Finally, we shall have to show how this sexual perversion was integrated with the neurotic structure of the case.

During the first year of Yves' analysis, we were able to collect information showing the origins of his voyeuristic fantasies: he recounted how, towards the age of thirteen, he had adopted the habit of masturbating whilst watching pictures of women in pornographic magazines. To do this, he locked himself up in the WC of the family cafe. At other times, at his grandfather's place, he aroused himself by looking at etchings in medical books. Later, he adopted the habit of looking for obscene descriptions in public urinals, those of cafes and cinemas. Let us recall that Yves had masturbated whilst dressing up as a woman and that he had the habit of hiding under the table in order to look underneath the skirt of his cousin. At his grandfather's place he also took a neighbourhood girl with him to the back of the garden, where the two children played the game of showing each other their genitals.

After the interpretation of the fundamental dream of the woman with the three penises, Yves spoke abundantly of his masturbatory fantasies, based on the stories and the drawings he invented. The principal themes were the following: a mature woman initiates a young girl; a crouching woman urinates in the street; a man urinates in a urinal; the subject is in a urinal, masturbates and is being seen by a woman hiding behind a latch, she is aroused by the sight and invites him to have sexual intercourse with her. He will explain later that these sexual relations were imagined as only via the mouth. He soon demonstrates a desire to see women urinating in toilets, and later to drink their urine.

During the second year of the treatment, a dream announces the emergence of the voyeuristic desires within the transference. The dream: it is morning, we offer him a bowl of cider, soon replaced with coffee, then we propose to him to buy us wine; he will ask his mother's permission; he then goes into a cellar where he urinates. We arrive, he ejaculates and we say to him: "masturbating that early in the morning is really no good". In his associations he talks about the lower cellars in L: he masturbated whilst watching women's legs, preferably those in high-heeled shoes. On different occasions, he tells us that he was tempted to look at our legs when lying down.

He thereupon continues to express the same desires. He often talks in particular about his desire to know of a toilet where he would have been able to watch a woman urinating and to masturbate. When he went to sit his exam, after he had assumed that our spouse might have died, and risking success in being considered virile by us, he noticed during a session the smell of urine, which he attributed to us. Let us repeat that after his success in the exam he discovered, in a cinema on the Champs-Elysées, the WC he wanted. From then on, he frequented the cinema on a regular basis.

The analytic work led him to elaborate the memories of his early childhood, in which his maid in the blue blouse appeared as she was cleaning the floorboards. We thought that this relived memory was very important because at first he did not remember the existence of this housekeeper at all. Yet his mother had always repeated to him that he had much preferred her to his parents.[5]

The end of the treatment announced itself: Yves was now looking at our legs without guilt. When he was surprised by an usherette entering the women's toilets, he gave up this habit without regrets, and he did not find himself drawn back into it for quite a while.

In order to situate these clinical facts, which were clustered around voyeuristic fantasies and perverse practices, in terms of the general theory of perversions, we can offer the following overall picture. First of all, the infantile sexuality, as we were able to reconstruct it during the psychoanalytic treatment, does not seem to have been profoundly perturbed. The sexual curiosity about the little girl with whom he engaged in reciprocal displays, as well as his desire to look underneath the skirt of his cousin seem very ordinary. Interpretive elaboration led to the comprehension of relived memories of being curious about the maid to whom he was very attached in his childhood. We have seen that this sexual curiosity led him to a phallic conception of a woman's anatomy. The importance of these pre-genital fantasies relived in the transferential situation justifies the hypothesis of the importance of pre-genital fixations at this period of his development. Insofar as it is possible to reconstruct the life of the drive during this period, it thus does not seem to be particularly marginal to mainstream sexuality, which is very polymorphous at this age. Nonetheless, we could talk about real fixations at this stage, which may explain the pathological aspect of the adult subject's sexual life.

During adolescence, Yves went through a fairly obvious period of Oedipal guilt, since he lived alone with his mother and slept in the conjugal bed, as he revealed at the end of the treatment. His sexual life does not seem to have had anything immediately abnormal during this period. It was essentially marked by masturbatory practices accompanied by fairly insignificant fantasies. Nonetheless, we can note that at a certain moment Yves dressed up as a woman. There were no voyeuristic fantasies during adolescence. At the most, the reading of pornographic magazines during masturbation could be considered as a preliminary sketch of voyeurism, although this practice was not particular to him, since these magazines travelled from hand to hand in secondary school.

During adulthood, when he left the sailing business, he had a mistress, but his sexual life did not satisfy him. He preferred masturbating. He revealed after several years of treatment that he would have contented himself happily with oral sex.

To sum up, Yves' infantile sexual life seems to have been coloured only by the awakening of the Oedipal situation. During adulthood, his sexual life was definitely not satisfying. Nonetheless, we can indeed say that before the psychoanalytic treatment there was no such thing as a distinct perversion. Yves' sexual life, as we were able to reconstruct it before the treatment, was much more that of a neurotic than that of a pervert. The absence of satisfaction in normal sexual intercourse and the preference for masturbation with perverse fantasies by no means characterises a genuine sexual perversion, in which the fantasies are acted out and the perverse practices represent the only possibilities of sexual realisation.

In our opinion, the voyeuristic perversion thus appeared during the course of the treatment itself, and it has developed within the framework of the transference neurosis. It is remarkable that this transference neurosis was essentially structured around the displacement of the maternal imago onto the analyst, yet it appears clearly enough that the patient did not talk about his perverse fantasies until his transference onto the analyst had been interpreted to him in terms of the displacement of the phallic mother onto her (as an identification of the man in armour with the phallic woman analyst). These fantasies were essentially interpreted during this period as the expression of a retreat from a dangerous Oedipal situation. But the interpretation most frequently given to him was that he was in regression before the terrifying image of the phallic mother. The fundamentally voyeuristic relation was conceived as less dangerous than even a passive oral relation with a woman who had three penises or had incorporated the paternal penis (dream of the engine). Until then, the fantasies had not been aimed directly at the analyst. The situation was transformed, starting from the dream in which the analyst proposed to him various drinks and in which the patient urinated in the cellar.

From this moment onwards, he has a desire and a fear of urinating on the analytic couch and in the toilet of the analyst and he imagines urinating on the remnants of her excrement. The voyeuristic fantasies are multiplied. This situation develops within the framework of the therapeutic situation. But at a period when he felt particularly frustrated by the analytic situation and when he declared incessantly that it was necessary to finish by having sexual intercourse with the analyst, we believed it appropriate to denounce this game and to tell him that he knew very well that this would not happen. After the holiday period that followed, he proclaimed his desire to be independent, and to court young girls. But in fact he really started developing an interest in voyeuristic practices in public toilets. He was afraid, he said, of being aggressive with the women he would have sex with. He wanted to avoid making them dirty and in particular he was afraid of being rejected by us because of this physical dirtiness.

We might wonder whether our intervention was justified, at least during this period of the treatment. In our mind it was destined to avoid an intellectual game that we thought we noticed in Yves. We had the impression that he was staging a situation in which he did not believe himself and which nonetheless terrified him. However, it is probable that the patient felt this warning as a prohibition of contact, not only on the genital level, but also on the pre-genital and aggressive level to which he was fixated. We can see the proof of it in the fact that, from then on, his perverse tendencies mark a very clear propensity to realise themselves outside the transference. One will actually recall that during this period his mother appeared to him as infinitely more tolerant than ourselves.

But the distance vis-à-vis the analyst was considerably reduced when, after having assumed that the analyst's husband was dead, he noticed a smell of urine during the session. It was then that he finally found the toilet which he had desired so much, in the cinema of the Champs-Elysées. Soon after, we could interpret his oral aggressivity and show to him that watching people urinate, and drinking urine was like incorporating the contents coming from the analyst's interior. In return he was afraid of being devoured, and this also explained the difficulties he had with speaking.

One thus sees that it is not until the moment that these perverse fantasies were brought back from extra-transferential action to desires lived in the transference and that they were analysed at the level of their signification as an exchange of partial objects with the analyst, that they started losing their intensity and became disinvested.

We know that at the end of the psychoanalytic treatment Yves looked at our legs without guilt and stopped being interested in the toilets in the cinema.

It seems easy enough to show how this perversion is integrated with the neurotic structure of this case. At the end of the treatment, it seems possible to define this structure as follows. The obsessive worry for which Yves had consulted seems indeed to enter the framework of the phobias, in particular because all anxiety is displaced onto the idea of height and because it is not annulled by a series of obsessional mechanisms. Nonetheless, in mainstream phobias, the anxiety is displaced onto an external phobogenic object. In this case here, the phobia seems very close to certain serious personality disorders. Moreover, as we have seen, some smaller phobias existed concerning the fear of wearing inadequate shoes and clothes. Yet there it concerns phenomena that are very akin to rites that are frequently observed in obsessionals. Some childhood phobias, although without absolute diagnostic value, would support the diagnostic hypothesis of phobia (disgust of red meat, fear of suffocating in the coverings).

The character structure is difficult to define. It shows a certain kinship with the obsessional type: emotional coldness which actually made contact within the transference difficult; the ritualisation of all behaviour, in external life as well as in analysis; fear of anything new. These tendencies were so profoundly bound up with his character traits that they allowed the anxiety to be camouflaged. Yves had attained the stage of Oedipal relations, but not without difficulties, because of the inverted structure of the parental couple. The regression before the Oedipus is no doubt explained by the importance of pre-genital fixations, which this inversion itself has favoured, and by the historical circumstances which, with the father being absent, have made every identification with him difficult.

From the perspective of psychical agencies, the importance of oral fixations, which seemed fairly evident given the intricate connection between the fantasies of watching people urinate and of drinking urine, seems to be confirmed by numerous arguments. Very often, Yves had a desire to suck breasts and to have his own sucked. He only desired sexual intercourse via the mouth. This erotism was intricately linked to aggressive drives, which clearly manifested themselves at the end of the treatment, when he was afraid of wrecking his mistress's vagina. The struggle against this oral aggressive erotism elicited a structuration of the Ego (*Moi*) of which the principal defence mechanisms were the tendency to rationalisation and emotional coldness. As for the Superego, it was essentially based on identification with a virile, demanding (and even devouring) mother. The paternal images were far less terrifying: the father was conceived as a weak person, only capable of making anal jokes. The uncle and the grandfather were stronger images, but without real importance.

The importance of the oral fixations is likewise certainly explained by the patient's entire past experience, at least as it had been elaborated during the psychoanalytic treatment. His Oedipus was reactivated during adolescence through his life with his mother in the absence of the father, but one can talk here about the pre-genital structure of his Oedipus. His mother wanted to prevent him from being virile, as he seemed to think was indicated by, for instance, the above mentioned memories of alimentary coercions, wrappings, enemas etc. Similarly, he remembered his childhood housekeeper as being harsh with him. It is probable that, on the dynamic level, these frustrations awakened aggressive drives, which expressed themselves in the transference in the form of voyeuristic drives, whose significance we have noted.

The perverse fantasies of this patient can also be explained in terms of the economic structure of the neurosis. On a superficial level we have seen that it was less dangerous for Yves to watch than to exercise his virile force with a penis so big that it might wreck the woman's insides. The phobia for which Yves consulted me certainly finds an important explanatory element there.[6] Furthermore, his fantasies undoubtedly had the value of narcissistic reassurance: the patient, in identifying with a young girl, avoided the attack from the phallic mother and the exchanges of incorporated partial objects were made less dangerous.

At the end of the treatment, the healing of the symptom seemed ensured. Yves had got rid of his phobia concerning his size; he had stopped walking with his head bent towards the ground. His minor phobias concerning his clothes and his shoes had disappeared. At the same time, genital pleasure was much more valued. The length of the psychoanalytic treatment perhaps explains partly why the subject contented himself for so long with his transferential investments.

This happy ending of the psychoanalytic treatment coincides with the cooling of voyeuristic perverse tendencies. For a long time, Yves had continued to occupy his observation post in the cinema toilets, but he was doing it without real pleasure. The compulsive aspect of this behaviour had disappeared, and the practice ceased by virtue of the chance incident mentioned above.

According to us, this happy development can be explained in the following way: it was only by virtue of his perverse fantasies, expressed in the transference, that Yves could make real contact with the analyst. In this way he could relive the realisation of his drives at the level of his pre-genital fixations. Similarly, when Yves discovered the cinema toilets on the Champs-Elysées, he declared to us that for the first time he felt that he was no longer living as an automaton. The disinvestment of his perverse tendencies required a long analysis of his pre-genital aggressivity. This analysis was first of all carried out within the framework of the presence of the transference, and then brought back to the historical frame of his relations with his mother and his childhood maid. We can estimate that the culminating point was situated at the moment when Yves gained insight into his retreat from the danger he was putting women in, and in particular his mistress, because of his aggressive drives. The interpretation according to which he contents himself more by his fantasies and his perverse practices than by his usual sexual relationships, because he fears the aggressive gift, seems essential.

To this point of view one can add that these perverse practices are essentially situated in the framework of an extra-transferential *passage-à-l'acte*. Therefore they do not deserve to be entered within the frame of the sexual perversions, on the one hand because they do not represent the only possibility of sexual realisation, on the other because they had a transient character.

Besides, one knows that amongst the sexual perversions, voyeurism has quite a singular significance. Let us bring to mind that Fain has shown that

> voyeurism is a normal moment of the development of the pre-genital stages, which allows, if it stays within its limits, a very developed approach to the Oedipal

conflict. Its transformation into a perversion is paradoxically the result of its failure in its function of protection against the possible destruction of the object.[7]

The psychoanalytic work on pathological voyeurism, of which we have been able to acquire knowledge, shows in any case that the voyeur seeks to have an object-relation that provokes little anxiety, through an avoidance of castration, and by reassuring himself against his own aggressive drives. The structure is often marked by pre-genital fixations, which explain the importance of urethral erotism.

It is therefore possible to conclude that the appearance of these tendencies and perverse practices within the transference and within extra-transferential acts has by itself allowed for the investment of the pre-genital, aggressive and erotic drives. Yves found in psychoanalysis the possibility of human contact he had never experienced because of defences against these drives. Their explanation has allowed for the mobilisation of these defences and for the gradual development of a genitalisation, which he seems to have attained.[8]

Notes

1 Originally published in *Bulletin d'activités de l'Association des Psychanalystes de Belgique*, 1956, 25, pp. 1 -16. Translation by Dany Nobus. Comments in square brackets in the bibliography and the notes, are by the translator. Although the references in the bibliography of the original paper are incomplete and inconsistent, I have refrained from adding the missing details and rendering the style consistent, because the reader should still be able to locate the source materials without difficulty. (Translator's note)

2 We want to express our great thanks, here, to Dr Bouvet, for agreeing to supervise this long treatment and for inspiring this work through his precious advice.

3 A general anti-government strike initiated by workers across the country and subsequently supported by the farmers, which brought France to a complete standstill. (Translator's note)

4 Named after the small town in North Vietnam where the conflict occurred, this battle took place from 13 March to 7 May 1954. Ho Chi Minh's unexpected victory over the French led to the withdrawal of French troops from Vietnam and effectively ended French colonial rule in Indochina. (Translator's Note)

5 One might think that we have here an analogy with the scene of the Wolf Man (in *Cinq psychanalyses* – Freud, p. 450) where Grouscha is doing washing on the floor whilst the little boy urinates. [The book to which Lebovici refers, here, is S. Freud, *Cinq psychanalyses*, trad. Marie Bonaparte & Rudolph Loewenstein, Paris: Denoël et Steele, 1935 – reprinted, Paris: Presses Universitaires de France, 1954.]

6 This explanation is certainly only one of the mechanisms, amongst the most profound ones, of the symptom, which is overdetermined. In particular, the fear of being tall may correspond in this way to the fear of rivalry with the father, who was short and stocky, or with the uncle, whereas the regressive situation is eroticised by the different masochistic components we have isolated in this case.

7 M. Fain, *Contribution à l'étude du voyeurisme, RFP*, XVIII, *avril* 1954.

8 Since writing this paper, reports have been presented at the *Congrès International de Psychanalyse* (Genève 1955) [the 19th Congress of the International Psychoanalytic Association] on the problem of perversions. The works of Gillespie, Phyllis Greenacre, Nacht, Diatkine and Favreau have contributed numerous historical and technical remarks confirming the few conclusions we thought we could present here.

Bibliography

Ey, H. (1951). *Les Perversions sexuelles. Etudes psychiatriques (II)*. Desclée de Brouwer.

Freud, S. (1932). *Trois Essais sur la Théorie de la Sexualité*. B. Reverchon (Trans.). Gallimard.

Fenichel, O. (1953). *La Théorie Psychanalytique des Névroses* (p. 835). M. Schlumberger & Coll. (Trans.). Paris: Presses Universitaires.

Gillespie, W. H. (1952). Notes on the Analysis of Sexual Perversions. *International Journal of Psychoanalysis*, 33: 397–402.

Nacht, S., Diatkine, R. & Favreau, J. (1955). Rapport sur les Perversions au Congrès International de Psychanalyse. (Le Moi dans la Relation perverse) à paraître dans la Revue française de Psychanalyse. [This paper was indeed published as: S. Nacht, R. Diatkine & J. Favreau (1956). Le Moi dans la Relation perverse. *Revue Française de Psychanalyse*, 20: 457–478. An English translation by Joyce McDougall (1956) appeared in *The International Journal of Psycho-Analysis*, 37: 404–413.]

Saul, L.J. (1952). A Note on Exhibition and Scoptophilia. *The Psychoanalytic Quarterly*, 21(2): 224–227.

INDEX

For Product Safety Concerns and Information please contact our
EU representative GPSR@taylorandfrancis.com Taylor & Francis
Verlag GmbH, Kaufingerstraße 24, 80331 München, Germany